Ergonomics

DATE DUE

Ergonomics
Body Mechanics and Self-Care for Bodyworkers

DIANE REDMAN, CMT, BA, CEAS

*Northern Wyoming Community College District,
Sheridan College*

ARDATH L. LUNBECK, MS

*Northern Wyoming Community College District,
Sheridan College*

PEARSON

Boston Columbus Indianapolis New York San Francisco Upper Saddle River
Amsterdam Cape Town Dubai London Madrid Milan Munich Paris Montreal Toronto
Delhi Mexico City Sao Paulo Sydney Hong Kong Seoul Singapore Taipei Tokyo

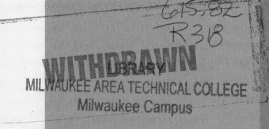

Cataloging-in-Publication Data on file with the Library of Congress

Publisher: Julie Levin Alexander
Assistant to Publisher: Regina Bruno
Editor-in-Chief: Mark Cohen
Executive Editor: John Goucher
Associate Editor: Melissa Kerian
Assistant Editor: Nicole Ragonese
Editorial Assistant: Rosalie Hawley
Senior Media Editor: Amy Peltier
Media Project Managers: Lorena Cerisano, and Julita Navarro
Managing Production Editor: Patrick Walsh
Production Liaison: Christina Zingone
Production Editor: Karen Berry, Laserwords Maine

Manufacturing Manager: Alan Fischer
Creative Director: Jayne Conte
Cover Designer: Suzanne Duda
Cover Image Photographer: Adam Jahiel
Director of Marketing: David Gesell
Executive Marketing Manager: Katrin Beacom
Marketing Specialist: Michael Sirinides
Composition: Laserwords, Maine
Printer/Binder: Courier/Kendallville
Cover Printer: Lehigh Phoenix Color/Hagerstown

10 9 8 7 6 5 4 3 2 1

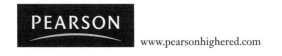

www.pearsonhighered.com

ISBN-13: 978-0-13-802485-7
ISBN-10:   0-13-802485-5

I dedicate this book to the memory of my beloved mother, Myrtle Redman Cuda,
and my wonderful father, James J. Cuda, for his love and support, and to my son, Brandon S. Kim,
for his encouragement and love.

Diane Redman

This book is dedicated to the memory of my mother, Thelma Shell, my father, Lewis Shell,
who have always encouraged me in my educational and professional endeavors, and my husband,
John, for his unwavering support and love.

Ardath Lunbeck

Brief Contents

Acknowledgments

We wholeheartedly thank the Pearson Health Science team for making this book a reality. We especially want to thank Mark Cohen, Editor-in-Chief, for taking a risk on us newbies; Nikki Ragonese, Assistant Editor, for her continual assistance; John Goucher, our Executive Editor, for insightful recommendations and guidance; and JaNoel Lowe for copyediting. We are grateful to our past, present, and future students for their enthusiasm, curiosity, and questions and for showing us the importance of this book. It would not be possible without the guidance, teachings, knowledge, wisdom, and practices of our previous mentors. Special thanks goes to Betsy Pearson for being instrumental in the early inception of this book and her continued support and enthusiasm.

We are greatly indebted to Adam Jahiel for his genius with a camera. His patience, experience, camaraderie, and great music during our photo shoot made long hours bearable. Many thanks to Laura Jahiel for feeding us exceptional food during the photo shoot. We appreciate Ashli Filkins and Erika Roman for their beauty, grace, and hard work as models for the book. Thanks to Courtney Green for her expertise and contribution to the chapter on exercise. We also want to thank Gayle Macdonald for her encouragement. Profound thanks to Thomas Myers for his generosity in writing the Foreword.

Reviewers

Rabia Bellante, LMT, RYT
HealthWorks Institute
Bozeman, Montana

Kathleen Crawford, LMT
Massage Shoppe
St. Charles, Missouri

Gabrielle J. Ham-Jones, BS, CMT
Massage Institute of Maryland
Catonsville, Maryland

Charles C. Houston Jr., B.MSC, LMT, MTI, MMP™
Amarillo Massage Therapy Institute
Amarillo, Texas

Kathy Hunt, LMT, NCTMB, MS
Elizabeth Grady School of Massage Therapy
Medford, Massachusetts

Cynthia Jaggers, MS, LMT, CNMT
Virginia College, School of Business and Health
Chattanooga, Tennessee

Tara McManaway, M. Div., LMT
College of Southern Maryland
La Plata, Maryland

Maj-Lis Nash, LMT
Mind Body Institute, LLC
Nashville, Tennessee

Teresa Patterson
Southwest Mississippi Community College
Summit, Mississippi

Teressa Sloan, PhD, DD, LMT, NCBTMB
Bluegrass Professional School of Massage Therapy
Lexington, Kentucky

Candy L. Washington, BA, LMT, NCTMB
National University of Health
Lombard, Illinois

Foreword

All across the manual therapy field—from physiotherapists to chiropractors to massage therapists to energy healers laying on hands—too little attention is paid to the issues related by F. M. Alexander, founder of the seminal *Alexander Technique,* regarding what he called "the use of the self." It is all too common for the manual therapist, a "giver" almost by definition by entering this field, to forget him- or herself in favor of the client's comfort. Thereby the manual therapist overreaches and bends in strange ways, causing him- or herself future injury, pain, or degeneration— a poor bargain indeed!

All too many therapists leave this work within the first decade after training in favor of something less grueling. Such statistics would understate the problem because many therapists cite growing children, aging parents, or the desire to be more "psychological" in their approach, or some other reason but never mention the pain in the back, neck, or knees, which is really the underlying cause of their exiting from this profession that provides the essential services of nurturing and providing informed contact in our touch-starved world.

As a profession, manual therapy cannot afford to lose practitioners just as they begin to put their training into effect and thrive in their practices. Training a good manual therapist is a labor-intensive task, and it takes a full decade in practice for most to achieve real competence in performing this complex set of skills. It is a poor return on everyone's investment if they leave the profession too soon after they begin. I have been working (overworking!) steadily over a treatment table since 1974, and I attribute my longevity in the field to a lucky encounter with Judith Aston, an early and ardent pioneer of the principles discussed in this book.

In fact, both client and therapist must be and can be served without compromising either. This book by Diane Redman and Ardath Lunbeck points to the salient factors necessary to achieve such easy balance. I especially appreciate the attention to both the "external" and "internal" approach to ergonomics because the best therapy—even self-therapy—is experienced from the inside, not imposed from the outside. In showing this compassion to yourself, you will, subtly but firmly, communicate this self-respect to your clients as well.

Although this book will primarily be introduced to students, I recommend keeping it on your shelf after you graduate because some of these issues do not arise immediately but come to the fore only when you have been working for a while (and have settled into your working habits—some good, some not so good).

A number of books on self-use in manual therapeutics are available. To say this one is good does not detract from the others. I would encourage any reader to find the book that best "fits your hand," much like finding the table or chair that fits your individual body and patterns of working. That said, the writers have ensured that this book is competent and thorough and provides a number of "ways in" for diverse readers.

In closing, I would also say that during their sessions, the clients have to be the primary focus— they are, after all, paying for the attention. To avoid overfocusing on the self, pick one or two of the suggestions herein each week, and pay attention to them until they are integrated into your work. Educate your clients with the same principles, and that will help you use them yourself. Do not be afraid to bend the rules a little to get something particular done, but in general, the guidelines here are solid.

You cannot violate the laws of physics with your body too often without getting caught. "Getting caught" in this case means pain, fatigue, and loss of concentration. Better to get started on the correct use of your body—it is, and always will be, your most proximate and important tool. This text is a guide on how to use your body well.

— Thomas Myers, author of *Anatomy Trains* (Elsevier 2001, 2009), and director of *Kinesis*, which offers continuing professional development worldwide.

Contents

Preface

Ergonomics: Body Mechanics and Self-Care for Bodyworkers is a practical guide for using ergonomics for students and practitioners in the field of bodywork. We use the word *bodyworker* because we felt it addresses practitioners using a broad range of modalities, from massage therapy to acupressure to energy work. In fact, the concepts of the book can be adapted to almost any care-giving field including nursing, dental hygiene, and physical therapy.

The book is grounded in our professional experience. Diane Redman is currently teaching and the Massage Therapy Program Director at Sheridan College of the Northern Wyoming Community College District (NWCCD) in Sheridan, Wyoming. Her career has spanned more than 30 years as a professional massage therapist including work on professional dancers and athletes. Years of study and observation of her clientele and the study of kinesiology led her to formulate a set of ergonomic principles for bodyworkers that she began teaching to students and practicing therapists. Diane is a certified massage therapist, holds certification as an ergonomic assessment specialist and fitness specialist, and has studied *tai chi* for the past 25 years and taught it for 15. She holds a Bachelor of Arts in Health, Arts, and Science from Goddard College in Plainfield, Vermont, and is currently working on a Masters of Arts in Community Health Education degree. She has taught therapeutic modalities for more than 20 years and has received the NWCCD's award for teaching excellence.

Ardath Lunbeck is currently the Dean of Arts and Sciences of NWCCD and brings 30 years of experience teaching human anatomy and physiology. She has developed and taught courses in medical terminology, microbiology, general pathology, and aging. Her ongoing commitment to developing methods to engage students in their learning has resulted in her receiving teaching awards at the district and state levels. She holds a BA in Zoology and a MS in Zoology and Physiology from the University of Wyoming. Ardath's avid interest in the field of bodywork and health led her to complete a massage therapy course and a fitness specialist course. She is certified in equine massage.

Diane moved to Wyoming with the intent of starting a proprietary massage school and met with Ardath with the intent of recruiting her to teach anatomy and physiology. With Ardath's background in curriculum development, she suggested establishing a program at the college. Our mutual vision to have a massage program supported by higher education science courses emerged. We became a team to develop the Sheridan College massage therapy program that enrolled its first students 1999.

PHILOSOPHY

The vision of this text was to provide a comprehensive look at the depth and breadth of elements that affect a bodyworker's physical ability to continue working. Ergonomics is much more than simply following good body mechanics in the work setting. Understanding ergonomics depends on knowledge of basic anatomy and kinesiology. Practicing good ergonomics depends on using proper technique and following a self-care regiment. Awareness of the mind-body connection strengthens the commitment of following good self-care practices.

Ergonomics applies to everything a person does at home, at play, and in the work place. The initial discussion of neutrality refers to both everyday activities and tasks performed by bodyworkers to emphasize the integration of ergonomics in all that we do. Later chapters directly address work in the office setting and the therapeutic environment.

Anatomy and kinesiology underlie proper body mechanics, and the authors believe it is imperative to have a good understanding of both to provide logic to the recommendations given. Programs vary in the amount of anatomy and kinesiology integrated within them. For some students, chapters covering these topics will serve as a review; for others they may serve as foundation material. Instructors can vary how they use these chapters and/or the sequence of the chapters to fit their program.

The self-care sections on exercise, stress, and self-massage have been incorporated to show how a practitioner can be proactive to reduce the risk of injury. The chapter on postural distortions is for the practitioners not only to assess their own deviations but also to enhance their understanding of postural distortions that their clients have.

EACH CHAPTER HELPS YOU LEARN THE PRINCIPLES AND PUT THEM INTO PRACTICE

Although primarily geared to students, *Ergonomics: Body Mechanics and Self-Care for Bodyworkers* is also appropriate for the working professional. It provides a strong foundation in basic body mechanics as well as techniques for self-assessment and reeducation. Practitioners can also apply these principles of ergonomics to their clients as part of their teaching for self-care.

The book is divided into two parts. Part I, Foundations of Ergonomics and Body Mechanics, provides a foundation for understanding the importance of ergonomics and avoiding postural distortion. Chapter 1 identifies the principles of ergonomics and discusses the relationship between ergonomics and injury, especially as they relate to bodywork. Chapters 2 and 3 provide techniques for maintaining neutral alignment when the body is stationary and when it is in motion. Chapter 4 describes nine common postural distortions and discusses their causes and effects.

Part II, Principles into Practice: Techniques, Environment, and Self-Care, provides strategies for incorporating ergonomic principles within and beyond the work environment. Chapter 5 identifies the best ergonomic alignment for work on specific regions. Chapter 6 addresses the work environment and gives recommendations for setting up the work space. Chapters 7–9 describe self-care through strengthening and stretching, self-massage, and stress management.

FEATURES AND PEDAGOGY ADDRESS A VARIETY OF LEARNING STYLES

Different learners take in, process, and master new information in different ways. Some learners are more visually oriented; others are more aural or kinesthetic students. Others learn best by reading and writing. This textbook includes elements and suggested activities to assist learners of all styles to comprehend the principles and guidelines, apply them, and develop them until they become engrained ergonomic habits.

Visual learners will find the book's generous and beautiful illustrations and photographs most beneficial. The photographs are designed to compare proper and improper ergonomics. The color format helps to visually guide the reader and emphasize key points.

The read/write learner will find the text-based learning aids most useful. These include chapter opening learning objectives and key terms that appear in boldface within the chapter and are defined in the Glossary at the end of the book. Each chapter concludes with a summary that identifies the key points addressed and a set of review questions

that readers can use to check their learning. Lists of references cited and suggested readings provide sources of further information for the read/write learner.

Text-based instruction always challenges the aural learner; for these learners, lecture and discussion are useful. When faced with nongroup learning situations, tape recording and playing back the information while practicing technique are advantageous.

Those who gravitate to the field of bodywork tend to be kinesthetic learners; that is, they prefer to learn by doing. All learners need to apply a kinesthetic style when practicing the techniques in this text. The book's design facilitates use during hands-on practice.

Several special boxes within the text are designed to serve all styles of learner. These include:

Helpful Hints

These provide a short synopsis to draw the reader's attention to key points and engage them in activities.

Case Studies

These features describe stories characteristic of bodyworkers with work-related injuries. They include accompanying critical thinking exercises to help learners apply the cases to their own work.

Worksheets

Worksheets are designed for self-assessments. These assessments provide personal engagement in practicing the principles being taught.

WE WELCOME YOUR COMMENTS

This book identifies the principles of ergonomics and describes straightforward techniques to help learners transfer those principles into sound ergonomic practice. We welcome your responses to the material including confirmation of where we have succeeded and suggestions for improving the next edition. We would also like to know how implementing the principles and techniques in this book affected your practice. Comments can be sent to dredman@sheridan.edu and alunbeck@sheridan.edu. We thank you and wish you a long, healthy, prosperous, and satisfying career.

Ergonomics

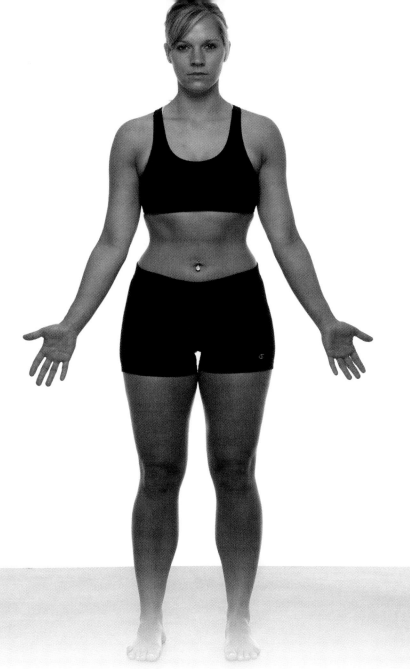

PART

1

Foundations
of Ergonomics and
Body Mechanics

CHAPTER 1

Introduction to Ergonomics

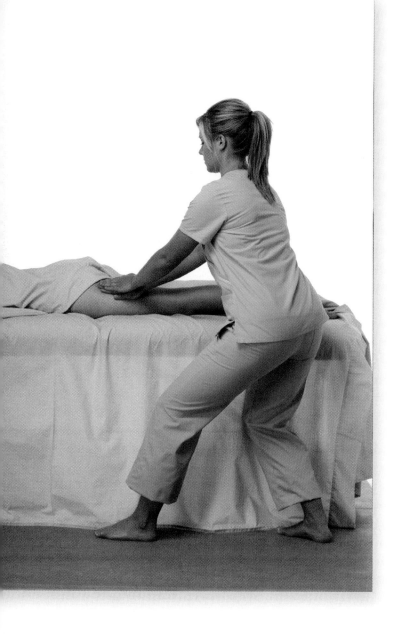

 CHAPTER OUTLINE

Defining Ergonomics

How the Body Moves

Injuries Related to Movement

Basis for Occupational Injuries

Ergonomics Principles to Prevent Injury

Summary

Review Questions

LEARNING OBJECTIVES

Upon successfully completing this chapter, you will be able to:

1. Describe the evolution of the field of ergonomics.
2. Correlate anatomical structure to movement.
3. Relate the process of inflammation to injury and repair.
4. Explain how repetitive motion can lead to postural distortion.
5. Discuss the contribution of body mechanics to occupational injury.
6. Explain the role of the physical work environment in the development of occupational injury.
7. Identify several risks factors for injury specific to the field of bodywork.
8. Identify the repetitive motion syndromes that most commonly affect bodyworkers.
9. Explain how ergonomics assessment and implementation help prevent and reduce occupational injury.
10. Describe the concept of neutrality and its contribution to musculoskeletal health.
11. List the keys to maintaining good posture.

KEY TERMS

Career choices are made for a variety of reasons including interest, opportunity, and aptitude. Seldom do we consider the risk of injury before we decide on a career choice. In reality, every career choice involves at least some injury risk. With expanded understanding and recognition of ergonomics, more massage programs have begun to teach injury prevention. The vision of this text is to provide a comprehensive look at the breadth of factors that affect a bodyworker's physical ability to continue to work. Understanding ergonomics depends on understanding basic anatomy and kinesiology as well as the mind-body connection. Practicing good ergonomics depends on using proper technique and following a self-care regiment.

Applying proper ergonomics starts with self-assessment and self-awareness. The first consideration is where you are in regard to ergonomics: What physical conditions do you bring to your career that can affect your work? Does your work create physical conditions that affect your personal life? Let's start with a simple body scan to identify physical challenges. More thorough assessments will be identified throughout the text, but this simple scan can be used periodically to help prevent injury. Complete the activity in Helpful Hint 1.1 and record your challenges. At this time, you may not be able to distinguish which challenges result from improper work practices and which from other activities or conditions. Throughout

this book, you will learn techniques and practices to reverse or diminish your current condition and prevent the acquisition of new ones.

In this first chapter, we describe how the field of ergonomics has emerged to prevent and reduce the frequency of work-related injuries and identify its fundamental principles. We also review the anatomy, physiology, and underlying limitations of the musculoskeletal system leading to injuries. Finally, we introduce some simple ergonomic principles that can help you to avoid injury. These ergonomic principles along with others are expanded upon in later chapters.

DEFINING ERGONOMICS

The term **ergonomics** is a relatively new word that, according to the *American Heritage Dictionary*, 4th edition (2000), comes from the term *ergon,* meaning "work" and *nomics* derived from *oikos* meaning "house" and *nemein* meaning "manage." So ergonomics literally means the management of the workplace.

The science of ergonomics studies two aspects of how bodyworkers manage their work. The first is **biomechanics** (see Figure 1.1 ■), which deals with the action of physical forces on the body and the actions of muscles and gravity

---

HELPFUL HINT 1.1
Preliminary Body Scan

A quick bodyscan helps to recognize physical conditions which we may have been oblivious to or ignored. A scan should achieve two things: Make us aware of our outward appearance and increase the inner awareness of our body. Learning to listen to our body is a skill that is built over time. We should note our observations for future discussions; all of them can relate back to an underlying problem of ergonomics in our work or daily activities and/or to a factor that leads to poor ergonomics.

Step 1: Stand relaxed in front of a mirror. What features
do you notice?
- Is your body alignment straight?
- How does your head line up with your torso?
- Are your shoulders level?
- Do both arms hang equally?
- Are your hips level?
- Are you overweight or underweight?
- Do you carry more weight in a given area
  of the body?

Step 2: Assess your awareness of your body. As you go through
the day, keep these items in mind and note the
conditions you notice.

- When you are rested and relaxed, do you notice any of the following?
  a. Any muscle tightness or pain?
  b Any joint pain?
  c. Any general feeling of discomfort?
- How does your body feel at the start of the day versus the end of the day?
  a. Are there areas of the body, such as your feet, that are noticeably tired and sore by the end of the day?
- When you are active, or after you are active, do you notice any of the following?
  a. Limited range of motion?
  b. Joint pain?
  c. Imbalance of muscle tension/strength?
- Do you tend to experience any of the following on a routine basis?
  a. Headaches?
  b. Anxiety or frustrations?
  c. Fatigue?

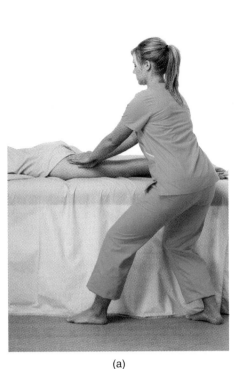
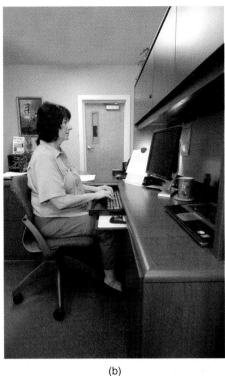

(a)   (b)

FIGURE 1.1

The science of ergonomics studies worker biomechanics as well as equipment and workspace design. (a) An ergonomically appropriate stance helps maintain the bodyworker's productivity and health. (b) An ergonomically designed workstation.

on bones and joints. A common example of biomechanics addressed in ergonomics is proper lifting techniques to prevent injury. However, biomechanics applies both when the body is in motion and when it is at rest. For example, sleeping on your stomach with your head turned to one side will reduce your range of motion on the opposite side the next day. In a similar fashion, proper support of the body during rest is important to recover from the effects of your work. Considering the importance of biomechanics, it is not surprising that many **ergonomists**—scientists in the field of ergonomics—have advanced training in **kinesiology**, the science that studies body movement.

The second aspect of ergonomics is the design of equipment and the workplace. From flints to looms to manual typewriters, tools have been developed over thousands of years of human history to help perform tasks more efficiently. As a field of study, however, ergonomics first came to the forefront as a result of World War II. This period is characterized by a tremendous upsurge of industrialization involving heavy equipment, machinery, and transport of supplies to meet the needs of the armed services. Injuries that resulted drew attention to the need to design safe products to protect workers. Dr. Lovesey of the Robens Centre for Health Ergonomics at the University of Surrey states that although ergonomics is based on long-established scientific disciplines, including engineering, physiology, and psychology, it became a separate field in 1949 (Dohrmann, 2004).

The field of ergonomics continued to develop postwar when industries began to see the benefits in reducing sick leave, workers' compensation claims, and lawsuits brought by employees with workplace injuries that were becoming increasingly expensive. Industry executives slowly began to appreciate the fact that such costs could be avoided and productivity increased by giving proper attention to ergonomics.

Perhaps the greatest boost to the field of ergonomics came when the U.S. government established the Occupational Safety and Health Administration (OSHA) in the early 1970s. OSHA regulations provide for safe and healthful working conditions and require stiff penalties for companies that fail to follow its regulations. Prior to the establishment of OSHA, more 2 million work-related injuries were reported annually. In the three decades since OSHA's implementation, workplace injuries and illnesses have dropped by 40% (U.S. Department of Labor, 2000; All about OSHA, 2006).

Ergonomists commonly work with engineers, psychologists, sociologists, applied physiologists, architects, and artists to develop equipment, furniture, and workspaces that ensure worker safety, reduce worker stress, and increase productivity. Some examples of ergonomically designed equipment include protective goggles for eye safety, push-button phones, and mouse pads with gel inserts that lift the wrist. Anyone who has held a desk job knows the importance of an adjustable "ergonomically designed" chair. A supported spine is more relaxed, and the proper chair can increase worker effectiveness. Proper musculoskeletal alignment reduces fatigue and improves circulation and respiration. This enhances worker health and thereby can reduce sick leave and health insurance claims.

Body shape and size play a key role in ergonomic design. **Anthropometry**, the study of human body measurement, is thus an important aspect of ergonomics. The design of devices and workstations that can adjust to fit their users must consider not only their height and weight but also the length of the neck, torso, limbs, and fingers. For example, a massage table that is raised to an appropriate height for one therapist would need to be adjusted for another therapist who is the same height but has different torso and limb proportions. The size of the client also affects how a table needs to be adjusted.

As part of workplace design, ergonomics also studies sensory input and the awareness of our body and our surroundings. Is the work area too noisy, too dark, or too cold? Are the ceilings too low or too high? Is the space cluttered? Does the room have an odd smell? Even the color chosen for the ceilings, walls, and floors of the work area can influence workers' senses and thereby their productivity and health.

In summary, then, ergonomics studies those factors that influence a person's capacity to work efficiently and effectively. It is a professional field that incorporates elements of kinesiology and body mechanics, and collaborates with a variety of related professional fields.

HOW THE BODY MOVES

We begin exploring ergonomics by examining how the body moves, making correlations to everyday experience and work practices common to the bodyworker. This foundation sets the stage for understanding how injury occurs and how to avoid it. The musculoskeletal system is the framework for body movement, which occurs when skeletal muscle contraction produces a force that is delivered to a system of levers formed by the skeleton. Both joints and muscles can be sites of injury.

Movement Occurs at Joints

The adult skeleton comprises 206 bones, organized and positioned to provide protection, support, and movement. The bones are held together to varying degrees from the tight ossification seen in the cranium to the looser articulation of knee, hip, and elbow joints. The joint structure and muscle attachments determine the type of lever created and the motion possible. The stability or lack of stability of the joint determines the risk for its injury.

STRUCTURE OF JOINTS

Although joints can be classified in different ways, one method considers the type of tissue that holds the articulation together. This method identifies three types: fibrous

joints, cartilaginous joints, and synovial joints (Figure 1.2 ■). **Fibrous joints** are held together by collagen fibers and allow very little movement. They include the cranial sutures and the tibiofibular joints. **Cartilaginous joints** are held together either by hyaline cartilage, such as that found between the ribs and sternum, or by a plate of fibrocartilage, such as the disc found between the bodies of two adjacent vertebrae. Some movement is possible with cartilaginous joints. If you compress your ribs, you will notice this slight movement. The third type of joint is the **synovial joint** (Figure 1.3 ■). Its complex structure imparts a freer attachment between the articulating bones and reduces friction to allow a wide range of movement. The joint capsule is lined with a synovial membrane that secrets a viscous synovial fluid for lubrication. In addition, the hyaline cartilage covering the articulating surfaces of the bones reduces friction. Ligaments assist in stabilizing the joint, and are potential sites for injury.

The point of movement along the skeletal framework is the synovial joint. The surrounding tissues need to be able to accommodate that movement. As a result, less muscle mass and other soft tissue (e.g., fat) are generally over the joint regions. Blood and lymphatic vessels and nerves lie close to the bones rather than being embedded in soft tissue. Injury to a joint can also damage these vulnerable structures. As bodyworkers, we need to be careful when working around joints to avoid impinging nerves and vessels.

TYPES OF SYNOVIAL JOINTS

Synovial joints are further classified by the shape of the articulating surfaces and the degree of movement as in Figure 1.4 ■. The degree of motion ranges from movement along one axis (**monoaxial**) to two axes (**biaxial**) or more (**multiaxial**). The six types of joints identified by the articular surface shape are plane, saddle, hinge, pivot, ball-and-socket, and ellipsoid. Check the range of motion from your fingers to your shoulder and from your head to your toes as each type of joint is described.

- The **plane joint** has two opposing, flat surfaces of equal size, and its ligaments and adjacent bones restrict its motion. Because plane joints allow some gliding action between the bones, they are also known as *gliding joints*. Degree of motion is slight as between two carpal bones, which are considered to be monoaxial because some rotation is possible. You probably cannot easily distinguish the movement between the carpel bones because the complexity of the wrist involves more than one type of joint, and the range of motion is attributed to all of them. However, pain in the wrist can stem from problems of the intercarpal joints, such as arthritis.
- The **saddle joint** has two concave, saddle-shaped bone surfaces fitted together at right angles. The thumb's carpometacarpal joint, which allows the thumb to oppose each of the fingers, is an example. Saddle joints are biaxial. Compare the range of motion of the

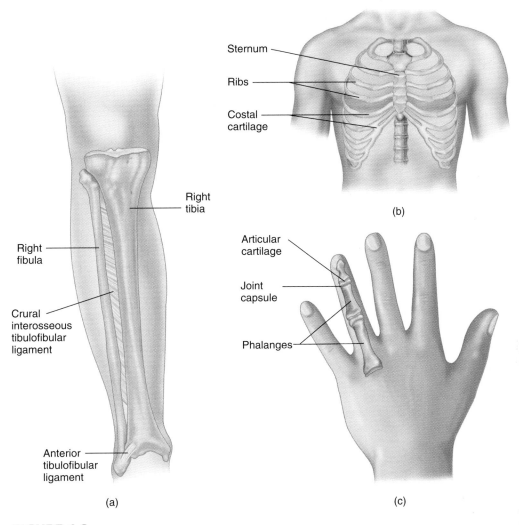

Sternum

Ribs

Costal cartilage

(b)

Right tibia

Right fibula

Crural interosseous tibulofibular ligament

Articular cartilage

Joint capsule

Phalanges

Anterior tibulofibular ligament

(a)   (c)

FIGURE 1.2

The three classes of joints are determined by how bones are held together. (a) The tibularfibular joint is a *fibrous joint* and is essentially nonmovable. (b) The costalsternal joint is a *cartilaginous joint*. It flexes during respiratory movement. (c) The interphalangeal joint is a *synovial joint* and is the most mobile joint of the three.

thumb to the fingers. Also check the hallux (big toe). It doesn't have the same range of motion as its equivalent, the thumb, because it is not a saddle joint. There is a tendency to use the thumb as a tool, but it is not designed to withstand the compressional forces that many bodyworkers use.

- The **hinge joint** has one cylindrical, convex articulating surface fitted into a corresponding concave articulating surface. It is monoaxial and works much like a door hinge; both the humeral-ulnar (elbow) and femoral-tibial (knee) joints are good examples. Starting at your finger tips and working to the torso and on down to your feet, how many hinge joints do you discover?

- The **pivot joint** is also a monoaxial joint, but it allows for rotation along the long axis of the bones involved. The pivot joint of the atlas-axis enables the head to turn from side to side. Supination/pronation of the forearm involves the pivot joint of the proximal end of the radius and ulna. An example of this in bodywork is applying a wringing stroke to the fingers.

- The **ball-and-socket joint** provides the greatest range of motion. The spherical end of one bone in this joint fits into the cuplike depression of the other. The two examples are the coxal (hip) and humeral (shoulder) joints. Check the range of motion of both your shoulder and hip joint. Notice that abduction, adduction, flexion, extension, circumduction, and rotation are all available. Of the two joints, in which do you have the best range of motion?

- The **ellipsoid joint** is similar to the ball-and-socket joint, but it has an oblong, ellipsoid surface instead of a round articulating surface. The shape restricts rotation but provides hingelike motion in two axes. Examples include the metacarpophalangeal joints (knuckles) and the radiocarpal joint of the wrist.

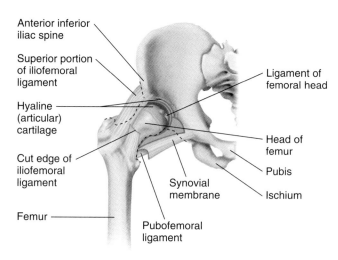

Anterior inferior iliac spine

Superior portion of iliofemoral ligament

Hyaline (articular) cartilage

Cut edge of iliofemoral ligament

Femur

Ligament of femoral head

Head of femur

Pubis

Ischium

Synovial membrane

Pubofemoral ligament

FIGURE 1.3

The synovial joint allows for movement and reduces friction. The joint capsule completely surrounds the articulation. It is lined with a synovial membrane which secretes a lubricating fluid into the joint. Hyaline cartilage covers the ends of the bones and provides for cushioning and lubrication. Ligaments stabilize the structure.

Compare the range of motion of the interphalangeal joint to the metacarpophalangeal joint. Notice the abduction of the fingers that the ellipsoid joint makes possible. Typically, when applying a stroke with the palms, the fingers are kept adducted. This position provides more support for the fingers and less risk for injury.

STABILITY OF SYNOVIAL JOINTS

The synovial joints' stability (or lack of it) significantly determines risk for injury. Stability is determined by (1) the shape, size, and arrangement of the articular surfaces, (2) ligaments, and (3) tone of the muscle around the joint. When stability is compromised, the joint structures and adjacent nerves and vessels can be damaged by stresses that otherwise would be no threat.

From reading the descriptions of the synovial joints, you might predict that ball-and-socket joints are more stable than hinge joints, and this is generally so. Within one class of joints, however, the stability provided by the articulation is often significantly different. One example of this is the coxal (hip) versus humeral (shoulder) joint: The coxal joint is extremely stable with the head of the femur inserted deep into the acetabulum. In contrast, the head of the humerus is smaller and the depression of the glenoid cavity much more shallow. As a result, the articulation of the humerus is less stable and much more prone to dislocation. To compensate for the reduced bony articulation, the humeral joint depends on muscles and ligaments to maintain stability.

Ligaments help to stabilize many of the body's joints. Within synovial joints, these strong bands of fibrous connective tissue can be part of the fibrous joint capsule

FIGURE 1.4

Each of the six types of synovial joints can be identified in the upper limb: ball and socket, pivot, hinge, plane, ellipsoid, and saddle.

Posterior View Right Arm

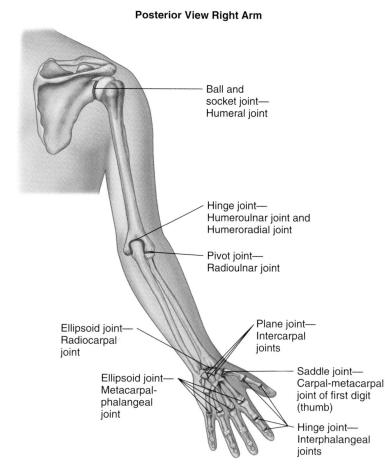

Ball and socket joint— Humeral joint

Hinge joint— Humeroulnar joint and Humeroradial joint

Pivot joint— Radioulnar joint

Ellipsoid joint— Radiocarpal joint

Ellipsoid joint— Metacarpal-phalangeal joint

Plane joint— Intercarpal joints

Saddle joint— Carpal-metacarpal joint of first digit (thumb)

Hinge joint— Interphalangeal joints

found outside the joint capsule or within it as with the cruciate ligaments of the knee. The tensile strength of ligaments allows them to withstand great force; however, with sufficient impact, they can be stretched or torn, which is known as a **sprain.** Bodyworkers commonly stand for extended periods and can tend to hyperextend the knees. This also put stress on the ligaments.

Well-toned muscle also supports joint stability. This is probably best noted in the case of the humeral joint, which is the most commonly dislocated joint of the body. The rotator cuff muscles play an important role in the stability of this joint; however, there are no muscles or ligaments on the side inferior to the axilla, which is the region where the joint is most often dislocated (Figure 1.5 ■). Poor muscle tone increases the risk for injury. Muscle fatigue also can put ligaments at risk. For example, ligaments of the joints in the feet cannot by themselves support the body's weight. Should the tone of the muscle that supports the arches become fatigued, the ligaments will stretch, leading to flat feet. The value of an exercise program for a bodyworker is to strengthen muscles to reduce the risk for injury. Programs can be developed to strengthen specific muscles that are necessary for work tasks.

Muscle and Connective Tissue Provide the Force for Movement

Muscle and connective tissue provide not only stability but also force. Each skeletal muscle, such as the quadriceps femoris or biceps brachii, is specialized to provide a selected body movement. At the gross anatomy level, a muscle is attached to the bones on either side of the joint (Figure 1.6 ■). Generally, a muscle originates on one bone and extends across the joint, typically by means of a

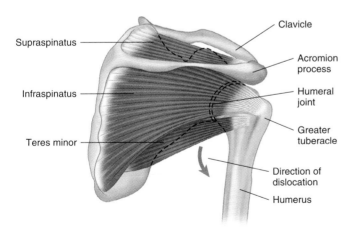

Supraspinatus

Infraspinatus

Teres minor

Clavicle

Acromion process

Humeral joint

Greater tuberacle

Direction of dislocation

Humerus

Posterior View of Scapula

FIGURE 1.5

The humeral joint is well stabilized superiorly; however, inferiorly it lacks stabilization. Thus, the majority of dislocations occur inferiorly, as shown by the direction of the arrow.

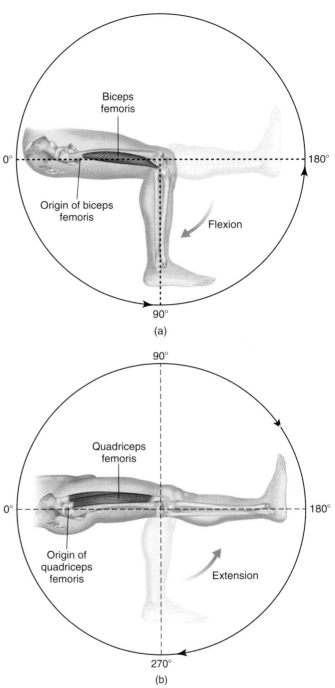

Biceps femoris

0°

180°

Origin of biceps femoris

Flexion

90°

(a)

90°

Quadriceps femoris

0°

180°

Origin of quadriceps femoris

Extension

270°

(b)

FIGURE 1.6

A muscle will span across an articulation. As the muscle contracts, force is applied to the insertion and the angle of the joint decreases in the direction of the force. (a) Contraction of the biceps femoris, which inserts on the posterior side of the tibia, causes flexion at the knee. With the origin of the biceps considered to be 0°, the fully extended tibia is at 180° and with flexion would be less than 180°. A 90° flexion is shown. (b) Contraction of the quadriceps femoris causes extension of the knee. Now the origin of the quadriceps is 0°. The flexed position earlier becomes 270° and full extension is 180°. Again, contraction of the muscle decreases the angle at the joint.

tendon, to insert on the other bone. As the muscle contracts, the force is directed onto the insertion point, causing the angle of the joint to change.

Muscle tissue is embedded in a connective tissue scaffolding (Figure 1.7 ■). Muscle fibers are organized into bundles, and connective tissue surrounds the individual fibers, bundles, and entire muscle. Collagen fibers from each layer become intertwined, and some extend into the tendon that attaches the muscle securely to bone. Thus, the muscle fiber is responsible for contraction, but the connective tissue is responsible for transmitting the force to the bone for movement. Without the connective tissue, the muscle would contract without creating movement, much like a car spinning its tires on ice. The connective tissue layers also create a pathway for blood and lymphatic vessels and nerves.

With physical conditioning, the muscle fiber becomes more developed and the connective tissue stronger. Stretching improves flexibility of connective tissue and makes it more resistant to damage. Nevertheless, there is always a limit to the capacity of any muscle. When a muscle is overextended, its fibers and/or connective tissue, including the tendon, can tear. This injury is known as a **strain.**

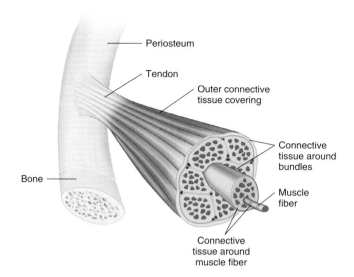

FIGURE 1.7

The muscle fibers are embedded in connective tissue scaffolding. The muscle fiber (or myofiber) generates the force of contraction and the connective tissue transmits the force.

INJURIES RELATED TO MOVEMENT

Understanding how to prevent movement-related injuries starts by understanding why they occur. In the realm of ergonomics, injuries occur from trauma when demands placed on the body exceed the physical capabilities of the musculoskeletal system and/or its accessory tissues. The result is tissue damage, inflammation, and loss of function. The body's ability to repair the injury depends on its degree and type, the individual's health, and whether the area is subjected to further trauma.

Inflammation and Healing

Inflammation is a part of the body's response to injury and is necessary for healing. The five most likely signs and symptoms of inflammation probably are redness, warmth, pain, edema (swelling), and loss of function. They occur as a result of vasodilation to the area and an increase in capillary permeability. Together, these responses bring more nutrients and white blood cells to the area and dilute the toxins. Pain and loss of function triggers a protective response to reduce the chance of reinjury. When the white blood cells remove the dead tissue materials from the area, tissue regeneration and repair can take place.

Although inflammation is normal and necessary, if it becomes excessive, it can actually cause further tissue trauma. The edema can cause **pressure atrophy,** degeneration of the tissue from the pressure of the excess interstitial fluid. The traditional prescription of rest, ice (a cold pack), compression, and elevation (RICE) can offset this process. Excessive inflammation often occurs when an injury is ignored and the area continues to be used. When an injury is ongoing, recurring, or the normal body's response is delayed or inadequate, chronic inflammation is triggered and healing is slowed or prevented. Chronic inflammation is a medical concern that leads to further injury.

Osteoarthritis, bursitis, tendonitis, and carpal tunnel syndrome are common work-related inflammatory disorders. As discussed, the relatively friction-free environment of the synovial joint is maintained in part by the presence of hyaline cartilage. The condition **osteoarthritis** wears this cartilage down; thus, friction increases and movement becomes more difficult. This sets a cycle in which more friction creates more damage, and more damage creates more friction. Improper ergonomics can set the stage for work-related osteoarthritis. Although it depends on the type of work, the bodyworker's highest risks for osteoarthritis are commonly the hands, wrists, elbows, shoulders, lower back, and knees.

Friction is also dissipated by **bursae,** fibrous, synovial-lined sacs that provide a fluid-filled cushion protecting tendons where they pass along bone, ligaments, or other tendons, usually in the area around a joint. The cavity of a bursa can communicate with the synovial joint cavity, as in the case of the suprapatellar bursa, which cushions the quadriceps movement over the distal end of the femur. However, bursae frequently are separate sacs, as in the case of the prepatellar bursa, which forms a cushion between the skin and the front of the patella (Figure 1.8 ■). Bursae are prone to injury and inflammation with excessive pressure or repetitive motion. For example, prolonged work performed while people are on their hands and knees can lead to **bursitis** of the prepatellar bursa, a condition commonly known as "housemaid's knee."

Where a tendon passes under ligaments or retinacula, or through osseofibrous tunnels, a tubular-shaped bursa,

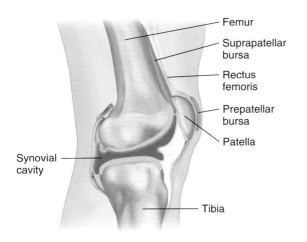

Labels: Femur, Suprapatellar bursa, Rectus femoris, Prepatellar bursa, Patella, Synovial cavity, Tibia

FIGURE 1.8

Two bursae are associated with the knee. The suprapatellar bursa lies between the quadriceps and the femur. Its cavity directly opens into the synovial joint. The prepatellar bursa forms a cushion between the skin and the front of the patella (kneecap).

known as a **tendon sheath,** surrounds the tendon to create a friction-free tunnel for movement. **Tendonitis,** clinically defined as an inflammation of the tendon sheath, is one of the most common causes of acute shoulder pain. Persistent abduction of the brachium while working puts the bodyworker at risk for this injury. It can occur with any tendon but usually in proximity to a joint as a result of friction.

Numerous tendon sheaths are found in the hand to accommodate the transit of the tendons of the extrinsic muscles of the hand to their insertion sites on the phalanges (Figure 1.9 ▪). A relatively common condition that can lead

Palmer View of Left Hand

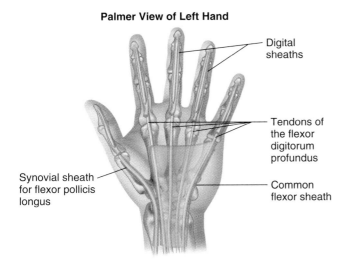

Labels: Digital sheaths, Tendons of the flexor digitorum profundus, Common flexor sheath, Synovial sheath for flexor pollicis longus

FIGURE 1.9

The extrinsic muscles of the hand transmit their forces for movement of the fingers through long tendons. The tendons are protected by tendon sheaths, which are tubular-shaped bursae.

to bodyworkers' need to give up their practice or cut back substantially is **carpal tunnel syndrome.** It is a group of characteristic signs and symptoms including pain, numbness, and reduced strength and motion of the hand. One explanation for carpal tunnel syndrome is that repetitive motion leads to inflammation of the common flexor sheath as it passes under the flexor retinaculum along with the median nerve (Figure 1.10 ▪). This puts pressure on the median nerve.

Strains and Sprains

As noted earlier, sprains often occur as a result of acute trauma such as a fall or blow to the body that knocks the joint out of position. However, continued, excessive stress can cause the fibrous ligaments to gradually stretch. For example, deliberate attempts to increase range of motion by a gymnast or ballet dancer can result in a stretch to the point that the ligament becomes more lax. Hypermobility (increased mobility) is achieved but involves decreased stability and associated risk for injury. There is also the potential for **subluxation** (misalignment of a joint) and even degenerative changes because of improper alignment of the articulating surfaces. In the workplace, any activity in which a joint is chronically or repeatedly moved to its physical extreme can have a similar effect on its stability and health. Bodyworkers tend to hyperextend the knee, which puts it at risk for injury. Being aware of stance and of keeping the knees slightly flexed can remove the risk.

Recall that a strain is a tear in the muscle fibers and/or connective tissue including the tendon. Acute strains can result from a direct blow to the body, overstretching, or excessive muscle contraction. On the other hand, chronic strains typically result from prolonged, repetitive movement or inadequate rest breaks during intense muscle use. One type of injury caused by chronic strain is **fibrositis,** inflammation of fibrous connective tissue. It occurs when muscles chronically worked beyond their capacity become fatigued. Repeated muscle fatigue prompts inflammation. This creates a reflex reaction causing a hypertonic condition in the muscle. The most severe form of hypertonicity of the muscle is a muscle cramp or "charley horse," but muscle spasms can be more insidious. Over time, spasms build up, and the muscle fibers involved become tighter until pain and stiffness occur. The pain is often noticed at the muscle's insertion point, which is typically in the vicinity of a joint. Diagnosis can be a joint injury when in reality it is a repetitive strain injury.

BASIS FOR OCCUPATIONAL INJURIES

Occupational injuries most commonly develop when the work activity requires repetitive motion. Improper body mechanics and a variety of factors in the work environment increase the risk. The U.S. Department of Labor defines a **musculoskeletal disorder (MSD)** as any injury or disorder of the muscles, nerves, tendons, joints, cartilage, and/or

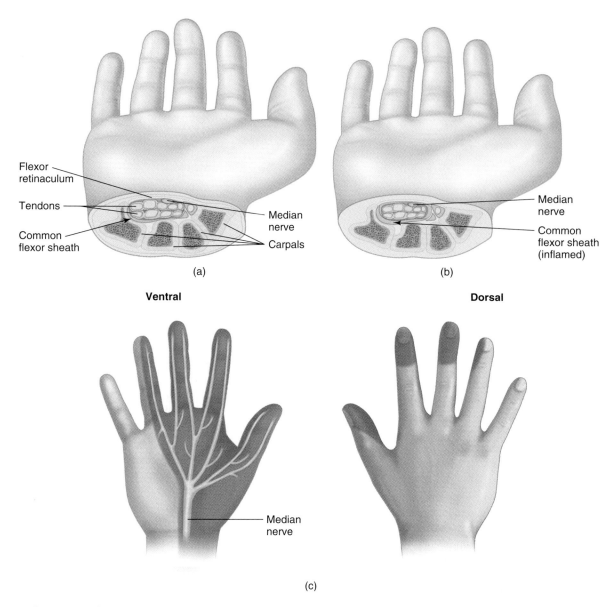

FIGURE 1.10

The carpal tunnel is formed by the carpal bones and flexor retinaculum. Tendons passing through the carpal tunnel are wrapped by the common flexor sheath. CTS involves inflammation of the common flexor sheath, which puts pressure on the median nerve. (a) Normal anatomy. (b) Inflammation. (c) Areas affected by nerve compression.

spinal discs not caused by slips, trips, falls, motor vehicle accidents, or similar accidents. MSDs account for 29% of work-related injuries and the highest percentage of workers' compensation claims filed per year (Department of Labor, 2009).

In 2002, the Department of Labor proposed a four-pronged strategy to address the problem of work-related MSDs including guidelines, enforcement, outreach, and assistance, as well as the creation of a national advisory committee on ergonomics with a research-based focus.

Repetitive Motion Syndromes

Motions that are repetitive—including many of the motions performed during bodywork—require the bones, muscles, nerves, and connective tissues to experience identical forces again and again. This continual repetition causes trauma to all of the associated structures, triggering inflammation, pain, and the potential for postural distortion.

The stress of performing the same activity over weeks, months, and years commonly leads to a group of characteristic symptoms collectively known as **repetitive motion syndrome** (also referred to as *cumulative trauma disorder, repetitive stress injury,* and *overuse syndrome*). The following is a list of these characteristic symptoms:

- Tingling, cold, or numbness because of reduced blood flow or nerve impingement
- Tightness, stiffness, soreness, burning, or discomfort because of hypertonic muscles, inflammation, or nerve impingement

- Loss of strength or coordination because of muscle weakness or nerve impingement
- Pain at night resulting from inflammation, hypertonicity, or nerve impingement

Common repetitive motion syndromes include the inflammatory disorders discussed earlier (osteoarthritis, bursitis, tendonitis, and carpal tunnel syndrome) as well as back injury, headaches, sprains, strains, tears, and simply chronic pain.

Any occupation that requires a person to move in a repetitive manner, such as sorting mail, lifting boxes, punching tickets, or performing deep tissue massage, increases the risk of developing a repetitive motion syndrome. Vibration, actions that create friction and uninterrupted repetitions, are particularly harmful. Excessively forceful moves or awkward positions (torque or twisting) significantly increase stress and the risk of injury. A common example of this in health care professions is lifting and turning immobilized patients. Bodyworkers do not typically lift patients but, depending on their practice, can lift and carry massage tables and massage chairs. Bodyworkers performing techniques that create friction or require deep pressure are also at risk for injury. When injury does occur, sometimes it is essential to take time off to heal and learn to use safe, effective ways to work that are ergonomically sound.

Repetitive Motion and Postural Distortion

The body's attempt to adapt to repetitive motion can lead to **postural distortion**. From time to time, you could meet people who look like what they do. For example, someone who uses a phone all day exhibits a lateral head tilt; someone bent over a microscope all day develops a more concave spinal flexure. For the bodyworker, improper attention to ergonomics commonly leads to elevated and/or protracted shoulders. Some postural distortions, such as club foot, are congenital, and others, such as kyphosis ("dowager's hump") result from degenerative disease. But many are acquired conditions related to occupation. Ergonomic principles can help people correct or reduce work-related postural distortions. The primary focus of this book is to educate you to avoid acquiring them in the first place. The secondary focus is to identify ways to compensate for postural distortions.

Postural distortion can also develop when the body attempts to compensate for repetitive motion. Most people have had the experience of buying a pair of shoes that don't fit properly. In the beginning the feet feel sore, but eventually a blister and ultimately a callus form. In the time it takes for the callus to form, the person's gait and stance will have changed to compensate for the stress of improper fit. In a similar way, people tend to compensate for repeated movements of one body limb or region and consequently stress other areas. In addition to causing postural distortion, compensation stresses body mechanics, leading the body to develop a restricted range of motion or inefficient pattern of movement.

Improper Body Mechanics and Injury

Without proper body mechanics, repeated movements can place undue stress on joints. Proper body mechanics also involves using the most efficient motion for the task. For example, using wrist action to swing a hammer to pound a nail creates much more stress than full arm movement. Wrist action is not as effective in delivering the blow to the head of the nail; thus, the action requires harder work. In a similar fashion, using the arms to deliver an effleurage stroke is not efficient use of the body. Rather, good technique is to use the gravity of the body in motion to deliver the force.

Body mechanics addresses body alignment. Joints not only allow for movement but also stabilize the body to maintain alignment, which is especially important for people who work with their hands whether playing piano, writing, typing, or performing a massage. During such tasks, it is not uncommon to hyperextend the wrist, stressing the joint and surrounding structures. This is a classic scenario for developing carpal tunnel syndrome. Keeping the wrist or any joint in proper alignment to minimize trauma is referred to as maintaining **neutral alignment**. Neutral identifies the angle during movement and rest that is most favorable to joint function and health. All synovial joints have only one position in which the articulating surfaces are precisely aligned for best joint stability. Neutrality is discussed thoroughly in Chapters 2 and 3, and is the subject of the accompanying Helpful Hint 1.2.

Work Environment and Risk of Injury

Environmental factors can compromise the body, resulting in fatigue, headache, and vision and hearing problems. Poor air quality, odors, and the presence of allergens can affect workers' health, as can an environment that is too hot or too cold. Inadequate lighting can cause eyestrain whereas lighting that is too bright can cause headaches. Background noise from jackhammers to traffic can cause distraction and subconscious tension. The distance between the work equipment and the worker's body, limbs, and fingers is an extremely important consideration in ergonomic design. Distances between the equipment and the worker must be precisely correlated to help the worker maintain neutral alignment.

As mentioned earlier, one result of poor ergonomics is an increase in workers' compensation claims and loss of work time. However, chronic low-grade stress and discomfort also affect workers' performance, relationships with colleagues, and general well-being and reduce workplace morale. As discussed in Case Study 1.1, the social and psychological implications of occupational injury, even for bodyworkers in independent practice, can be extensive.

Summary for the Bodyworker

The adage "Physician, heal thyself" applies to bodyworkers as well: As we treat clients' injured tissues, we put ourselves at risk for developing musculoskeletal disorders.

HELPFUL HINT 1.2
Finding Neutral

One of the most important aspects of ergonomics is maintaining a neutral alignment; that is, the place exactly intermediate between extreme flexion and extreme extension. To see this kinesthetically and visually, perform the following exercise:

Rest the olecranon (elbow) on a table with the hand and forearm extended upward. Observe the position of the wrist in neutral position identified by the absence of any crease at the wrist. In this position, a smooth line goes from the elbow to the fingertips. Now hyperextend the wrist and observe the feeling as well as the deep creases on the dorsal side of the hand. Next hyperflex the wrist and observe the creases on the ventral side and note the feeling in the wrist. Then return to neutral and feel the easy relaxation of the joint.

To avoid injury, we need to assess our work environment and learn how to work safely. As you read this summary, check to see whether any of your earlier body scan observations appear.

Besides repetitive motion, all fields of bodywork share specific range-of-motion issues that can lead to MSDs and postural distortions. For most bodywork, the client is stationary. Target areas for treatment are usually the client's neck, back, shoulders, wrists, hands, legs, and feet. Most people tend to look at the surface on which they are working. For the therapist, this means looking down at the client on the table or in the chair. If the therapist is seated, the angle of the flexion is reduced but still is problematic. Constant neck flexion keeps the posterior neck muscles stretched and the anterior muscles contracted. Therapists who hunch forward instead of standing or sitting upright develop back tension. In addition, improperly aligned feet create stress on the knees and legs and ultimately affect the back. And as noted earlier, the wrists and hands are often problematic areas and are discussed in subsequent chapters.

Clients come in all shapes and sizes, and for this reason, adjusting the height of the treatment table to fit the anthropometrics of the client is very important. A man with a 42″ chest requires a different table height than one with a 38″ chest. Adjusting the table keeps the bodyworkers' shoulders from elevating to accommodate to the height of the table and the person lying on it. Chronically heightened shoulders cause the development of a holding pattern. Over time, they remain elevated even when the person isn't working. Notice that this is an example of a *postural distortion*. In addition, if a therapist specializes in deep tissue massage (e.g., neuromuscular work or Rolfing™), the table needs to be lower to avoid compromising the arms, hands, shoulders, and neck. Whenever the treatment table is too high or too low, the stage is set for musculoskeletal problems.

The massage chair presents ergonomic challenges slightly different from those of the table. A therapist using a chair must use a greater degree of upper body flexion; therefore, if the stance is not the appropriate width and distance, the therapist's back will tire from the strain. This is

---

CASE FOR STUDY 1.1
Overuse Injury

Susan is a massage therapist who predominately uses her thumbs for deep tissue massage. She further exacerbates this overuse by hyperextending her wrists. The thumb is primarily for grasping, but this doesn't mean it can't be used to do deep tissue work; however, it needs to be used in moderation. Susan's physician tells her she has strained the intrinsic hand muscles controlling the thumb and has developed carpal tunnel syndrome. Because the recommended time off for recovery from this injury would hurt her financially, she continues to work, compromising by cutting back on the number of massages she does per day and working more superficially. Some of her clients who like deep tissue work are no longer satisfied and switch to other therapists. The loss of income compounds the stress Susan is under because of her pain. As this pattern continues, she becomes depressed and withdrawn. Her attitude becomes negative and begins to affect all of her relationships.

The future for Susan could take several routes. Consider her challenges and options in discussing the following questions.

1. With this scenario, what is the potential long-term outcome to Susan's career?
2. As Susan's co-worker or therapist, what would you recommend to her?

just one example of how injury can develop while doing chair massage work.

Carpal tunnel syndrome, discussed earlier, is one of the most common repetitive motion syndromes affecting bodyworkers. It often is a result of chronic hyperextension. The work situation always needs to be considered. For example, if a client of a reflexologist displays an exaggerated external rotation of the feet (abduction), the reflexologist needs to modify position and use props to reduce injury. Two definitive tests for carpal tunnel syndrome are *Phalen's test* and *Tinel's sign*. Both are described in Worksheet 1.1.

The therapist's physical condition influences body mechanics and in turn the potential for injury. For example, an overweight therapist who carries the weight predominately in the abdominal region will strain the dorsal muscles. Obviously, the combination of this compromised physical

condition and repetitive movement, especially if the equipment is inadequate or improperly adjusted, takes a heavy toll on the body. The use of props such as step stools, bolsters, and adjustable features on equipment are important.

Another consideration specific to bodyworkers is the variety of locations in which they work. Although body therapists traditionally have worked independently, the increased demand for their work has led to employment in increasingly diverse establishments: at spas, salons, health clubs, offices, resorts, and hotels, medical facilities, and sporting events—even on cruise ships. In such settings, therapists have little control over the work environment, and the risk of injury subsequently increases. In addition, the "have table, will travel" industry is on the rise with bodyworkers carrying their massage tables and chairs into businesses, airports, and malls, risking injury from the continual setup, breakdown, and transport of their equipment.

WORKSHEET 1.1
Phalen's Test and Tinel's Sign

Phalen's test and Tinel's sign are quick, simple assessments for carpal tunnel syndrome. To perform Phalen's test (a):

1. Put the backs of the hands together, keeping arms parallel to the floor and fingers pointing down.
2. Hold hands firmly together.
3. If within 1 minute, pain, tingling, or numbness of the hand and wrist, or a combination of these symptoms, is experienced, the disorder is probably the diagnosis. (Don't hold this position for more then the required minute.)

To check for Tinel's sign (b):

1. Rest the hand on a flat surface with the wrist in a neutral position.
2. Tap with fingers or reflex hammer at the sight over the median nerve and carpal tunnel. If pain, tingling, and/or numbness of the hand and wrist are experienced, the test is positive.

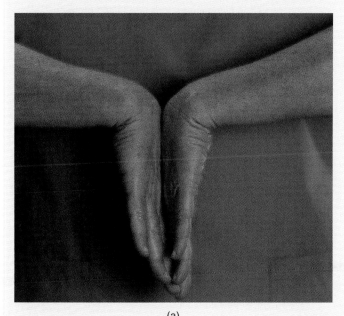

(a)

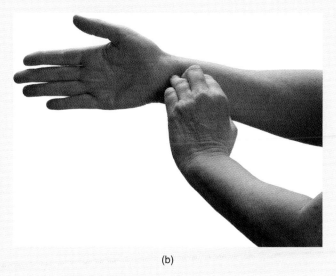

(b)

Phalen's test and Tinel's sign

ERGONOMICS PRINCIPLES TO PREVENT INJURY

Ergonomics begins with the appropriate assessment of a worker, the activity(ies) performed, and the workspace. These assessments can then be used to design equipment and work environments and prescribe body mechanics that protect worker health. The following are some guidelines for helping bodyworkers prevent occupational injury; they are further explored in later chapters.

Maintain Neutral Alignment

As noted earlier, neutrality identifies the joint angle that is most favorable to joint function and health. Chapters 2 and 3 provide a thorough discussion of techniques for maintaining neutral alignment in stationary position and in motion. In addition, Helpful Hint 1.3 discusses how the study of *tai chi* can increase kinesthetic awareness.

Maintain a Healthful Posture

Good posture has many benefits; it keeps the joints in alignment with minimum stress on muscles and supporting tissues. Consequently, it reduces postural distortions and the risk of injury. Perhaps most important, attention to posture tends to lead quite naturally to appropriate body mechanics during movement. The keys to learning how to maintain healthful posture are:

- Keep objects within range.
- Don't slump when sitting; looking down creates strain in the neck and back.
- Pivot and turn with the entire body, especially when carrying something heavy. Remember the motto: Nose with the toes.
- When lifting, bend at the knees and lift with the legs rather than the back, and contract the abdominals for support and stabilization.

Assessing posture daily helps to define areas of concern and allows for an action plan to address these areas before they develop into chronic conditions or acute injuries.

Use Proper Body Mechanics

During massage and other bodywork, using proper body mechanics alleviates stress and minimizes injury, improving

HELPFUL HINT 1.3
Using *Tai Chi* to Increase Kinesthetic Awareness

This text often refers to kinesthetic awareness. It is the ability of the senses to detect and be aware of body position and movement. People who practice the ancient martial art of *tai chi* develop increased kinesthetic awareness as they focus on their balance and weight distribution and learn how to direct their breath to areas of the body. In its name, **chi** is life force, or vitality, and is driven by breath. Thus, breath is the equivalent of force. Being aware of breath and focusing it is not a common skill in the Western world. The following two activities demonstrate practices that will hone these skills. *Tai chi* works in parallel with the Western approach to ergonomics in teaching how to maintain a relaxed torso that supports the natural spinal curves and a stable stance from the feet to the pelvic floor. Uniting Eastern and Western approaches is useful for the therapist to establish healthy body mechanics for career longevity.

Activities

1. This activity can be done sitting upright, standing or lying down. It is beneficial to practice it lying down the first time and progress to the other positions.

   Begin by lying comfortably and covered with a blanket on the massage table. Use a bolster under the knees if needed. Place your hands on your lower abdomen. The upper arms should be relaxed and resting on the table with the palms of your hands resting comfortably on your abdomen, just

below anterior superior iliac spine (ASIS). Inhale through the nose and exhale from the mouth. If you need to inhale through the mouth, do so. The most efficient way to breathe is diaphragmatically so that your abdomen rises on the inhalation filling your hands and falling on the exhalation. Become aware of the rhythm of breathing and the movement of the body. With each repetition, you will find the breath naturally deepening and encompassing more of the torso. You will likely find this activity relaxing. Once you are proficient at this technique while lying down, performing it either seated or standing will be easier. This is a recommended technique for relaxation and focusing on body movement.

2. Once you are comfortable using breathing to focus on body movement and develop kinesthetic awareness, you are ready to begin to visualize breath movement. In a relaxed state, close your eyes, take a deep breath, and, as you exhale, visualize the breath and energy flowing down your arm and out through your fingers. This visualization can take time to develop. As you practice the exercise, notice that you become aware of muscle tone, limb position, and cutaneous sensations. This improves your kinesthetic awareness, and from that, you develop the skills to be conscious of your body. This awareness helps develop better ergonomic practice.

efficiency and extending careers. Chapter 5 discusses these techniques in detail.

Take Breaks

Taking breaks throughout an activity is also important to prevent problems. Even a few moments of rest, such as glancing out the window or shaking out the hands, can be therapeutic. Stretching, using focused breathing, taking short walks, scanning the body for tension and visualizing letting it go are all tools.

Additionally, consider whether leisure activities are actually exacerbating the stress the body experiences at work. For example, it is possible to undo good posture during the day by yielding to poor habits during rest, whether during sleeping, reclining, reading, and so on. Chapter 9 discusses strategies for enhancing career longevity through appropriate rest and relaxation in detail.

Perform Frequent Work Self-Assessment

Self-assessment is critical to continuing good health and productivity in bodywork. Important questions to ask regarding this follow:

- What motions are required to complete the task?
- Does the task require standing or sitting, or both?
- What postures are required for the task?
- How far are horizontal or vertical reaches?
- Do any sensory aspects (e.g., color, clutter, temperature, sound, smell) have the potential to provoke stress?
- Is the space adequate for performing the task with proper body mechanics?

Self-assessment and self-care are discussed in much more detail in later chapters, which will also include the needed tools to answer these questions in regard to specific work situations.

CHAPTER SUMMARY

- The field of ergonomics deals with safety in the work environment by addressing issues of biomechanics and the design of equipment and workspaces. It also considers numerous environmental factors, such as noise, light, temperature, and vibration.
- The field of ergonomics expanded rapidly following World War II, especially after the establishment of the Occupational Safety and Health Administration.
- Attention to ergonomics is financially prudent because this can improve productivity and reduce lost work time and wages, workers' compensation claims, and lawsuits.
- Consequences of poor ergonomics include MSDs, which can develop in an insidious manner as a result of repetitive motion.
- Injuries occur when demands placed on the body exceed the physical capabilities of the musculoskeletal system and/or its accessory tissues. Both the physical work environment and the body's limitations play a role in risk for injury.
- The stability of joints is an important factor for identifying potential risk for injury and is determined by the type of joint; shape, size, and arrangement of

- the articulation of synovial joints; support by ligaments; and tone of the surrounding muscle.
- Friction is reduced in the musculoskeletal system by the synovial fluid of the joint capsule, cartilage surface of the articulations, bursae, and tendon sheaths. However, repetitive action increases friction and can lead to injury.
- Injuries commonly related to movement include inflammatory disorders such as osteoarthritis, bursitis, tendonitis, carpal tunnel syndrome, strains, and sprains.
- The proper alignment of joints, known as *neutral,* reduces the risk for injury.
- Adaptation to or compensation for repetitive movement leads to postural distortions and ultimately injuries.
- The various disciplines in the field of bodywork share common ergonomic issues that later chapters address more fully.
- Ergonomics principles that help bodyworkers prevent injury include maintaining neutral alignment, maintaining healthful posture, using proper body mechanics, taking breaks, and performing self-assessment.

REVIEW QUESTIONS

1. The historical event that prompted the development of the field of ergonomics was
   a. The establishment of the U.S. Department of Labor
   b. World War II
   c. The invention of the typewriter
   d. The invention of the conveyor belt
2. The study of human body measurement is called:
   a. anthropometrics
   b. kinesiology
   c. osteopathy
   d. ergonomics
3. The most freely movable joint type is the:
   a. fibrous joint
   b. plane joint
   c. cartilaginous joint
   d. ball-and-socket joint
4. True or false? Pain, numbness, stiffness, and loss of strength are symptoms of repetitive motion syndrome.
5. True or false? Compensation is a mechanism by which the body avoids postural distortion by adapting to repetitive motion.
6. True or false? It is possible to undo good posture during the day by poor positioning during sleep.
7. Identify three ways a joint is stabilized.
8. Name each of the types of synovial joints and the direction(s) of motion of which they are capable.
9. Identify the five signs of inflammation.
10. Define *neutrality* and explain its role in preventing occupational injury.

REFERENCES

All about OSHA (2006). U.S. Department of Labor, OSHA 3302, 2006. Retrieved August 29, 2010, from http://www.osha.gov/Publications/3302-06N-2006-English.html#Introduction

Department of Labor. (2000, December 22). OSHA lists highlights of three decades—Meeting the mandate: Saving lives, preventing injury, preserving health. OSHA National News Release. USDL:00-376. Retrieved January 15, 2005, from http://www.osha.gov/pls/oshaweb/owadisp.show_document?p_table=NEWS_RELEASES&p_id=445.

Department of Labor. (2009, November 24). Nonfatal occupational injuries and illnesses requiring day away from work, 2008. Bureau of Labor Statistics News Release. USDL-09-1454. Retrieved August 29, 2010, from http://stats.bls.gov/iif/oshwc/osh/case/osnr0033.pdf.

Dohrmann, M. General Information about ergonomics. Retrieved March 13, 2004, from http://www.ergonomics.com.au.

SUGGESTED READINGS

Hendrikson T. (2003). *Massage for orthopedic conditions.* Baltimore, MD: Lippincott Williams & Wilkins.

Lippert, L. S. (2000). *Clinical kinesiology for physical therapist assistants.* Philadelphia: F. A. Davis Company.

McAndrew, M., and Lezak. A. OSHA's new ergonomics regulations. 15 minutes of fame. Retrieved June 27, 2004, from http://www.dcba.org/legal/artindex.htm

Molleson, T. (1994, August). The eloquent bones of Abu Hureyra. *Scientific American*, pp. 70–75.

Occupational Health and Safety Administration. Retrieved June 22, 2004, from http://www.oshsa.gov.htm.

Seeley, R. R., Stephens, T. D., and Tate, P. (2000). *Anatomy and physiology* (5th ed.). Boston: McGraw Hill.

Snell, R. S. (1992). *Clinical anatomy for medical students* (4th ed.). Boston: Little, Brown.

U.S. Department of Labor. (2002). Lost-worktime injuries and illnesses: Characteristics and resulting days away from work. June 27, 2004, from http://www.bls.gov/iif/home.htm.

U.S. Department of Labor. (1970). OSHA Act of 1970 Section 2 Congressional findings and purpose. Retrieved August 29, 2010, from http://osha.gov/pls/oshaweb/owadisp.show_document?p_table=OSHACT&p_id=3356

Van de Graaff, K. (2000). *Human anatomy*. (5th ed.). Boston: McGraw Hill.

2 Postural Assessment

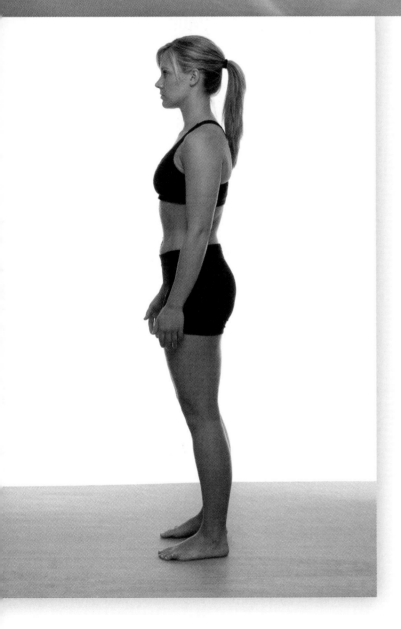

CHAPTER OUTLINE

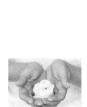

LEARNING OBJECTIVES

Upon successfully completing this chapter, you will be able to:

1. Compare and contrast the external and internal approaches to neutral alignment.
2. Describe the anatomical position and relate it to neutrality.
3. Explain how the center of gravity and base of support relate to balance.
4. Assess body alignment when standing from the anterior, posterior, and lateral views.
5. Identify the ideal seated position for neutral alignment.

6. Explain the relationship between flow and awareness.
7. Differentiate between adaptation and compensation relative to posture, and explain how the internal approach can reverse their effects.
8. Discuss the role of sensory awareness and energy awareness in the internal approach.
9. Describe the balanced approach and how it can be used to develop desirable muscle memory.

KEY TERMS

Maintaining neutral alignment is essential to preventing injury. In Chapter 1, we defined neutrality as the angle of any joint during movement or rest that is most favorable to joint function and health. Neutral alignment places the least amount of stress on the joints, ligaments, and supporting muscles. Maintenance of the neutral position begins with awareness, and because awareness is more easily accomplished when we are still, this chapter explains and explores a variety of approaches to neutral alignment in stationary positions. We begin with the external approach, which requires a person to look objectively at the body to determine whether or not it is physically balanced. In everyday life, people do not have the luxury of always being able to assess their posture in an objective manner. Thus, we next explore the internal approach, which provides a subjective means of becoming aware of the body and its alignment. In truth, both approaches are necessary: We develop and learn to maintain neutral alignment by a combination of knowing what proper alignment should be and becoming familiar with how it feels. We call this the *balanced approach.*

EXTERNAL APPROACH

The **external approach to neutral alignment** is achieved through attention to two components: posture and balance. Posture is the alignment of the body's parts, especially the components of the axial skeleton. The **anatomical position** is the traditional means of looking at posture. It is a standing position with feet parallel, arms at the side with palms forward and fingers pointed straight down, and head facing forward (Figure 2.1 ■). Few people find the anatomical position relaxed or neutral; however, from this position, alignment can be evaluated by looking at the person from anterior, posterior, and lateral views. We explain how to evaluate posture from each of these views shortly. In a view of the skeleton in anatomical position, the bones can appear to be strategically placed on top of one another like a stack of balanced blocks. However, the joints and supporting ligaments are insufficient to maintain such an alignment very long. If the joints and ligaments could, it would be possible to sleep while standing up! Thus, posture depends not only on bones but also on muscle tone with agonists and antagonists working in concert to maintain the position. A continuous pull on the skeleton from opposite directions counters the effect of gravity.

Balance keeps the body in alignment. It is a complex body process in which the vestibular apparatus of the inner ear, visual input from the eyes, and proprioceptors throughout the body detect changes in position and send information to the brain, which in turn signals to correct the muscle tone. This mechanism is continuously at work to keep the body's center of gravity within the bounds of the **base of support**. When we are standing upright, the base of support is our stance, which is influenced by the distance our feet are apart from each other. This exercise demonstrates the importance of the base of support: Stand with your feet close together and have someone push you from

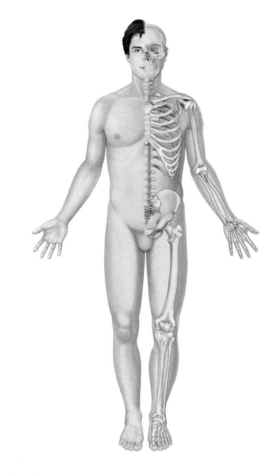

FIGURE 2.1

The anatomical position is an upright position with feet flat on the ground and positioned in alignment with the hips. Arms are at the side with palms facing forward. Note that the ulna and radius are lying parallel with one another in this position. Head is facing forward. The underlying skeletal view shows bone alignment for the position.

the side at shoulder level. It is very difficult to keep your balance when this occurs. Next repeat the action with your feet separated to shoulder or hip width. Notice how much easier it is to stand with the wider base of support; your torso has more room to change position before your center of gravity is compromised to the point that you must take a step to avoid falling.

Continual postural adjustment occurs involuntarily when we are in a stationary position. Good posture, with all skeletal components in their optimal, balanced position, reduces the neuromuscular effort needed to stay in position. When we assume an unbalanced position, muscles need to tighten to compensate for the effect of gravity. It should also be noted that both overly tight muscles and weak muscles change the forces placed on the skeleton and can cause poor posture.

"Normal" posture is difficult to define because each person has unique anthropometric and physiological characteristics. Body type, whether long and lean (ectomorphs), short and fat (endomorphs), or athletic and muscular (mesomorphs), influences alignment and the center of gravity. For example, the ectomorph often demonstrates drooped shoulders, and the endomorph has a tendency to gain weight in the abdominal area, which promotes lordosis (excessive lumbar curve). The characteristics of a person's bone structure and ligaments also play a role in posture and body mechanics. Loose ligaments cause a person to exhibit more exaggerated spinal curves and hyperextended knees and hips. Health and illness also affect posture. A person in good physical condition has better muscle tone to maintain proper posture than someone who is not. In contrast, neuro-muscular, respiratory, and bone diseases can manifest in postural distortion. Long-term habits, from watching television to doing desk work, dramatically influence posture as the common slouching seen in our society demonstrates. Also, our posture changes throughout the day as we become tired. Our emotional state also influences our posture: Compare the posture of someone cheerful and confident to someone who is depressed. A person's emotional state often can be read by studying his or her posture.

The next sections of this chapter explain how to evaluate your own or a client's posture while standing in anterior, posterior, and lateral views. Self-evaluation requires standing in front of a full-length mirror. A mirror is also helpful for pointing out observations to clients. Regardless of the direction of the view (anterior, posterior, or lateral), compare each side of the body by imagining a vertical line (or plumb line) running down the mid-axis (Figure 2.2 ■).

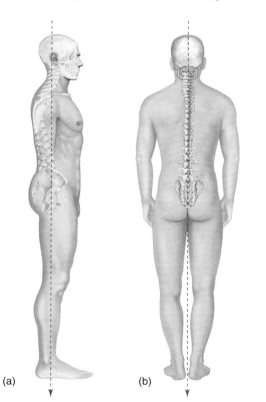

(a)　　　　　(b)

FIGURE 2.2

The lateral (a) and anterior (b) views show a well-aligned posture by the balance on either side of the imaginary vertical axis.

Strategic points on either side can be observed for alignment with each other along a horizontal line perpendicular to the axis. When checking for alignment, it is important that the person is barefoot because shoes will vary weight distribution on the feet.

Evaluating Standing Posture: Anterior View

Stand in the anatomical position and check for the following alignments.

- Legs parallel
- Coxal joints straight
- Knees level and not rotated
- Feet straight with no inversion or eversion
- Head level, not rotated
- Torso straight
- Shoulders level
- Pelvis level and not rotated
- Arms equal distance from the torso and of equal length

The feet form the base of support and should be about hip-width apart, placed below the centers of the quadriceps rather than their lateral extremes, which are approximately 8 centimeters apart. As in Figure 2.3 ■, an imaginary line drawn from the anterior superior iliac spine (ASIS) through the top of the arch of the foot (approximately the second metatarsal) should be parallel for neutral leg alignment. This creates a feeling of standing firm and connecting strongly to the ground.

The coxal (hip) joint is straight without any lateral or medial rotation. A lateral rotation results in a bow-leg effect and a medial rotation in a knock-kneed effect. The knees should be level, not rotated. Level exists only if the coxal joint is straight. Because the knee joint is a hinge joint, its most common deviation from neutral alignment is hyperextension, which is not readily observed from the anterior view. Slight rotation of the knee is possible only when it is flexed.

The talocrural (ankle) joint is also a hinge joint. It involves articulation of three bones, the tibia, fibula, and talus, in one joint capsule. It is supported on the lateral surface by the strong deltoid ligament and on the medial surface by four smaller ligaments: the lateral collateral ligaments, anterior talofibular ligament, posterior talofibular ligament, and calcaneofibular ligament. Ankle sprains often involve tearing one or more of these ligaments. Just distal to the talocrural joint are the intertarsal joints. They are responsible for inversion and eversion of the foot and if misaligned, can prevent a solid stance and alter the straight alignment of the legs.

The head and torso should be in neutral alignment with normal spinal curves. Check to see that the eyes and ears are level to determine whether there is any lateral flexion of the neck. A lateral tilt of the head affects the alignment of the ears as does the rotation of the head: When the head rotates to the right, the left ear moves forward and appears to be more elevated than the right ear from the anterior

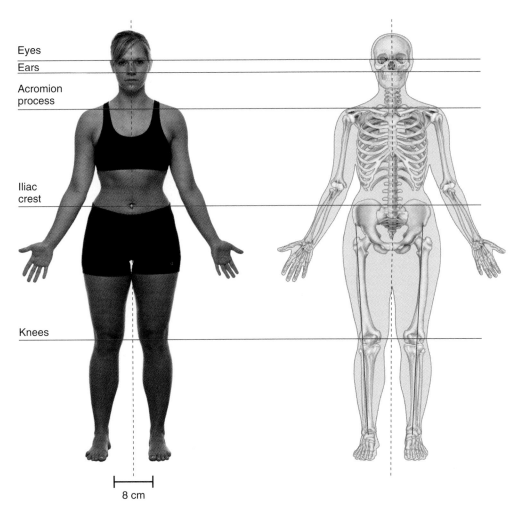

Eyes
Ears
Acromion process
Iliac crest
Knees

8 cm

FIGURE 2.3

The body should be symmetrical on either side of the mid-axis that extends down the middle to the vertebral column. The underlying skeletal and ligament structures are illustrated to demonstrate the proper alignments.

view. Shoulders should be level and neither protracted nor retracted. Protraction and retraction are easier to observe from a lateral view; however, protraction or retraction of one shoulder can manifest as the shoulders not being level. This state can also be characterized by a general twist to the entire torso.

The skin at the waist should have an equal crease on either side. The pelvis should be level, not rotated. Comparing the positions of the ASIS on either side can assess rotation. As with the shoulders, a twist to the torso could show a misalignment of the ASIS. Because the femur articulates with the pelvis, misalignment of the ASIS commonly correlates to misalignment of the legs as discussed previously.

In a full anatomical position, the arms are at the side with fingers pointing down and palms facing forward. Notice in this supine position that the radius and ulna run parallel. With both arms hanging from the shoulders an equal distance from the torso, you can check alignment of the hands and the elbows to confirm shoulder alignment.

The distance between the antebrachium (lower arm) and the torso referred to as the **carrying angle,** varies from one person to another. The carrying angle measures the antebrachial deviation from a line running straight with the axis of the humerus (Figure 2.4 ■). A normal carrying angle, which is approximately 5 degrees in males and between 10 and 15 degrees in females, allows the elbow to rest against the depression at the waist above the iliac crest. The carrying angle is a congenital anatomical trait and cannot be changed. A carrying angle outside the normal ranges can limit some people's ability to place the elbow in the optimal position for certain tasks. Techniques described later include ways to accommodate the carrying angle.

As stated earlier, a relaxed position differs from the true anatomical position. Most people find that when they relax, their forearms rotate with the palms turning in toward the body. This movement should involve only the forearm. Any rotation of the humerus results in the protraction of the shoulder. This misalignment impacts the torso.

Evaluating Standing Posture: Posterior View

A posterior view of the body in the anatomical position helps to confirm the assessments you made in the anterior view and to identify any lateral deviations of the spinal column.

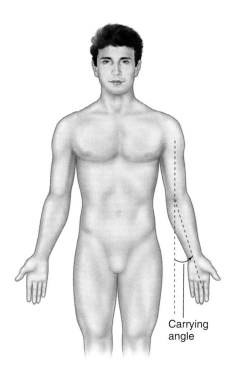

Carrying angle

FIGURE 2.4

The carrying angle is the angle the antebrachium deviates from the axis of the humerus. It varies between individuals and influences how they can position their arms or hands while performing some tasks.

The points to check for horizontal alignment (Figure 2.5 ■) include:

- Head straight with the midline
- Both acromion processes level
- Inferior angle of the scapulae level
- Iliac crests level
- Buttock creases level
- Knee creases level

The acromion processes should be level and the head straight with the midline. The shoulders should be of equal size and have the same angle. The inferior angles of the scapula should be level and the medial borders of the scapula equidistant from the spine. As explained for the anterior view, if one shoulder is protracted or retracted, the shoulders are not level. In addition, the scapulae change position. In protraction, the shoulder moves forward, and the scapula rotates, moves away from the spine, and tips out. This is called *winging*. Shoulder retraction causes the medial border to move toward the spine, becoming more prominent.

A common individual difference that influences posture is handedness (i.e. right or left handed). As in Figure 2.6 ■, the shoulder on the dominant side is often lower. The hip deviates slightly to the dominant side, and the spine drifts to the opposite side. The opposite foot also is slightly more pronated.

From the posterior view, it is easier to determine whether weight distribution on both feet is equal by observing the position of the calcaneus and any difference in the

shape, size, and position of the calcaneal tendon. Also right and/or left flexion or hyperextension of the knees is more noticeable. If only one knee is misaligned, the pelvis shows a lateral tilt.

The vertebral column should appear straight. **Scoliosis** is an abnormal lateral curve anywhere along the spine. If it is severe enough, it is visible as a noticeable lateral tilt or flexion of the torso.

Evaluating Standing Posture: Lateral View

Whereas the anterior and posterior views look at symmetry on either side of a midline, the lateral view reference is the line of gravity dividing the body into anterior and posterior halves. This makes the lateral view slightly more difficult to evaluate. The view assesses the curves of the spine, angle of the pelvis, and flexion of the knees. The spinal curves depend on the tone of the abdominal, pectoral, and back muscles and general weight distribution.

The spinal column goes through a series of changes during development. At birth, it has a generally concave curvature. As the infant begins to raise his or her head, a convex cervical curve develops. Subsequently, as the child begins to stand and walk, a convex lumbar curve forms. A 6-year-old child's center of gravity lies at about the 12th thoracic vertebra. That, in addition to a relatively large abdominal mass, weak abdominal muscles, and small pelvis, causes the child to have a more exaggerated lumbar curve than an adult, whose center of gravity has moved to the first or second sacral vertebra.

Weight distribution and muscle tone also influence the development of postural distortions such as exaggerated cervical lordosis, kyphosis, and lumbar lordosis. The specialized structure of each vertebra (such as the heavier body of the lumbar vertebrae, as compared to the thoracic or cervical vertebra) as well as the alignment of adjacent vertebrae and the position of the intervertebral discs provides the weight-bearing, flexible support to the torso that is critical for our upright posture. Acute trauma or chronic change in weight distribution causes vertebrae to become misaligned and/or discs to become damaged. This occurs most often in the lumbar region and is the basis for many chronic back problems.

See Figure 2.7 ■ for the proper alignment of lateral standing posture. The arms can be relaxed at the side for this assessment. The ear lobe should be in line with the acromion process (tip of the shoulder) and the top of the iliac crest. If this imaginary line is extended downward, it passes just anterior to the lateral malleolus and should be perpendicular to the ground.

Use this imaginary line to make the following assessments along the vertical axis.

- Head alignment with ear lobe positioned superior to acromion process: neutral versus protracted/retracted or hyperextended/flexed
- Shoulders: neutral versus elevated/depressed or protracted/retracted
- Thoracic curve: neutral versus rounded or flattened

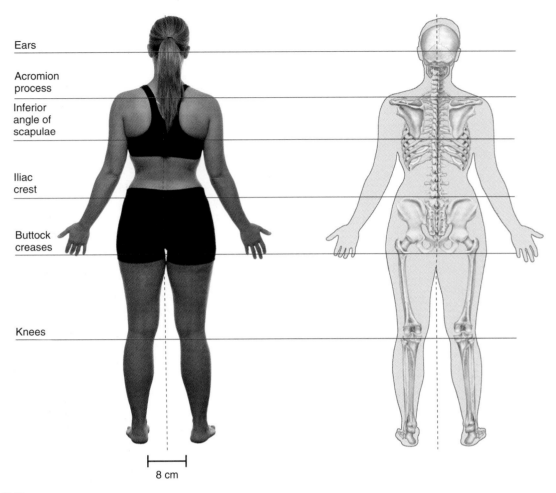

Ears

Acromion process

Inferior angle of scapulae

Iliac crest

Buttock creases

Knees

8 cm

FIGURE 2.5

Normal alignment shows a straight mid axis and level (horizontal) alignment of the acromion processes, scapula, iliac crests, and creases of the buttocks and knees.

- Lumbar curve: neutral versus exaggerated or flattened
- Pelvis: neutral (30 degree tilt) versus anterior tilt/posterior tilt
- Knee: neutral (0–5 degree flex) versus hyperextended/flexed

Evaluating Seated Posture

Because we perform many tasks while sitting, maintaining neutral alignment in the seated position is an important ergonomic goal. When we are seated, the ischial tuberosities and upper thighs are our base of support. A twist to the torso prevents equal weight distribution. The weight of the legs needs to be transferred to the feet and have direct contact with the floor. If there is not direct contact, a footrest needs to be used. With proper positioning, there is no undue pressure on the back of the knee joint.

If a backrest is used for support, it should provide a slight backward inclination. Forward flexion increases the weight load on the spinal column (Figure 2.8 ■). On the other hand, leaning back too far or slouching downward causes protraction of the head and affects the cervical spine. The position and range of motion of the arms need to be adjusted to avoid elevation or protraction of the shoulders. These considerations are important when choosing furniture.

INTERNAL APPROACH

An awareness of how your body alignment deviates from neutral is essential to developing and maintaining neutral alignment in stationary position; however, it is only one piece of the puzzle. Another piece, the **internal approach to neutral alignment**, is the ability to tune into the body through sensory awareness. Stationary neutrality at the internal level requires being present to whatever you are experiencing in your external environment. Becoming aware of what you are seeing, hearing, tasting, smelling, how hot or cold you are, and your body's position in your environment are all part of the internal approach to stationary neutrality.

Another requirement of the internal approach is to tune into your body internally throughout the day. This isn't difficult, but it does require practice if you are to develop the ability to sense in a moment that something has

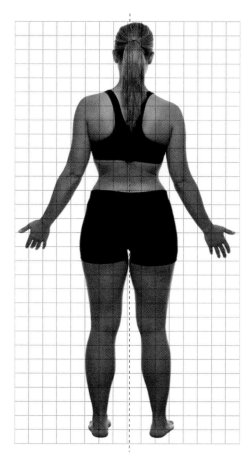

FIGURE 2.6

The greater use of the muscles on your dominant side causes an unequal development and alignment of the two sides of the body. This is a common cause of variation from what is considered to be *normal* alignment. Can you identify which side is dominant in the photo?

changed. Once developed, this internal sensing is tremendously empowering.

Personal experience can shape and define the level of internal awareness. For example, professional dancers, gymnasts, and many professional athletes typically have a high level of body awareness, feeling "tuned in" to every nuance their bodies. This tuning in is what the internal approach to neutral is all about.

Internal Awareness as Flow

Some writers refer to this constant internal awareness as **flow**. In his book *Flow: The Psychology of Optimal Experience*, Mihaly Csikzentmihalyi (1990, p. 4) states that flow merges awareness with action and leads to optimal experience. "We have all experienced times when, instead of being buffeted by anonymous forces, we feel in control of our actions, masters of our own fate." Being in tune and present sets the tone for flow and enhances our inner awareness.

To see how this applies to physical alignment or balance, consider the times when you catch yourself in a position of tension or discomfort. Awareness is the first

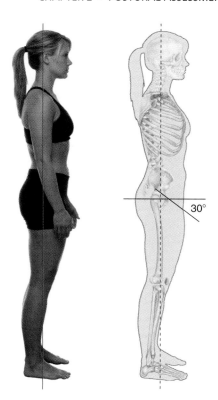

FIGURE 2.7

The lateral alignment determined from the vertical line of gravity. The spinal curves, pelvic tilt, and knee flexion/hyperextension are all assessed.

step in assessing tension and the catalyst for change. Consciously adjusting to become more comfortable is the second step. Consistently doing this is *flow*.

Challenges of the Internal Approach

The internal approach to neutral alignment can be extremely challenging, requiring us to move beyond our comfort zone. Over the years, most of us develop less than

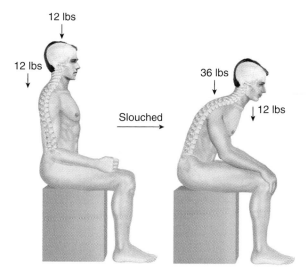

FIGURE 2.8

Proper sitting posture minimizes the weight load on the spine.

optimal patterns of posture and movement. For example, someone who works for 20 years hunched over a desk typically has chronically tightened muscles and ligaments involved in holding the spine erect. This process is called **adaptation.** As the muscles involved adapt to the positions required, the body takes on postural distortions, and both stationary and movement patterns deviate from neutral. This process is called **compensation.**

Compensation promotes patterns that become habitual and begin to feel normal. When this happens, a person's first few experiences of optimal alignment can feel foreign and uncomfortable. The discomfort can be so intense that the individual feels tempted to give up the attempt to develop more healthy neutral postures. Tremendous energy and effort, including a willingness to move through fatigue and discomfort, are required to break the old patterns and reeducate the body. Fortunately, experience suggests that, in time, most people can "reset their internal sensors" so that the compensatory patterns no longer feel comfortable, but the new, neutral patterns do.

Activities for Increasing Internal Awareness in Stationary Position

Begin your exploration of internal awareness in stationary position by directing your attention to the sensations you are currently experiencing in your body. These can include tension, pain, heat, cold, numbness, fluidity, lax muscles, or even the absence of sensation. If it is difficult to consciously feel your body or particular parts of your body, begin by asking yourself the following questions:

- Does any area of the body feel as if it's contracted or overworked, which are some descriptions of tension?
- Do any regions feel taut or tight, as though two opposing forces are pulling them? If so, they could be overstretched.
- Do you or any areas of your body feel fluid as though the energy is freely moving without blockage?
- Do you have areas of heat or coldness to the touch?
- Do you have areas where the muscle(s) feel lax or weak?

These general questions can help you choose a particular point in the body to focus on for further evaluation. Focus the mind's attention (mindfulness) on the point in question, and *feel* any and all sensations that arise. Sometimes touching the region in question can awaken awareness there. For example, to practice inner awareness of the left knee joint, pretend the mind has left the brain and taken up residence in your left knee. What does it feel like? Reach down and place your left hand over your knee and feel the sensations of something touching the knee. What other feelings are in that same location?

You can promote an even more subtle inner mindfulness by focusing on the presence and movement of *energy* within your body. Energy is transmitted by forces; two that transmit energy in our daily lives are electromagnetism (the attraction of electric charges) and gravity (the pull exerted by the mass of the earth). The following questions use the language of electromagnetism and gravity to help you locate energy and its movement throughout your body:

- Where does the body feel heavy? Where does it feel as if it's floating?
- Where does the body feel as if a current is being freely conducted? What parts of the body feel resistance to the current?

Other questions use imagery borrowed from studying the dynamics of work and fluids:

- Is there any place where the body has to overwork? Are some parts of the body simply not contributing to the work that is underway?
- Does the body feel as if it is open to flow?
- Do any regions feel as if they are under pressure or blocked?

Other ways to identify energy are more general and relate to inner awareness of daily physical sensations:

- What region has more general sensation (more feeling) or seems to be particularly engaged in the task about to be performed?
- Where does the body feel as if something is happening?

To practice awareness of energy, sit in a chair. In the sitting position, energy most noticeably moves down. Feel the presence of weight pushing down on the chair. It is also possible to feel the opposing force from the chair pushing up. Imagining a silk thread suspended from the ceiling and attached to the mid-saggital line can encourage this feeling. Feel the lift from the string gently elongating the spine. Some energy is rising. A mid-point exists approximately 1 or 2 inches below the navel where the body energetically separates from the downward motion into the chair. Notice that your mere imagining of lifting and elongating the spine directs your energy to rise.

Similarly, a body therapist's intention affects the energy available for performing bodywork. For example, a therapist can plan to apply pressure along the length of a client's erector spinae to lengthen those muscles and create a feeling of elongation in the spine. The therapist has two intentions: (1) to apply pressure and (2) to lengthen. For this to be accomplished, energy must move from the therapist's hands with some depth to the client's muscles and, simultaneously, in a superior direction along the client's body. When the therapist's attention focuses on the deep lengthening without simultaneously focusing on the superior direction, sustaining the pressure is more difficult. Holding both produces a more fluid stroke for the therapist and client. Helpful Hint 2.1 leads you through a related activity, the power of intention.

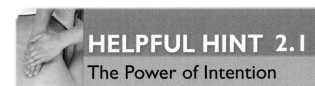

HELPFUL HINT 2.1
The Power of Intention

This exercise works and effectively demonstrates *the power of intention,* although it can seem impossible, by enabling you to compare the effect when two people share an intention or have different intentions. Choose a partner fairly equal in height and weight and have him or her stand facing you and gently place his or her stocking feet on top of your feet (the balls of the feet work best).

Activities

1. *Shared intention:*   Intend to walk forward and do so. The other person intends to be light while standing on your feet. Now try to walk backward.

2. *Changed intention:*   The passenger decides to become heavy and not move by focusing his or her weight into the feet as if they are nailed to the floor. When both partners are ready, try to move; notice how difficult it has become.

BALANCED APPROACH

The **balanced approach to neutral alignment** integrates the external and internal approaches. It requires knowledge of both the anatomically correct neutral positions and a keen awareness of our own body's sensations and energy flow. We are born with this natural awareness but learn to ignore it. In a similar way, we learn to ignore thirst, resulting in dehydration; satiety, resulting in overeating; and the need to void the bladder, increasing the incidence of urinary tract infections. Through daily practice and subtle, deliberate mindfulness of the body at all times, you can reduce your risk of somatic dysfunction and potential injury. Helpful Hint 2.2 discusses the value of *tai chi* in improving awareness.

We all have a distinct physical makeup reflecting not only what we are born with but also what we have acquired through life. Thus, each of us faces unique challenges in

striving to reach neutral alignment. Rather than requiring that we place our body directly into an objective neutral position, the balanced approach allows us to begin at whatever position our body currently accepts as normal. From this position, we can assess external alignment and attempt to move into neutral alignment. We observe and identify changes in muscle tension, weight distribution, and body balance. Identify the changes. We note which position is more (or less) comfortable. Throughout the day, we need to schedule quiet intervals to internally check alignment and make corrections to establish neutral alignment. When the normal position is not neutral, we should try moving the body to the extreme opposite position to help find neutral. For example, if we slouch (i.e., shoulders protracted and increased kyphosis), we can hyperextend the neck and spine, retract the shoulders, and then relax. The returned position will be closer to neutral alignment. Worksheet 2.1 is a guide for making external and internal assessments.

HELPFUL HINT 2.2
Applying *Tai Chi* to Neutral Alignment in the Stationary Position

Practicing *tai chi* can increase your internal awareness of neutral alignment in a stationary position. It not only promotes a sense of internal well-being but also provides instruction in breath control, focus, and intention. These in turn are integral to cultivating energy, or *chi*, which can then be used to increase your stability, strength, and balance.

The neutral body is a state of awareness, of inner and outer quality, of effort and ease, and of many other apparently opposite subjective conditions. Ideally, each one in any pair of

opposite body states balances the other. For example, a hard, muscular body is balanced by softness (i.e., flexibility). Softness needs to overcome hardness without eliminating it. In the same way, the stationary body in neutral alignment can encompass both relaxation and tension and has the immediate potential for both extension and flexion. Neither opposite is dominant. By teaching the concept of the interdependence of opposites, *tai chi* assists the body in reaching a stationary position to achieve and maintain neutral alignment, or balance.

WORKSHEET 2.1
Assessment for Neutral Alignment

Instructions: Assess your physical alignment, preferably with the help of a partner. Indicate on the diagram any area not in a neutral position and, in the column on the left, place a checkmark for the alignments observed. During or following the external assessment, assess each region again using the internal approach and record your observations. If you are not in neutral alignment, make the best adjustment that you can and comment on any changes of which you are internally aware. This worksheet can also be used to assess yourself while you are doing daily activities such as, cooking, reading, and showering.

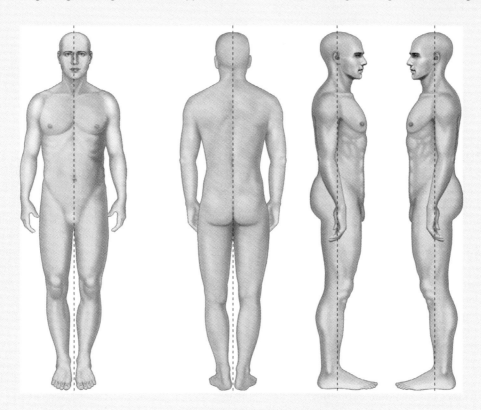

External Assessment

Head/Neck

_____ Neutral _____ Flexed _____ Hyperextended

Shoulders

_____ Neutral _____ Protracted _____ Retracted

_____ Neutral _____ Elevated _____ Depressed

Torso

_____ Neutral _____ Lateral Tilt (direction _____)

Thoracic region

_____ Neutral _____ Kyphosis _____ Flattened

Internal Assessment

Feels

_____ Balanced _____ Unbalanced _____ Tight _____ Relaxed

Comments

Feels

_____ Balanced _____ Unbalanced _____ Tight _____ Relaxed

Comments

Feels

_____ Balanced _____ Unbalanced _____ Tight _____ Relaxed

Comments

Feels

_____ Balanced _____ Unbalanced _____ Tight _____ Relaxed

Comments

WORKSHEET 2.1 (CONTINUED)

Lumbar region

_____ Neutral _____ Lordosis _____ Flattened

Pelvis

_____ Neutral _____ Lateral Tilt (direction _____)

_____ Neutral _____ Anterior Tilt _____ Posterior Tilt

Knees

_____ Neutral _____ Flexed _____ Hyperextended

_____ Straight _____ Unlevel

_____ Straight _____ Rotated (direction _____)

Feels

_____ Balanced _____ Unbalanced _____ Tight _____ Relaxed

Comments

Feels

_____ Balanced _____ Unbalanced _____ Tight _____ Relaxed

Comments

Feels

_____ Balanced _____ Unbalanced _____ Tight _____ Relaxed

Comments

Feels

_____ Balanced _____ Unbalanced _____ Tight _____ Relaxed

Comments

Feels

_____ Balanced _____ Unbalanced _____ Tight _____ Relaxed

Comments

Feels

_____ Balanced _____ Unbalanced _____ Tight _____ Relaxed

Comments

Your goal for this chapter is to be able to identify external neutral alignment and recognize your postural problems. Use the internal approach to help you distinguish between when you are in neutral alignment and when you are not. But understand that sometimes neutral feels normal and other times it does not.

The balanced approach requires patience. Keep in mind that lifelong habits build **muscle memory**, or tensions that are stored within the neuromuscular system. It takes time to retrain the body to develop new muscle memories that bring it into neutrality, so give yourself time to apply the external and internal approaches. We suggest that you establish a daily practice appropriate to the challenges you face. Case Study 2.1 illustrates how you can apply the balanced approach to help you with your practice.

The balanced approach quickly and powerfully sustains, nourishes, and assists you in maintaining neutrality in a stationary position, thereby maintaining a pain-free practice. Once your body experiences the benefits of these gentle attentions, it will begin to relax, and you will enjoy more and more rejuvenating moments in neutral. Indeed, your body can actually change over time, moving closer to objective neutral and requiring fewer environmental adaptations. As your body becomes more optimally aligned and your inner awareness expands, you can even find that you are better able to pay attention to the external world, including being more authentically attentive to your clients, which will enhance the massages that you give, allowing you to better nurture yourself and your clients. These are only a few of the rewards that come from attention to healthy ergonomics.

CASE FOR STUDY 2.1
Protracted Shoulders

Angie is a bodyworker who also enjoys making pottery. She complains of tension in her pectoral muscles. A postural evaluation identifies her shoulders as protracted (rounded).

1. What factors have contributed to Angie's condition?
2. How can she, by following the balanced approach alleviate, her tension?

CHAPTER SUMMARY

- The external approach to the stationary neutral position assesses the objective alignment of the body based on posture and balance. To do so, view the body in the anatomical position from the anterior, posterior, and lateral views.
- To remain upright, the body's center of gravity must be maintained within the base of support. Good posture reduces the work required for maintaining a position whereas poor posture creates muscle tension.
- The standing position in the anterior, posterior, and lateral views can be assessed by determining the balance on either side of an imaginary vertical axis running with the midline. Key anatomical points on either side of the midline can be evaluated to determine whether they are level. Congenital and acquired misalignments can be identified.

- In the seated position in neutral alignment, the ischial tuberosity forms the base of support with the thighs adding stability. Seated posture also determines the weight load on the spine.
- The internal approach to the stationary neutral position is subjective, requiring sensory and energy awareness.
- Challenges to the internal approach include adaptation and compensation.
- The balanced approach to the stationary neutral position integrates the external and internal approaches.
- Challenges to the balanced approach include individual physical attributes, both congenital and acquired. To achieve neutral requires reeducating the muscles in combination with ongoing sensory awareness.

REVIEW QUESTIONS

1. Physical alignment of the body (the external approach to neutral) is achieved through _____ and _____.
2. The following is(are) part(s) of the complex process of balance.
   a. vestibular apparatus (inner ear)
   b. vision
   c. proprieoceptors and brain
   d. all of the above
3. A person's posture is influenced by:
   a. the body type
   b. the physical condition
   c. the emotional state
   d. all of the above
4. Which is best assessed from the anterior view?
   a. head straight, not rotated
   b. spine straight, not curved
   c. knees slightly flexed
   d. pelvic angle at 30 degrees
5. Why is the base of support important?
6. What are the three body types?
7. Sensory awareness is essential to what approach?
8. True or false? The carrying angle is congenital.
9. True or false? The anatomical position is assessed in three views.
10. True or false? Muscle tone is a factor in posture.
11. True or false? For most people their normal position is neutral alignment.

REFERENCE

Csikszentmihalyi, M. (1990). *FLOW: The psychology of optimal experience*. New York: Harper & Row.

SUGGESTED READINGS

Man Ch'ing, C. (1985). *Cheng Tzu's thirteen treatises on t'ai chi ch'uan* (B. Lo and M. Inn, Trans.) Berkeley, CA: North Atlantic Books.

Seeley, R. R., Stephens, T. D., & Tate, P. (2005). *Anatomy and physiology* (7th ed.). Boston: McGraw-Hill.

Snell, R. S. (2000). *Clinical anatomy* (7th ed.). Boston: Little, Brown.

Tolle, E. (1999). *The power of now*. Novato, CA: New World Library.

Trew, M., and Everett, T. (2001). *Human movement: An introductory text* (4th ed.). London: Harcourt.

Van de Graaff, K. (2000). *Human anatomy* (5th ed.). Boston: McGraw-Hill.

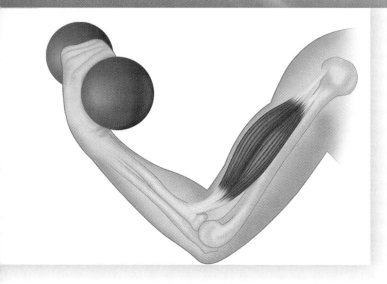

CHAPTER OUTLINE

External Approach

Internal Approach

Balanced Approach

Summary

Review Questions

LEARNING OBJECTIVES

Upon successfully completing this chapter, you will be able to:

1. Compare and contrast the external and internal approaches to neutral alignment in motion.
2. Distinguish among three classes of levers involved in movement.
3. Explain how each of the three force systems contributes to body movement.
4. Discuss the roles of prime mover, antagonist, fixator, and synergist muscles in achieving movement.
5. Identify five externally based activities for maintaining neutral alignment in motion.
6. Describe four sensory-awareness tools for neutral alignment in motion.
7. Perform internal assessments of your head and torso, upper limbs, and lower limbs in motion.
8. Describe the balanced approach to neutral alignment in motion.

KEY TERMS

Antagonist 39

Body scanning 43

Contract/relax technique 44

First-class lever 36

Fixator 40

Focused breathing 43

Force system 37

Fulcrum 36

Isometric contraction 37

Isotonic contraction 37

Kinesthetic awareness 36

Prime mover 39

Second-class lever 37

Synergist 40

Third-class lever 37

Vector 37

Visualization 43

In Chapter 2, we established the importance of maintaining neutral alignment in a stationary position; here we address the essential task of maintaining neutral alignment while in motion. Again, our topic is presented from the external (objective) to the internal (subjective) approaches, consolidating the material into a balanced technique. The external approach requires an understanding of the physics of movement, including principles related to classes of levers, force, and the changing roles and relationships of working muscles. The internal approach challenges you to maintain your **kinesthetic awareness;** that is, your sensory awareness of your body while it is moving. A body in motion is ever changing; thus, this chapter empowers you to tune into your body moment by moment to assess, achieve, and maintain healthful neutral alignment.

EXTERNAL APPROACH

As we mentioned in Chapter 1, body movement is achieved by muscle force acting on the lever system of the skeleton. Thus, an understanding of some principles of body mechanics is essential if you are to develop the ability to maintain neutral alignment in motion.

Classes of Levers

Recall from Chapter 1 that some joints show a wide range of motion, such as abduction, adduction, flexion, extension, and rotation of the glenohumeral joint. Nevertheless, each individual motion is achieved by a unique physical interaction of muscle on bone. When studying the mechanics behind any body movement, one of the first tasks is to identify where the muscle force is applied along the length of the bone in relationship to the resistance and the **fulcrum** (i.e., the pivot point of the joint). The relationship of the force, resistance, and fulcrum determines the class of lever of a specific joint.

Understanding the three classes of levers will increase your awareness of the types of actions for which the body is best designed. In the **first-class lever,** the fulcrum is located between the force and resistance. This relationship has a mechanical advantage: It reduces the amount of force that would otherwise be needed. The first-class lever is found in many simple devices including a seesaw and a pair of scissors. If you have ever used a screwdriver to open a can of paint, you have employed a first-class lever. A downward force on the screwdriver handle is transmitted to an upward force against the lid rim (see Figure 3.1a ■). Anatomical examples of first-class levers include the triceps brachii extension of the forearm against resistance or during a pushup when raising the body. Another example is extension of the head by the splenius capitis and semispinalis capitis, muscles that insert on the occipital bone at the skull. As the muscles contract, the weight of the head is overcome, and the face lifts upward. The movement occurs at the atlanto-occipital joint. Using the mechanical advantage

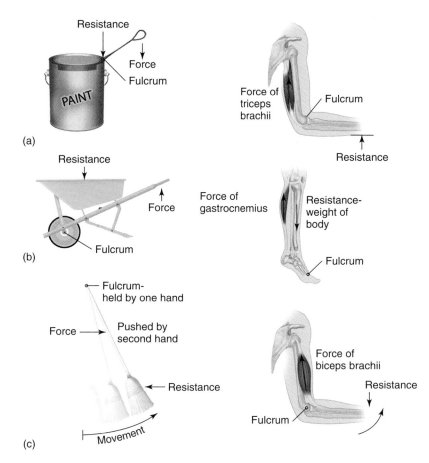

(a)

(b)

(c)

FIGURE 3.1

(a) Examples of first-class levers include a screwdriver opening a can of paint and the triceps brachii extending the arm against resistance. Notice the triceps brachii is inserted on the olecranon process, proximal to the trochlea, which is the fulcrum point. (b) Examples of second-class levers include a wheelbarrow lifting a load and the gastrocnemius raising the body up onto its tiptoes. The gastrocnemius is inserted on the calcaneous and the distal end of the metacarpals is the fulcrum point. (c) Examples of third-class levers include a broom sweeping a floor and the biceps brachii flexion of the forearm. The biceps brachii is inserted on the radius, distal to the fulcrum point, but proximal to the distal end of the forearm.

of a first-class lever is important here because the weight of the head (approximately 8% of the body mass) is significant.

A **second-class lever** places the resistance between the force and the fulcrum. A second-class lever also provides a mechanical advantage and is effective for lifting heavy loads as the wheelbarrow (Figure 3.1b) demonstrates. Your ability to stand on your tiptoes and lift the entire weight of your body upward exemplifies the efficiency of a second-class lever. The fulcrum point is the metatarsal head, or ball of the foot. The gastrocnemius of the calf applies its force on the calcaneus, much like lifting the handles of a wheelbarrow.

By far the most common type of lever found in the body is the **third-class lever**. This system applies the force to the middle of the lever with the fulcrum and resistance to each end. Third-class levers do not have the mechanical advantage of load lifting as the other levers do but instead have the advantage of the distance and velocity at which the lever can be moved. The leverage created when sweeping with a broom demonstrates this advantage (Figure 3.1c). When the upper end of a broom is stabilized with one hand and the other hand applies a force along the length of the broom, the distance and speed at which the head of the broom can be moved is significant. In the body, the muscle attachment usually is closer to the fulcrum point than to the load. This maximizes the speed and distance of travel that can be achieved. Good examples include the biceps brachii insertion on the radius for flexion at the elbow, the quadriceps femoris insertion on the tibia for extension at the knee, and the deltoid insertion on the humerus for abduction of the arm.

Force and Force Systems

To recognize how the body moves and how external factors influence it, *force* needs to be further described. Force has a **vector** quality (i.e., it has both *magnitude* and *direction*). For example, a muscle contraction results in a force with a magnitude that depends on the strength of contraction and a direction based on the position of the muscle in the body.

Usually forces occur in combinations. In the body, forces typically involve a combination of muscles associated with one action. Combinations can include not only muscles but also the external resistance (force) against which they are working. Ergonomics addresses both forces created in the body as well as external resistance forces. The sum of all forces involved in any particular movement can be referred to as a **force system**. Force systems can involve forces that act in (Figure 3.2 ■):

- The same plane and direction
- The same plane but opposite direction
- More than one plane and direction simultaneously.

Each of these force systems occurs with body movement.

A force system in which forces work together in the same plane and direction of movement can make a physical task easier or more effective. For example, consider the action of pushing against a surface (Figure 3.3 ■). Extension of the arm provides the force of pushing; however, the action of leaning forward can distribute the weight of the body in the same direction. Body weight provides force as does the muscle contraction. The force generated by combining the two is greater than either one individually.

When we attempt to pick up a heavy object, forces are acting in the same plane but opposite direction (Figure 3.4 ■). If the force of the muscle exceeds that of the force created by the object's mass and inertia, the object is moved in the direction in which the muscle force is exerted. To achieve such movement, the muscle must contract to the degree that its force exceeds that of the object. This is the *isometric period of contraction.* Once the object's force has been exceeded, the muscle shortens and is said to be in an **isotonic contraction**. On the other hand, if the object's mass and inertia exceed those of the force that can be created by the muscle, the object does not move. The muscle remains in an **isometric contraction**. The tension in a muscle in isometric contraction can become significant and deplete the muscle's energy stores and/or result in tissue trauma. Thus, when considering a task that requires overcoming significant resistance, you need to assess your muscle strength realistically. Even if you can lift a heavy object, the great exertion needed during the isometric phase can cause tissue injury. The ability to perform tasks is related to physical condition. As discussed in Chapter 1, overexertion of muscles beyond that for which you are conditioned is a common cause of occupational injury.

Forces can act in more than one plane and direction simultaneously, either within a single muscle or when multiple muscles work collectively. The trapezius is a good example of a single muscle in which forces can act in more than one plane and direction (Figure 3.5 ■). The trapezius muscle originates broadly from the occipital bone and the spines of the cervical and thoracic vertebrae. The muscle fibers converge and insert narrowly on the spine and acromion process of the scapula. Muscle control allows for selected contraction within the muscle so that if the superior portion of the muscle contracts, the scapula is adducted and elevated whereas if the inferior portion contracts, it is adducted and depressed. However, if the entire muscle is contracted, the force vector is directed medially. This means that the forces created by the superior and inferior regions are summed with the medial portion and the force vector adducts the scapula medially toward the vertebrae.

As just noted, forces can act in more than one plane and direction when several muscles work together. The earlier example of the splenius capitis and semispinalis capitis causing extension of the head illustrates this action. These muscles are on both sides of the body. All four insert on the occipital bone; however, each has its own point of origin (see Figure 3.6 ■). When the muscles contract in unison, they extend the head at the neck. One of the muscles acting alone rotates the head to its side.

Roles of Muscles Involved in Movement

Muscles play a significant role not only in force systems but also in stabilization of the skeleton. Its stabilization is important for posture and facilitation of muscle actions.

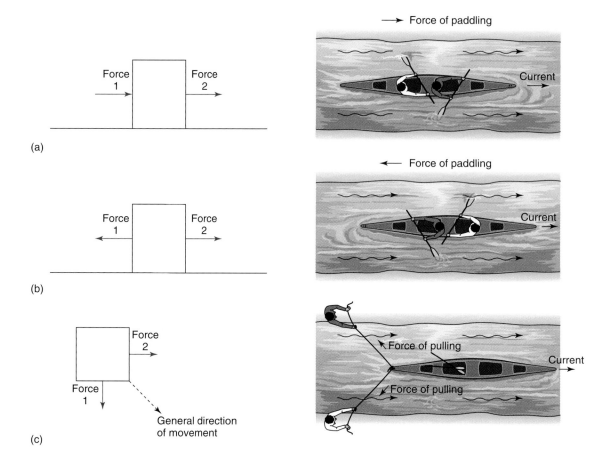

FIGURE 3.2

Force systems are the sum of forces applied in one situation. (a) Forces may act in the same plane and direction, for an additive effect. An example would be paddling downstream with the current. The force of paddling and the force of the current have an additive effect. (b) Forces may act in the same plane, but in opposite directions, counteracting one another. The final direction and magnitude of movement is determined by which force is greater and by how much. Paddling upstream against the current would be an example. The rate of moving upstream depends on by how much the canoer can overcome the force of the current. (c) Forces may be applied from several planes and directions simultaneously. The magnitude and direction is the sum of the forces applied. An example would be having ropes from both banks of a river attached to an object out in the current, which would be a total of three forces acting on the object. Pulling the object directly upstream would require both ropes being pulled with equal force and the sum of their forces being greater than the current.

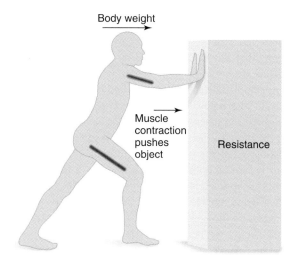

FIGURE 3.3

The effect of using body weight to complement the action of pushing.

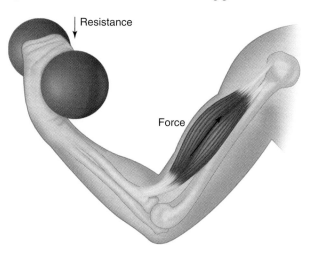

FIGURE 3.4

The object represents resistance that the muscle needs to work against. If the force of the muscle is greater than the mass of the object, it will be raised. If it is not, the object is not moved even though the muscle is exerting force.

FIGURE 3.5

The trapezius has a broad origin and relatively narrow insertion point. Contraction of the entire muscle results in the scapulae moving medially.

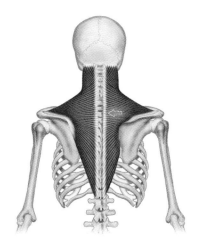

Each action in the body depends on a combination of muscles in which each has a specific role. For any given action, muscles work as prime movers, antagonists, fixators, or synergists.

A muscle is the **prime mover** when it is the principal muscle or one of a group of principal muscles responsible for the action. An example is the quadriceps femoris during the extension of the knee.

A muscle acts as an **antagonist** when it opposes a motion. An example is the biceps femoris opposing the action of the quadriceps femoris during the extension of the knee. As the prime mover contracts, the antagonist must relax to an equal degree to allow for the movement.

FIGURE 3.6

(a) The combined action of the splenius capitus and semispinalis capitus results in extension of the head. (b) If muscles on one side of the body are contracted, the result is extension and rotation to that side.

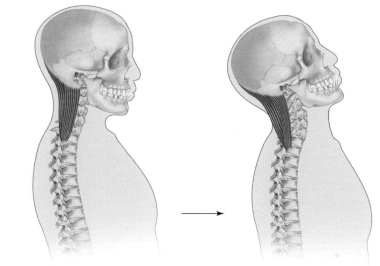

Contraction of the splenius
capitus and semispinalis capitus

(a)

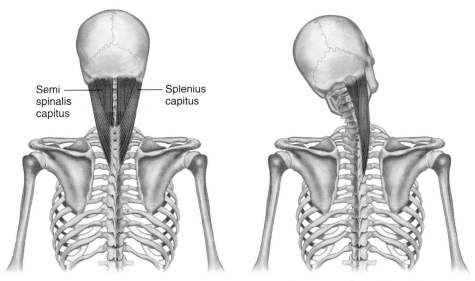

Contraction of the right splenius
capitus and semispinalis capitus

(b)

The **fixator** muscles contract isometrically to stabilize the origin of the prime mover. For example, abduction of the arm by the deltoid muscle requires the stabilization of both the scapula and clavicle (Figure 3.7 ■). This is so because the deltoid originates from the lateral portion of the clavicle and the acromion process and spine of the scapula. Muscles around the shoulder girdle that connect the scapulae to the vertebral column and sternum act as fixators that include the subclavius, trapezius, rhomboids, and serratus anterior. If the deltoid muscle has to contract with more force to overcome a resistance to abduction, the tension generated in the fixator muscle increases. Chronic or repetitive movements requiring such tension can become a basis for hypertonic contraction or spasm.

Considering the fact that much of the body's action entails the movement of the limbs and that such movement requires significant stabilization, it is not surprising that major groupings of fixator muscles occur in the torso (Figure 3.8 ■). For example, arm movement requires stabilization of the pectoral girdle (scapulae and clavicle), and leg movement requires stabilization of the pelvic girdle. In turn, either movement or stabilization of the girdles requires stabilization of the vertebral column. This "domino effect" helps explain why so many occupational injuries involve the back. With repetitive movement in poor alignment, muscle stress can extend from the site of action to the stabilization of the girdle and then to the stabilization of the vertebral column. An over-stressed back muscle can go into a hypertonic contraction, increasing the risk for misalignment of the vertebral column. Thus, an important aspect of neutrality during limb movement is to keep the supporting structures in their neutral position.

The center of gravity and the base of support (BOS) are also important to consider for minimizing the impact of movement on fixator muscles. If the center of gravity is shifted away from the core of the body, fixator muscles attempt to compensate. For example, a task performed with the arms fully extended in the front of the body causes the center of gravity to shift forward. The muscles along the length of the vertebral column contract to compensate for this anterior shift to keep the body in balance.

Synergist muscles come into play when the prime mover muscle crosses more than one joint before it reaches its insertion point where the action occurs. Their role is to prevent unwanted movement at the joints between them. This helps to make movements more efficient and to keep joints in neutral alignment. Important synergists of the carpus are the extensor muscles (extensor carpi radialis longus and extensor carpi radialis brevis) and flexor muscles (palmaris longus, flexor carpi ulnaris, and flexor carpi radialis), which contract together to fix the wrist joint (see Figure 3.9 ■). These muscles insert on the metacarpals. Their collective contractions stabilize the wrist and allow the long flexor and extensor muscle of the fingers to work efficiently. The fingers' long flexors and extensors also originate from the humerus, radius, and ulna, but they insert on the digits. As a result, they act to move the wrist and/or the digits. Examples of these muscles are the flexor digitorum profundus and the extensor digitorum. If the wrist is not stabilized, contraction of the extensor digitorum causes extension of both the fingers and wrist. However, when the synergist muscles stabilize the wrist, the entire force of contraction is delivered to the digits to cause extension of the fingers.

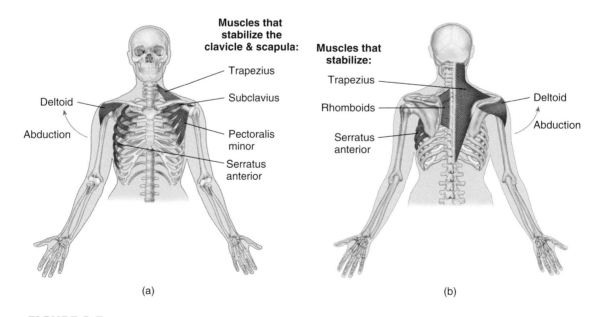

(a)   (b)

FIGURE 3.7

The abduction of the arm by the deltoid muscle requires fixator muscles to stabilize the scapulae and clavicle. (a) Anterior view. (b) Posterior view.

FIGURE 3.8

Stabilization of the girdles facilitates limb movement. Many of the fixator muscles extend from the vertebral column to the girdles. In turn, the vertebral column is stabilized by muscles extending along the length of the column.

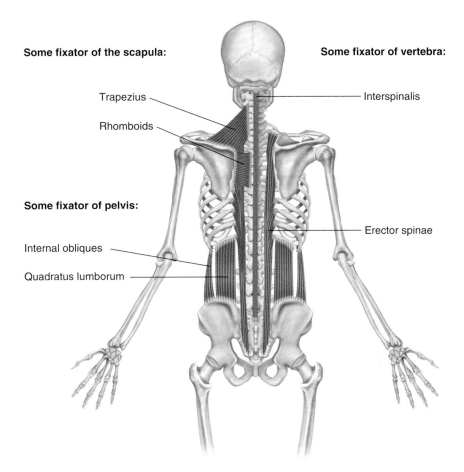

Some fixator of the scapula:
Trapezius
Rhomboids

Some fixator of vertebra:
Interspinalis
Erector spinae

Some fixator of pelvis:
Internal obliques
Quadratus lumborum

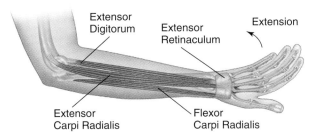

Extensor Digitorum
Extensor Retinaculum
Extension
Extensor Carpi Radialis
Flexor Carpi Radialis

FIGURE 3.9

Extensor and flexor muscles of the carpus contract to fix the wrist joint. This allows the long flexor and extensor muscles of the fingers to work more efficiently. Illustrated is a medial view of the left arm and hand showing the extension of the fingers by the extensor digitorum. Without the stabilization of the wrist, a portion of the force created by the extensor digitorum would result in extending the wrist.

Keep in mind that the roles of prime mover, antagonist, fixator, and synergist are applied to particular muscles only for particular movements. The same muscle can play a different role in different movements. For example, the triceps brachii is a prime mover for extending the forearm, is an antagonist for flexion of the forearm, and can assist in stabilizing the glenohumeral joint (shoulder joint).

Role of Reflex Patterns in Complex Motor Skills

During complex movements, the center of gravity and the BOS are in an almost constant state of flux. Walking, which is one of the most fundamental and complex body motions, involves the process of balancing on one leg at a time with the center of gravity continually shifting and the BOS changing (Figure 3.10 ■). If you have ever watched children learning to walk, you can appreciate the complexity of the movements required as they lean forward on one leg and then catch themselves with the other leg to avoid falling. Children learning to walk are unable to carry an object while they walk because any weight changes their center of gravity. To be able to walk and carry an object requires a compensation of muscle action that they have not yet mastered. Only with development of the nervous system, practice, and establishing reflex patterns will walking become automatic and routine.

Whenever we learn a new physical task, whether in sports, work, or recreation, we undergo a learning process similar to that for walking before that task can become routine. In the process, we establish a reflex pattern for the movement. Recent research suggests that these reflex patterns of motor skills are stored as memory separately from cognitive memory, primarily in the cerebellum and the premotor cortex of the cerebrum. The fact that cognitive memory and motor skill are stored in separate locations in the

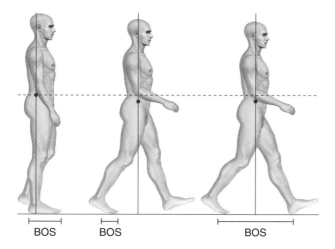

FIGURE 3.10

During walking, the center of gravity moves vertically as well as in relationship to the base of support. While stepping forward, there is a moment just before setting the forward foot down when the center of gravity is in front of the base of support.

brain explains why individuals with cognitive memory loss, such as Alzheimer's disease and other forms of dementia, are still able to perform learned motor skills. The specific storage of skilled movement indicates the importance of using proper ergonomics when learning a new skill. Changing a habitual pattern of movement is more difficult than learning it correctly the first time. Thus, it is important to know and maintain the proper ergonomic alignment when approaching any new task.

External Activities for Maintaining Neutral Alignment in Motion

The external approach to remaining neutral while in motion requires application of the principles of body mechanics discussed thus far to repetitive movements performed daily. Chapter 2 introduced several activities for maintaining neutral alignment in a stationary position, and many of these apply to the body in motion. Perhaps the greatest difference between the two states is the increased workload placed on muscles while in motion. As a body moves, forces change and alter the center of gravity. Muscle dynamics keep the body in balance and provide for movement. The following are some practical approaches that can help to maintain neutrality during motion:

- Maintain the best center of gravity possible to minimize the impact on fixator muscles and trauma to joints and ligaments. This includes maintaining proper postural alignment and doing manual tasks within safe zones and at the correct distance from the body. A manual task should keep the forearm(s) at a 90 degree angle as much as possible (see Figure 3.11 ■). Minimize reaching whether you are seated or standing. When reaching for something, keep the items

within arm's reach to prevent the need to lean towards the object. Full range of flexion of the forearm is considered a safe zone. If you must hold something outside the zone, the lighter the object, the better. Any position outside these parameters puts you at risk. The following recommendations particularly apply to the traveling bodyworker who must lift, shift, and/or carry the massage table.

- Apply force efficiently and effectively. Use your own body weight to provide additional force when needed. Use muscles that are most appropriate for the action and force required. Adjust the task to use larger and more powerful muscles when more force is needed. For example, when lifting a heavy object from the floor, squat, grasp the object firmly and as close to the torso as possible, tighten your stomach muscles, and use your legs to lift the object. Avoid bending over the object and lifting it with the arms extended, which is a risk factor for back injury. Twisting while lifting also greatly increases the risk for injury.
- Recognize the limitation of muscle force and use alternate methods for a task to prevent injury. Plan ahead and test weight first before attempting something new.
- Keep proper joint alignment by using synergist muscles to make movement more effective and reduce joint trauma as has been explained for the wrist.
- Use appropriate ergonomic techniques when acquiring new skills to develop the proper motor skill memory.

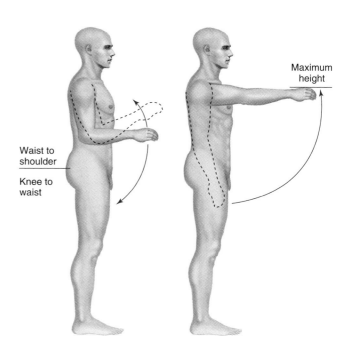

FIGURE 3.11

Keeping the forearm at a 90° angle is optimum, but any position ranging from the side to full flexion is considered safe. The upper arm should not extend above the shoulder level.

INTERNAL APPROACH

Even in the absence of pain or dysfunction, our moving bodies provide subtle signals when something is wrong, for example, a tension headache triggered in response to working with the head overflexed. Bodyworkers commonly look down at the client instead of keeping their head/neck in neutral alignment. An excellent activity to break this habit is to massage blindfolded. Another example is hand cramping in response to the repetitive motion of writing for a long time. The cramping communicates that it's time to stretch the hand and fingers. These cues left unattended create undue tension, which results in chronic conditions. As noted in Chapter 2, the ability to pick up these internal signals requires that we quiet our minds and focus on our senses, including our kinesthetic sense. However, maintaining sensory awareness during movement is more challenging than maintaining sensory awareness while sitting or standing still. Thus, in the following sections, we identify some tools and assessment skills specific to the internal approach to neutral alignment in motion.

Four Tools of Sensory Awareness in Motion

An understanding of the principles of body mechanics should help you to identify areas of your body that are at greatest risk for tension and injury. You can also evaluate and adapt your movement patterns with the internal approach by using four tools of sensory awareness in motion: body scanning, visualization, breath and focused breathing, and the contract/relax technique. Although discussed as separate techniques, these tools are interrelated.

BODY SCANNING

You can sense what occurs in your body while you move by monitoring your internal sensations of energy. One technique for doing so is called *body scanning.* As you know, energy can be static or moving. **Body scanning** tracks the flow or decrease of your internal energy and your state of balance in a sequential manner. A systematic approach that moves through specific body regions sequentially begins by becoming aware of the body area from which you want feedback and observing *all* to which you are attuned, such as temperature, tension, pulse, and vibration. Some people find scanning the body as a whole instead of one region at a time easier. Either approach is fine.

VISUALIZATION

You were performing **visualization** in Chapter 2 when you became aware of your energy while sitting in a chair. In that activity, you sensed the weight of your body pushing into the chair and then a string pulling you upward and elongating your spine. Visualization is useful for assessing and altering your postural alignment as well as in preparing you for a task.

Consider, for example, an assessment of the shoulders. First use body scanning to feel whether any tension is there and whether the shoulders are balanced. While holding your attention in the shoulders, note any image that comes to mind. These images can be used as a metaphor or serve as a catalyst for change. A potential image for tension in the shoulder might be the sensation of a solid mass. Visualize the mass dissolving and the arms as tubes through which the mass in fluid state is flowing. Feel the tubes (arms) extending downward as they fill with the heavy fluid. In the process, the shoulders relax and stretch. After working with this visualization while stationary, try the technique as you apply a long, smooth effleurage stroke so you can achieve relaxation of your own body as you treat your client.

Visualization can prepare you for a task as is common in sports. Slalom skiers visualize themselves completing the run down the slope before they push off the ramp. The visualization improves focus and provides a mental check on how the body should be positioned when the skiers move to complete the task.

BREATH AWARENESS AND FOCUSED BREATHING

Breath awareness and **focused breathing** are useful for both evaluating and adapting our alignment in motion. Breath is a source of information. It can tell us about the quality of our movement and reveal potential sources of tension, pain, and constrictions. Ideally, the breath is relaxed and flowing freely throughout our movement.

Reflexes from the respiratory center regulate breath; however, the conscious and subconscious can interrupt breathing patterns. Apprehension, anxiety, and similar states often block respiration and cause us to hold our breath, which causes more tension, which further inhibits breathing. If we work on a client while in this condition, our tension will be perceptible because our movement and strokes will not be fluid and smooth. By becoming aware of our breath, we can break down the tension-breath-holding cycle.

To apply these techniques, we make mental note of our breathing, especially when we begin a new task or one with which we are less comfortable. We should be aware of whether (1) our breathing pattern is smooth or we are holding our breath, (2) our depth of breath is sufficient, or (3) we are breathing. Once we note our breath and begin to breathe normally, our body tension dissipates.

The frequency needed to reappraise breathing depends on each situation and our comfort level. We should be aware that when we are least comfortable with a task, we begin to hold our breath, but during those times, we are also less aware of what is happening inside. That is why it is important to develop the habit of checking our respiration on a regular basis.

Focused breathing requires us to direct our attention not only on how we are breathing but also on the quality of our breath. Then we direct it to areas of our body and apply it to the mechanics and delivery of massage strokes. For example, we observe our breath in the abdomen, sensing the rise and fall of the belly. Next we direct our breath more fully and deeply, and with the next deep inhalation, we prepare to do an effleurage stroke and use the exhalation to deepen the stroke. If possible, we inhale through the nose and exhale through the mouth, directing our breath whenever a stroke requires more energy whether for depth or directional force. We revisit the topic of breath later to explain more about how to integrate it into practice.

CONTRACT/RELAX TECHNIQUE

Another tool to help achieve neutral alignment in motion is the **contract/relax technique** a simplified approach to positional release (counterstrain) and proprioceptor neuromuscular facilitation (PNF). We apply the contract/relax method by first going through the body scan to identify any areas of tension. When we identify a tight area, we complete an isotonic contraction of the antagonist muscles, followed by relaxation. We hold the specific muscle or groups of muscles in the contraction for 90 seconds; holding it for less than 90 seconds diminishes the result. Another variation is to contract for 90 seconds, relax, and then move into a stretch. These techniques not only release tension but also increase flexibility and, therefore, range of motion. If tightness in the upper back is identified, for example, we isotonically contract the pectoral muscles, hold for 90 seconds, then relax, and move into a stretch.

USE OF THE FOUR TOOLS WHILE PERFORMING ACTIVITIES

Knowing how to use these four tools of sensory awareness while performing any activity is important. Using them hones skills in internal sensing much as sharpening a knife allows a chef to prepare food more efficiently. Internal sensing becomes natural and instantaneous, guiding external adjustments such as postural refinements and leading to the optimum experience of moving harmoniously in neutral alignment. The following discussions provide help in developing an internal awareness of the alignment of specific regions of the body while it is in motion. Our recommended sequence moves from awareness of the head and torso to the upper and then lowers limbs; however, any sequence that seems most natural is appropriate. When evaluating each body region, you should try to sense the contrast between the old, habituated pattern and the new, healthier one. As you open new neural pathways by doing something in a new way, you will change your muscle memory. The goal is to reeducate your body until neutral alignment in motion feels entirely natural to you.

Head and Torso

You can increase your internal awareness of neutral alignment of the head while doing almost any activity. To begin, place your attention on the position of your head, and what your head is doing via sensation. Use your inner observer to assess the following:

- Observe sensations of the head at this moment (e.g., tension, weakness, discomfort, temperature). Can you visualize and use your breathing to change these sensations?
- Is the crown of your head suspended as though attached to a silk thread hanging from the ceiling?

This gives a feeling of openness to the cervical vertebral column.

- Internally scan the forehead and eyes; if the brows have a furrow between, visualize them relaxing. Imagine a horizon and feel the eyes relax as they go from observing a central point to an expanded scene on the horizon. Another tool is to close the eyes and focus toward the bridge of the nose and then laterally to the outer creases of the eyes.
- Does your head feel balanced on the torso?
- Be aware of the jaw; relax it by feeling a gentle space between the upper and lower teeth, as compared to clenched teeth, which creates tension. Experience the difference between the teeth touching and being slightly apart. The touching feeling relates to more tension in the temporal mandibular joint (TMJ). Teeth should be slightly apart when relaxed or at work except when chewing.
- As you move your head, do the muscles of your neck feel stretched, contracted, or balanced? Shift the head position as needed to achieve a more neutral, relaxed state for the neck muscles.

The torso is the easiest place in the body on which to focus internal awareness because it is the easiest place in the body to feel the flow of the breath, and, as discussed earlier, breath is a source of information.

- Internally observe the upper chest from the clavicles to the rib cage. Note any tension in the muscles of this area. Does this area feel open and relaxed, and when the breath is directed to the upper chest, do you feel it? (*Note:* Deviation of the natural spinal curves [e.g., hunching or slouching] while working can compromise the breath. Visualize the lungs opening and closing like a set of bellows.)
- Scan from the abdominal area to the pelvic girdle, observing the quality of the breath. Is it relaxed? What sensations do you feel in this area? If you feel tension, contract and then relax the muscle(s) while moving. Be aware of the sound and feeling of your breath both while you are moving and making subtle corrections. This awareness will help you begin to reestablish balance.
- Direct your attention to the muscles of your back, scanning from superior to inferior areas and noting areas of tension or areas where your breath seems restricted. Can you find a way to adjust while moving to ease the tension and restriction?
- Feel what is occurring in the pelvic girdle; using body scanning, observe any tilt: anterior, posterior, or lateral. For example, you will notice an anterior tilt from a more prominent lumbar curve and tightness in the lumbar muscles. As you move, is the pelvis flexible? Correct the tightness by using visualization and breath. Visualize the flexibility of the pelvis and soft, fluid movement of a belly dancer.

Upper Limbs

The metaphor about carrying the weight of the world on your shoulders is applicable to many body therapists. Several factors that contribute to upper limb problems are protraction of the shoulders while working, failure to maintain proper table height, and failure to adjust your own or your client's position according to the work being done.

- Using internal awareness, scan your shoulders. Are they up by your ears or relaxed? Stay mindful of both shoulders while working and, if you feel any tension, either contract/relax or elevate/depress to break the tension cycle. Sense whether one shoulder is more elevated than the other. If so, then contract/relax for 30–90 seconds, breathe and visualize the softening and relaxing and lowering of the elevated shoulder.
- Assess the upper limb from fingertips to shoulder. Scan intermediate points (e.g., knuckles, hand, wrist) for muscular tension by tuning in to each site separately. This will help you identify where tension is being created.

As students and practitioners, you will be doing computer work. As you type, scan the placement of your wrists and hands. If you feel fatigue in either, visually observe whether your wrists are in ulnar deviation, a common misalignment (Figure 3.12 ■). Next determine how best to correct it. This could require you simply to adjust the seat farther from the keyboard, visualizing your fingers bouncing on the keys while typing instead of pounding the keys. The correction should bring relief within moments.

Bodywork that presents a positional challenge provides an excellent opportunity for you to apply the internal approach to alignment of your upper limbs in motion. While engaging in the task, think, observe, and feel your way to the appropriate body mechanics. For example, a client needs to be moved into the side-lying position during a session. The table is at the correct height for the practitioner with a client in the prone or supine position; however, in the side-lying position, the client is higher on the table. This creates the need for the practitioner to modify posture and to be more attentive to maintaining neutral alignment to prevent the tendency to elevate the shoulders and hyperextend the wrists. The modifications needed depend on the region of the body being worked on.

Lower Limbs

In the *The Power of Now,* Eckhart Tolle (1999, p. 97) states, "The key is to be in a state of permanent connectedness with your inner body—to feel it at all times." The lower limbs are integral to establishing and maintaining good body mechanics, to experiencing the *"state of permanent connectedness with your inner body"* to which Tolle refers.

As discussed earlier, the BOS is that part of the body in contact with the surface that supports it. If you are standing, your feet are your BOS. During movement, you can't easily view your center of gravity and BOS externally, but you can sense them internally and integrate them kinesthetically. To remain stable during movement, the center of gravity must stay within the BOS. Recall from Chapter 2 that a wider BOS provides increased stability and the ability to move more freely and confidently.

- It is important to observe whether the stance or BOS is sufficient for the movement required. A feeling of imbalance indicates that the stance is insufficient and needs to be widened.
- If you still experience tension, use body scanning while moving to ascertain whether improper lower limb joint alignment and/or muscular tension are factors. For instance, hyperextended knees can shift the line of gravity, causing stress that often leads to the development of hypertonic hamstrings. If you experience misalignment or muscle tension, apply any or all of the four tools.

BALANCED APPROACH

The balanced approach to neutral alignment in motion integrates application of the principles of body mechanics with an inner awareness of and response to kinesthetics. This approach involves a constant observance of both and, when cultivated, maintains an awareness that allows you to recognize a disturbance in the equilibrium of the two. Kinesiologists and bodyworkers have developed a number of approaches for achieving this equilibrium. Several of these are discussed in Helpful Hint 3.1.

To achieve neutral alignment, we must start with knowledge of our physical alignment during a motion and be able to recognize when it is out of neutral. Visualizing the body in neutral while in motion is a tool of the internal approach, which depends on knowledge of the external. It can't be achieved without knowing what the external view

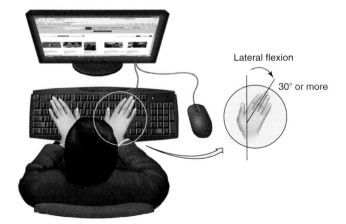

Lateral flexion

30° or more

FIGURE 3.12

This figure shows the typist too close to the keyboard, thereby causing the ulnar deviation. Ulnar deviation is considered to occur when the wrist is laterally flexed 30° or more.

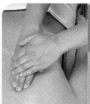

HELPFUL HINT 3.1

Using Complementary Modalities to Develop and Maintain Neutral Alignment in Motion

Thomas Hanna, founder of Hanna Somatics Education (HSE), says "the living body in its wholeness moves with grace, ease, and coordination." If you wish to further increase your kinesthetic awareness, HSE teaches a hands-on procedure for developing conscious control of the neuromuscular system. A superb example of a balanced approach, HSE integrates many of the principles of the external and internal approaches discussed in this chapter. Other excellent modalities for developing neutral alignment in motion are based the principles of gravity and stability, or *gravitational biology*. They include the following:

- Rolfing, developed by Ida Rolf, a biochemist and physiologist, is also referred to as structural integration. It involves deep tissue technique that improves anatomical and energy alignment with gravity. Rolf and her colleagues established a relationship between posture and psychological/emotional stress.

- The Feldenkrais Method, developed by Moshe Feldenkrais, a physicist and athlete, includes movement lessons known as Awareness Through Movement (ATM). The method involves taking complex movement and breaking it down to simple movement patterns to dissolve habitual patterns and replace them with more efficient ones.
- The Alexander Technique, developed by Mathias Alexander, an Australian stage actor, is one of the oldest movement therapies. The approach focuses on developing conscious control over postural habits by releasing holding patterns and facilitating correct posture.

In addition, we recommend studying the work of Wilhelm Reich, who first recognized that chronic holding patterns, which he referred to as "muscular armoring," have a psychological basis. His work supports the recognition that ergonomics needs to consider not only physical, but also psychological factors.

WORKSHEET 3.1

Walking Assessment

Instructions: Have someone videotape you in the frontal and lateral views for 30 to 60 seconds when you are walking. An outside observer can be used if a camera isn't available. After viewing the video, use the external assessment checklist and check the alignmnets observed. After noting any postural deviations, begin walking and internally sensing these deviations. Use one or all of the four tools to make corrections and then check the appropriate box. Make comments on what you feel and sense adjacent to the tool(s) used. Upon completion, compare your internal and external assessments.

External Assessment

Head/Neck:

___Neutral;___Lateral tilt

 (direction ____)

___Neutral;___Protracted

 ___Retracted

___Neutral;___Flexion___Extension

Shoulders:

___Neutral;___Protracted___Retracted

___Neutral;___Elevated___Depressed

Torso

___Neutral;___Lateral tilt, (direction__)

Internal Assessment

Feel/Sense: 4 Tools

_____ Body scanning

_____ Breath

_____ Visualize

_____ Contract/relax

_____ Body scanning

_____ Breath

_____ Visualize

_____Contract/relax

_____ Body scanning

_____ Breath

_____ Visualize

_____ Contract/relax

Pelvis

___Neutral;__Lateral tilt (direction__)

___Neutral;__Anterior tilt__Posterior tilt

Feet: Base of support (BOS)

(A neutral foot strike is heel to toe)

___Neutral__toes in__toes out

___Neutral__Balls (metatarsal head)

 ___ heels (calcaneus)

_____ Body scanning

_____ Breath

_____ Visualize

_____ Contract/relax

_____ Body scanning

_____ Breath

_____ Visualize

_____ Contract/relax

of neutral movement is and without being able to visualize how the body moves to stay in alignment. The fact that it is easier to learn a new task if it is first demonstrated to us verifies this principle. Learning a technique by reading how to do it is much more difficult. Even after watching a technique demonstrated, when we first attempt it, we often feel awkward and may or may not achieve correct body alignment. Feedback from our instructor helps us adjust and find the neutral alignment and motion. In the process of learning a new technique, we create the motor skill memory and, with the use of body scanning, become mentally aware of the correct balance and muscle dynamics.

When body movements are not kept neutral or they exceed the limits of physical ability or are repetitive, muscle strain, tension, and joint and tendon injury occur. Optimum ergonomics is being aware of the proper external approach and avoiding any action that compromises the body. Being aware of the physical demand of a task and staying within our physical limits, visualizing our movement, and applying focused breath to place energy into a movement helps keep us neutral. However, to be realistic, we must realize that we can lapse into less than perfect body mechanics.

We use the balanced approach to assess our performance of habitual tasks to reeducate our body. As an example, Worksheet 3.1 leads us through an evaluation of our walk. When evaluating our performance of habitual—and especially complex—movements, keep in mind that recognizing an unhealthful pattern is the first step in changing it. We start small by assessing and adjusting just one aspect of the movement. Then we expand our awareness to include additional aspects, one at a time. With continual awareness and adjustment, directing our mind and senses to any point on the body becomes easier. The key to developing a safe practice is to practice!

CHAPTER SUMMARY

- The relationship of the force, resistance, and fulcrum determines the class of lever at a specific joint.
- The first-class lever locates the fulcrum between the force and resistance.
- A second-class lever places the resistance between the force and the fulcrum.
- The third-class lever, which places the force in between the fulcrum and resistance, is the most common type in the body. Third-class levers provide speed and distance rather than a mechanical advantage.
- Body movement is the result of force, which has a vector quality. The magnitude and direction of the force depends on the relationship of the muscles involved to the resistance encountered.
- A force system is the sum of all forces involved in any particular movement. Force systems can involve forces acting (1) in the same plane and direction, (2) in the same plane but opposite direction, or (3) in more than one plane of direction.
- Each action in the body can involve a number of muscles with each muscle taking on a different role. Roles include that of prime mover, antagonist, fixator, and synergist.
- The roles of prime mover, antagonist, fixator, and synergist are applied to particular muscles only for particular movements. The same muscle can play different roles in different movements.
- The body's center of gravity changes continually during motion. Appropriate muscle response is necessary to keep the center of gravity within the BOS.
- Motor skill memory develops as a complex task is learned and is stored in the cerebellum and premotor cortex of the cerebrum, separate from the brain areas involved in cognitive memory storage.
- External approaches to maintain neutral alignment during motion include keeping the appropriate center of gravity to minimize impact on fixator muscles, applying force efficiently and effectively including the use of body weight, using the most appropriate muscle for an action, avoiding activities beyond muscle capacity, preserving proper joint alignment, and using the proper ergonomic approach when first learning a new task.
- Tools for evaluating and adapting movement patterns using the internal approach to neutral alignment include: body scanning, visualization, breath awareness and focused breathing, and the contract/relax technique.
- Body scanning is mental imagery used throughout the body or a specific area.
- Visualization is a form of mental imagery with the specific intent.
- Focused breathing is awareness, enhancement, and direction of the breath.
- The contract/relax technique is the tensing of a specific muscle or group followed by relaxation to release tension.
- Observation of the torso and the breath while moving helps identify restricted patterns.
- Several factors that contribute to upper limb problems are protraction of the shoulders while working, failure to maintain proper massage table height, and failure to adjust the therapist's or the client's position according to the work being done.

- To remain stable during movement, the center of gravity must stay within the BOS. The wider the base of support, the more stability exists and is felt, and the more freely and confidently bodies can move.
- The position of the client and bodyworker relative to the task is an important consideration for ergonomic safety.

- The balanced approach to neutral alignment in motion integrates an application of the principles of body mechanics with an inner awareness of and response to kinesthetics.

REVIEW QUESTIONS

1. A first-class lever is:
   a. the most common lever in the human body
   b. a lever in which the fulcrum is located between the force and the resistance
   c. exemplified by a wheelbarrow
   d. exemplified by the biceps brachii insertion on the radius for flexion at the elbow
2. When we attempt to pick up a heavy object, forces are acting:
   a. in the same plane but opposite direction
   b. in the same plane and direction
   c. in more than one plane and direction simultaneously
   d. in the opposite plane but the same direction
3. During extension of the forearm, the triceps brachii is:
   a. a prime mover
   b. an agonist
   c. a fixator
   d. a synergist

4. A tool useful for the internal approach is:
   a. a mirror
   b. an instructor or peer to provide feedback
   c. body scanning
   d. armoring
5. True or false? While you are lifting a carton of milk, your muscles are in an isometric contraction.
6. True or false? The torso is the easiest place in the body on which to focus your internal awareness.
7. True or false? Our memory for reflex patterns of complex movements is stored separately from our cognitive memory, primarily in the cerebellum and the premotor cortex of the cerebrum.
8. Give an example of how a change in the client's position on the table affects the therapist's ergonomics.
9. Explain the importance of the center of gravity and BOS to maintaining neutral position while in motion.
10. Apply the balanced approach to learning a new skill.

REFERENCE

Tolle, E. (1999). *The power of now*. Novato, California: New World Library.

SUGGESTED READINGS

Bowden, B., & Bowden, J. (2002). *An illustrated atlas of the skeletal muscles.* Englewood, CO: Morton Publishing.

Lippert, S. L. (2000). *Clinical kinesiology for physical therapist assistants* (3rd ed.). Philadelphia: F. A. Davis.

Oschman, J. L. (2000). *Energy medicine: The scientific basis.* New York: Churchill Livingstone.

Seeley, R. R., Stephens, T. D., and Tate, P. (2005). *Anatomy and physiology* (7th ed.). Boston: McGraw-Hill.

Snell, R. S. (2000). *Clinical anatomy* (7th ed.). Boston: Little, Brown.

Trew, M., & Everett, T. (2001). *Human movement: An introductory text* (4th ed.) London: Harcourt.

Van de Graaff, K. (2000). *Human anatomy* (4th ed.) Boston: McGraw Hill, 2000.

Common Postural Distortions

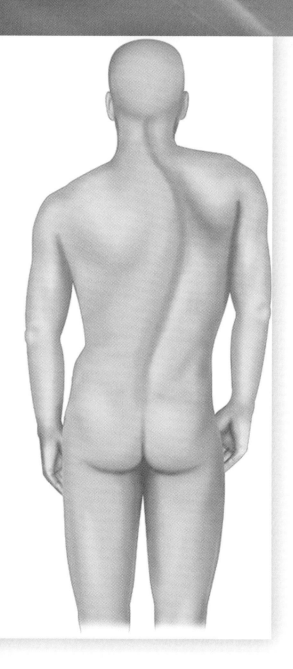

CHAPTER OUTLINE

LEARNING OBJECTIVES

Upon successful completion of the chapter, you will be able to:

1. Discuss how postural distortions occur.
2. Identify the common postural distortions.
3. Explain how each of the common postural distortions affects body mechanics.
4. Evaluate and assess your own and your clients' posture for postural distortions.

KEY TERMS

Postural distortions (PDs), commonly called *misalignments,* are chronic deviations from neutral alignment. Because they reduce the efficiency of body mechanics, developing the ability to recognize them in yourself and your clients is essential. Full explanation of the causes of all PDs falls outside the scope of this book; instead, we provide a general overview, emphasizing PDs that develop as a result from a postural or ergonomic habit. For each body region, we discuss neutral alignment; identify the most common deviations for bodyworkers, their causes and impact; and then give preventive measures. Worksheet 4.1 is intended only as a checklist to help you: diagnosing disorders is beyond the therapist's scope of practice. If you or your clients show signs of a distortion that cannot be explained by poor postural or ergonomic habits, seek medical advice.

THE CAUSES AND EFFECTS OF POSTURAL DISTORTIONS

Before covering specific PDs, let's discuss the three mechanisms that cause them as well as their general effects on the body.

How Postural Distortions Occur

PDs can be genetic, congenital, or acquired. A genetic basis involves inheritance of the condition. An X-linked genetic disease that distorts posture is Deuchenne's muscular dystrophy. It severely compromises muscle function, which commonly begins to appear during early childhood as muscle weakness. More common and less severe are PDs related to general familial body anthropometrics, such as an altered carrying angle.

Congenital defects are present at birth and can result from inherited genetic abnormalities or new mutations occurring within the fertilized egg, or they can be acquired during fetal development because of the intrauterine environment. Intrauterine factors known to cause congenital defects include the mother's use of alcohol or other drugs, inadequate intake of folic acid, or viruses as well as an inadequate oxygen supply to the fetus. For example, cerebral palsy is a motor disorder that can result from fetal brain damage occurring as a result of maternal anemia, infections including rubella, or drug or alcohol abuse. The resulting damage to the brain's motor control regions is reflected in postural and locomotion problems. Talipes equinovarus (club foot) results from arrested growth of the feet during fetal development, causing the feet to be twisted in and downward. Two suggested causes for the condition are genetic and insufficient amniotic fluid (oligohydramnios.)

Acquired conditions arise after birth and can be attributed to disease, injury, or chronic misuse. For example, a stroke patient could lose motor control to a part of the body,

perhaps leading to an imbalance of muscle tone resulting in distortion. Traumatic injury commonly causes a PD; for example, a hip or leg fracture can cause one limb to be shorter than the other.

However, the acquisition of postural distortions usually is more insidious. Habitual misuse and poor ergonomic practice often underlie postural distortions. Results from habitually working outside neutral alignment range from tightened muscles to acute and/or repetitive injury to muscle, ligaments, and cartilage, which culminates in perpetual PDs.

To avoid work related acquisition of injury and risk for postural distortion, the Occupational Safety and Health Administration (OSHA) has established *safe zones* for working while lifting or moving an object and has set a maximum weight of objects to be moved within each zone (Porter, 2005). The safe zones consider the distance from the body and the height at which the task is performed (see Figure 4.1 ■). The working distance from the body that an object is being maneuvered are *primary* (0–7 inches), *secondary* (7–12 inches) and *tertiary* (12 inches or more). Note that heavier objects should be moved within the

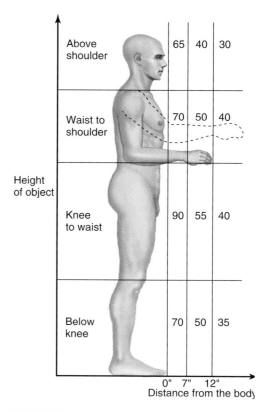

FIGURE 4.1

The safe zone for lifting established by OSHA takes into account the weight of the object and its relative position to the body. The recommended weights in pounds is given within each grid. However, these weights would vary with differences in body size and physical condition.

WORKSHEET 4.1
Assessment for Postural Distortions

Instructions: This worksheet is a refinement of the Worksheet 2.1 in Chapter 2. The assessment here focuses on identifying PDs and determining muscle imbalances and other distortions that could be involved. This is best done with the help of a partner. This worksheet should alert you to possible underlying challenges for performing ergonomically correct technique.

Area Assessment

Head/Neck:

__ Neutral; _____ Lateral tilt (Rt or Lf)

_____ Rotation (Rt or Lt)

__ Neutral; _____ Protracted _____ Retracted

__ Neutral; _____ Flexed;

_____ Cervical lordosis

Shoulders:

__ Neutral; _____ Protracted; _____ Retracted

__ Neutral; _____ Elevated; _____ Depressed

_____ Unbalanced

(Rt or Lf elevation)

Comments/Notes: (Identify muscles with associated tightness/weakness or other predisposing factors.)

Head/Neck:

Shoulders:

Area Assessment

Torso-Posterior View

__ Neutral; _____ Scoliosis (Rt or Lf curve)

_____ Region of the scoliosis

Cervical Regions

__ Neutral; _____ Lordosis; _____ Flattened

Thoracic Region

__ Neutral; _____ Kyphosis; _____ Flattened

Lumbar Region

__ Neutral _____ Lordosis; _____ Flattened

Pelvis:

__ Neutral; _____ Lateral tilt (Rt. / Lf tilt)

__Neutral; _____ Anterior tilt;   Pelvis:

_____ Posterior tilt

Knees:

__ Neutral; _____ Flexed;

_____ Genu recurvatum   Knees:

__ Level; _____ Unlevel (Rt. / Lf high)

__ Straight; _____ Genu varus (medial)

_____ Genu valgus (lateral)

Comments/Notes: Muscles with associated tightness/weakness or other predisposing factors.

Torso

Pelvis

Knees

Area Assessment

Ankles (calcaneal tendon) Posterior View

__ Straight; _____ Calcaneovarus;

_____ Calcaneovalgus

Feet - Lateral view (just prior to ground contact)

__ Straight; _____ Forefoot varus;

_____ Forefoot valgus

Feet - Medial View

__ Neutral; _____ Pes cavus;

_____ Pes planus

Comments/Notes: Muscles with associated tightness/weakness or other predisposing factors.

primary zone because in that position the body is within neutral alignment and has its greatest weight-bearing ability. Working in the tertiary zone forces the body out of neutral alignment, impairing body mechanics and increasing injury risk.

Pathology Underlying Postural Distortions

Regardless of the cause (genetic, congenital, or acquired), the pathology underlying most PDs includes one or more of the following problems:

- Skeletal malformations or misalignments. For example, degeneration of the vertebral body during osteoporosis can lead to kyphosis of the thoracic spine.
- Muscle imbalance between the agonist and antagonist muscles can lead to either loss of balance of muscle tone or of eccentric and concentric contraction. For example, weakening the muscles on one side of the body following a stroke could result in a drooped shoulder, and overtraining one muscle group in relation to its antagonists can result in an imbalance, such as improper sit-ups (abdominal crunches), overly tightened hip flexors, and the predisposition to lordosis.
- Loss of stability of joints, commonly seen as tightening or stretching/weakening the supporting ligaments and muscles. Loss of stability of the shoulder girdle can be attributed to chronic irritation or injury of the rotator cuff muscles. In addition to overall loss of stability of the glenohumeral joint, other changes associated with the condition include a superior displacement of the humeral head, which limits abduction of the arm, and tightening of the subscapularis, which causes a medial rotation of the arm.

Effects of Postural Distortions

The primary PD can be localized to one area, but it commonly has a wide impact on the body, including:

- Increased risk of injury to other joints, tendons, and ligaments
- Reduced range of motion
- Altered muscle tone in other areas, including tight and/or stretched muscles
- Pain because of inflammation or nerve impingement

Noting the wide range of signs and symptoms of PDs serves several purposes. First, recognizing that PDs can be the underlying cause of these complications can help you identify them when they are presented. Ergonomic steps can be taken to correct a diagnosed PD.

Second, notice that the preceding list repeats many of the same factors that initially cause PDs. In general, an injury can cause a PD, which in turn can lead to further injury. This reciprocating process has a broad, cumulative effect on the body and can be resolved only when the underlying cause is corrected.

Third, recognizing the wide impact of PDs makes us more acutely aware of the importance of avoiding ergonomic habits that lead to them. Because bodywork is a physically demanding career, lessening the risk for injury is important. Reduced range of motion impairs the bodyworkers effectiveness, such as the ability to deliver a full stroke during massage. Accumulating effects of injury make maintaining proper ergonomic posture more difficult, and the reciprocating process further complicates the condition. Injury and pain can compromise the bodyworker's ability to work and decrease the person's quality of life.

Correction of Postural Distortions

Clinicians classify PDs as structural (fixed) or functional (mobile or nonstructural) based on the underlying abnormality. Scoliosis is a good example of this classification. Structural scoliosis involves a bone deformity of the vertebrae causing the vertebral column to rotate. Its origin can be genetic, congenital, or acquired and it can be progressive. Structural scoliosis does not disappear with alterations of posture (i.e., there is no way to correct this structural defect by altering the posture). Normal posture can be accomplished only by surgically correcting the bone deformity.

In contrast, functional scoliosis does not involve vertebral bone deformity, is not progressive, and can be reversed by compensating for the underlying cause. A leg length discrepancy, for instance, can cause a functional scoliosis. Because the vertebral structure is normal, correction of the discrepancy as with an orthotic causes the scoliosis to disappear.

Scoliosis exemplifies how treatment of a PD starts by identifying the underlying cause. If a structural PD exists, surgery could be an option. When it is not, the modification of movement and use of props can reduce the impact of the distortions. Many of the PDs discussed in this chapter are related to persistent poor posture to which bodyworkers are prone and thus are functional conditions that can be corrected. Initially preventing the development of poor postural habits is an even better option.

POSTURAL DISTORTIONS BY BODY REGION

Recognizing that postural distortions are present is the first step in reducing their impact. Because a distortion in one area of the body typically affects other areas, therapy should begin with an assessment of the body as a whole.

Feet and Ankles

The feet form the base of support (BOS) while standing and moving. The complex structure of arches of the foot formed by the tarsal bones of the ankle, metatarsal of the foot, the plantar fascia, and ligaments provide:

- Stability on a variety of surfaces
- Ability to handle significant weight-bearing stress on a relatively small surface area
- Propulsion to initiate each step

The transverse arch allows the foot to adjust from side to side to provide stability on uneven surfaces. The longitudinal arches are largely responsible for acting as shock absorbers, which allow the feet to handle the weight-bearing stress placed on them. Walking creates a weight-bearing stress of 1.2 times the body weight, whereas jumping from a height of 2 feet creates a weight loading of 5 times the body weight (Magee, 2006). The longitudinal arches depress with weight (with the greatest range of motion applying to the medial arch) and spring back when the weight is released. The arches' adjustment to the weight load provides shock absorption. As weight is removed, the springing back of the arches aids the propulsion of each step.

NEUTRAL ALIGNMENT

Together, the feet form the BOS for the body. Each foot assumes a slight toe-out position at about a 12–18 degree angle, which is known as the *Fick angle*. This occurs because the tibia is normally rotated slightly in a lateral direction. The first through fifth metatarsals of the foot and the base of the calcaneus (heel) form a triangular base (see Figure 4.2 ■). The tibia, the key weight-bearing bone of the leg, articulates with the talus. When the ankle is neutral, the tibia, talus, and calcaneus are vertically aligned (Figure 4.3 ■). While standing, 50–60% of the weight is normally distributed to the calcaneus, and 40–50% to the metatarsal heads with all metatarsal heads bearing weight. The first metatarsal head (hallux) carries half of the forward weight and the four lateral toes carry the other half. Two sesamoid bones within the first metatarsal joint help distribute pressure and serve as attachment points for the adductor hallucis muscle. Shoes reflect the weight distribution on the

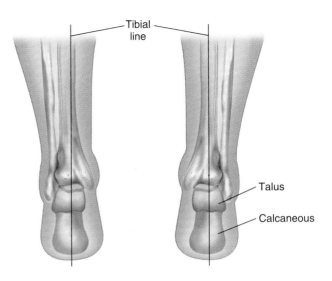

FIGURE 4.3

The tibia, calcaneous, and talus should align in a vertical axis, known as the tibial line.

feet. The most wear typically is on the balls of the feet and slightly to the lateral side.

Neutral alignment of the feet also relates to the stability of the arches, which are maintained by the wedging of the interlocking tarsal and metatarsal bones, the plantar fascia, ligaments and intrinsic and extrinsic muscles of the foot (see Figure 4.4 ■).

THE CAUSES AND IMPACT OF DEVIATIONS

A variety of factors can lead to deviations of the foot and ultimately pain in the feet and/or legs including:

- Leg length differences
- Pelvis out of neutral position
- Genu varus and genu valgus
- Altered gait because of structural defects or habit
- Muscle imbalance
- Fatigue
- Obesity

Six deviations of the feet can be differentiated. The first four involve the foot's alignment with the axis of the tibia (varus and valgus conditions.) The terms *varus* and *valgus* describe alignment along the vertical axis of the limb; **varus** indicates that the distal component is positioned toward the midline from the vertical axis. **Valgus** indicates that the distal component is lateral from the axis. These two PD conditions involve the stability of the arches. They change the BOS, as you can experience for yourself by performing the activity in Helpful Hint 4.1. The changes in base of support and weight distribution have an effect on the body both when standing and while in motion.

Calcaneovarus Calcaneovarus (hindfoot varus) occurs when the distal portion of the calcaneous lies medial to the tibial line (Figure 4.5a ■). It is an inversion of the hindfoot

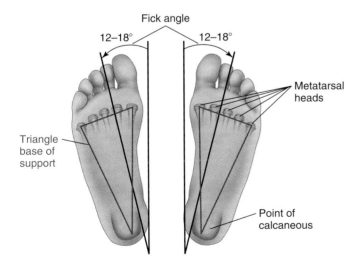

FIGURE 4.2

The feet normally turn out equally at an angle ranging between 12 and 18°, known as the Fick angle. There should be equal weight distribution between the two feet, with each foot having support points delineated as a triangle formed by the five metatarsal heads and the calcaneous.

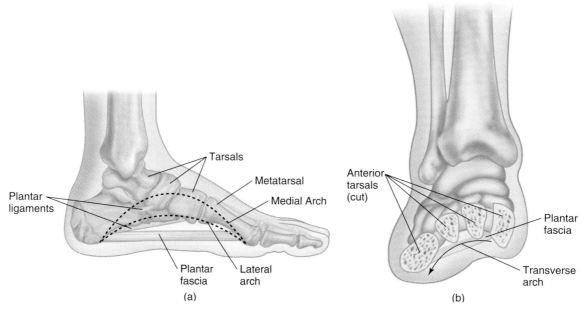

Tarsals

Metatarsal

Medial Arch

Plantar
ligaments

Plantar
fascia

Lateral
arch

(a)

Anterior
tarsals
(cut)

Plantar
fascia

Transverse
arch

(b)

FIGURE 4.4

The arches of the foot are maintained by the interlocking of tarsal and metatarsal bones, the plantar fascia, plantar ligaments, and intrinsic and extrinsic muscles of the foot. (a) Medial view of the longitudinal arches of the right foot. (b) Anterior view of a cross section of the transverse arch.

that some pathologists refer to as *supination*. Excessive bulging and wear on the lateral side of the heel of the shoes suggest that inversion is occurring. The condition exaggerates the medial longitudinal arch, giving the appearance of a high arch. It reduces the foot's pronation mobility and can contribute to shin splints, plantar fasciitis, hamstring strains, and further injury to the ankle and knees. Genu varus can be a contributing factor in its development.

Calcaneovalgus Calcaneovalgus, the reverse of calcaneovarus, is an eversion of the hindfoot and is associated with pronation (Figure 4.5b). Shoes likely show excessive bulging and wear on the medial side of the heel. The medial longitudinal arch appears flattened. Calcaneovalgus can create an eversion of the forefoot along with a lateral deviation of the large toe (hallux valgus). Pain under the large toe is often experienced because of inflammation of the joint and its

HELPFUL HINT 4.1

Experience the Change of Pressure on the Feet as You Rotate Your Torso

Use body awareness to evaluate the force against the plantar surface of the foot. You'll be able to feel the force best when you are either barefoot or in socks and standing on a noncarpeted floor. While standing in a neutral position, you should be able to sense an equal force across the ball (forefoot) and the calcaneous (heel) of each foot as well as an equal force between both feet. Change in the force against the feet occurs as you rotate your torso. This also reflects a change in the base of support.

From the neutral anatomical position, rotate your torso to the right. What changes in force do you sense? Compare the forefoot to the calcaneous of the right foot and compare the right foot to the left foot. You will likely experience an inversion of the right forefoot with more pressure on the lateral surface. You can also experience more pressure on the calcaneous than the forefoot. The left forefoot usually retains equal pressure,

although it can feel lighter than the right foot. What you are experiencing is the dynamic change in your base of support. If you were to move to the right, your weight distribution would be optimal for lifting the left leg to swing to the right while rotating the right leg.

Now consider what happens when you mimic a PD. Resume the anatomical position, feel the force against the plantar surface of the feet, rotate your torso approximately 45 degrees to the right, and then allow/cause the plantar surface to make contact with the floor. What happens to the alignment of the forefoot and calcaneous of each foot? As the right forefoot goes from supination to flat, you will likely experience a medial rotation of the right femur and the sensation of calcaneovalgus. Depending on your stance, you could sense a change in your left foot.

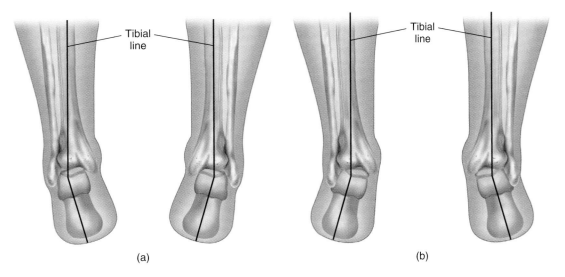

FIGURE 4.5

A posterior view of the ankle and foot is assessed. (a) Calcaneovarus is a condition in which the distal end of the calcaneous lies medial to the tibial line. (b) Calcaneovalgus is a condition in which the distal end of the calcaneous lies lateral to the tibial line.

sesamoid bones, a condition known as **sesamoiditis.** The altered structure within the foot causes the calcaneotendon to shift laterally and to shorten, resulting in a restriction of dorsiflexion. However, the overall mobility of the hindfoot remains unchanged and as a result, the condition has fewer complications than calcaneovarus. Weak supinator muscles or a tightening of the peroneus longus, a strong pronator muscle, can lead to calcaneovalgus. It can also result from genu valgus.

Forefoot Varus   The forefoot, which includes the metatarsal heads, can also show altered alignment. **Forefoot varus** involves inversion of the forefoot when the calcaneous is in neutral alignment. As in Figure 4.6a ■, forefoot varus decreases the medial longitudinal arch, thus resembling a flat foot. When bearing weight, the first metatarsal head must move farther to make contact with the surface, resulting in the midtarsal joint becoming pronated. Over time, this leads to a variety of complications, including tibialis posterior tendonitis, toe deformities, stress to the medial ligaments, shin splints, plantar fasciitis, postural fatigue, and Morton's neuroma, a compression of the medial plantar nerve causing tenderness and pain between the third and fourth metatarsal.

Forefoot Valgus   Forefoot valgus, essentially the reverse of forefoot varus, involves eversion of the forefoot when the

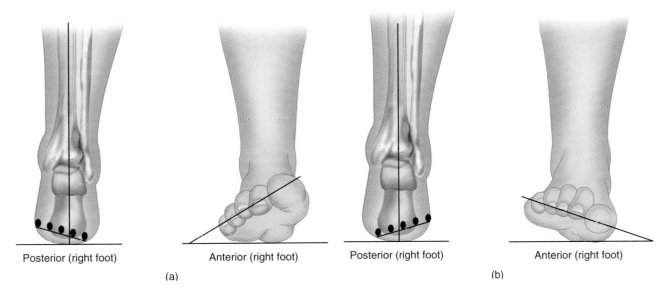

Posterior (right foot)   Anterior (right foot)   Posterior (right foot)   Anterior (right foot)

(a)   (b)

FIGURE 4.6

Posterior and anterior views of forefoot deformities are shown (a) Forefoot varus. (b) Forefoot valgus.

calcaneus is in neutral (Figure 4.6b). During the weight-bearing phase, the midtarsal joint has to become supinated so that the lateral border of the foot can contact the surface. Prolonged supination increases the risk for lateral ankle sprains, plantar fasciitis, toe deformities, sesamoiditis, and leg and thigh pain.

Pes Cavus Pes cavus (high arch) involves an exaggeration of both longitudinal arches, with the lateral arch potentially becoming visible from the side. The metatarsal heads are lower than normal to the hindfoot, and the soft tissues of the sole are shortened. Claw toes often develop and do not touch the ground. The deformity results in a rigid foot that is less capable of shock absorption and adaptation to the stresses placed on it. Individuals with pes cavus are also less able to tolerate repetitive activities. Tarsal pain often develops over time as osteoarthritis develops in these joints. Numerous causes of pes cavus include congenital problems, neurological problems including poliomyelitis, talipes equinovarus, and muscle imbalance, including tight intrinsic muscles of the sole or tight anterior or posterior tibialis muscles. Genetic factors are also thought to play a role because pes cavus commonly runs in families.

Pes Planus A depressed or collapsed medial longitudinal arch is referred to as **pes planus** (flatfoot), the condition in which the forefoot becomes everted and the body weight forces the talus between the calcaneous and navicular bones. Of the two types, the more infrequent form is the rigid (or congenital) flatfoot that has a combination of calcaneovalgus, a pronation of the midtarsal region, and bone changes of the tarsals as well as contracture of the soft tissues. The second type is the flexible (or acquired) flatfoot distinguished by the fact that the arch reappears when weight is removed. Soft tissue contracture and bony changes usually are not present with the flexible type. Flexible flatfoot can be caused by a variety of conditions, including:

- Tibial or femoral torsion (medial torsion of the tibia or medial rotation of the hip)
- Muscle weakness of the intrinsic plantar muscles, or the anterior or posterior tibialis
- Weakening of the plantar ligaments

Muscle tone plays a very important role in maintaining the arches. Excessive exercise, standing for long periods of time, and being overweight can cause muscle fatigue. As muscle support wanes, ligaments become stretched and the arches become compressed. Loss of the arches places more stress on the plantar fascia, increasing the risk for plantar fasciitis. Also, both pes cavus and pes planus require more muscle action during the propulsion phase of any gait, which in turn causes fatigue and pain to those muscles.

PREVENTIVE MEASURES

Assessment for distortions of the ankle is important because they can make a tremendous impact on the ability to work efficiently and without pain. If a condition has begun to manifest itself either as pain or as reduced function, consultation with a podiatrist can determine corrective measures. In addition bodyworkers' work habits need to be modified as follows:

- Work while seated, especially in areas conducive to seated work, such as the face and feet.
- Be mindful of the stance. Maintain foot distance approximately hip width apart and keep the ankle and heel in neutral alignment.
- Wear appropriate and supportive footwear. Custom-made orthotics can be necessary.

A more generalized way to prevent injury is by maintaining appropriate body weight. Losing excessive weight directly reduces the workload on the feet. Also, strengthening and stretching the muscles of the feet and ankles will help.

Shoes are critical to healthy, happy feet and can influence the ergonomics of other body regions. Select shoes that give proper support to the foot. Worn-out shoes do not provide the support needed, but shoes that are rigid limit the foot's normal movement and flexibility. Wearing shoes with pointed toes can lead to problems related to toe compression, such as Morton's neuroma. Wearing high heels can cause hallux valgus because of the increased weight bearing on the large toe. In addition, when their heels are raised, people tend to walk with their knees flexed, triggering knee pain. Over time, wearing high-heels also leads to the contracture of the calf muscles and an increase in lumbar lordosis to compensate for the change in the center of gravity. In contrast, shoes with a negative heel ("earth shoes") stretch the calf muscles and lead to hyperextension of the knees. We recommend a good-quality walking or running shoe; they can cost more, but the support they give will be worth the investment.

Knees

The knee is the largest joint in the body. Within it, the inferior end of the femur articulates with the patella (knee cap) and the tibia to form a structure that is capable of numerous functions:

- Assisting in forward motion of the tibia and foot clearance while a person walks or runs
- Stabilizing the body while a person stands in place
- Allowing for flexion, extension, and some medial and lateral rotation, enabling a person to sit, stand up, squat, kneel, and crawl
- Assisting in shock absorption

Knee stability is greatly influenced by the integrity of the muscles, tendons, and ligaments supporting the knee, which act together to "lock" the stationary joint and "unlock" it for movement. Given the complex anatomy of the knee, the physical demands placed on it, and the many factors—such as overweight, hip dysfunction—that can stress it, its dysfunction is probable in the course of a lifetime.

The phrase from the song about "the knee bone connected to the thigh bone" suggests that distortions of the knee can affect the thighs and hips. Knee distortions can also affect the feet. On the other hand, a distortion originating in the hips or feet can affect the knees. For this reason, assessment of the whole body is essential.

NEUTRAL ALIGNMENT

Identifying the range of motion and alignment of the knee can help the bodyworker to assess and correct postural distortions. If the deviation is congenital or genetic, applying the information offered here will not correct the deviation. However, many of the suggestions will be helpful.

Ideally, the knees should be level when standing with 0–5 degree of flexion. No visible rotation should be noted. The knees' greatest range of motion is flexion: From 0 degree of extension, they can flex to approximately 135 degrees. Internal and external rotation is approximately 10 degrees. The knee locks in the last 15 degrees of extension, via a mechanism referred to as the **screw-home mechanism** (Figure 4.7 ■). This mechanism enables people to stand upright with minimal use of muscles for long periods of time.

Another factor to assess for neutral alignment is the Q (quadriceps) angle. The Q angle (patellofemoral angle) in Figure 4.8 ■ is determined by establishing two lines as points of reference. One line is drawn from the anterior superior iliac spine (ASIS) through the center of the patella and the second from the tibial tuberosity to the midpoint of the patella and then extended superiorly. The angle between the two lines is the **Q (quadriceps) angle**. When the knee is extended, the normal Q angle ranges from 13 to 18 degrees. Angles that lie outside this range are associated with knee problems. Abnormal Q angles create excessive stress on the patella, leading to joint complications. This angle normally tends to be larger in females because of their wider pelvis. As a consequence, females are at increased risk for a variety of knee problems.

THE CAUSES AND IMPACT OF DEVIATIONS

Three PDs of the knees are common: **genu recurvatum,** commonly called *hyperextension,* **genu varus,** often known as *bowlegs,* and **genu valgus,** also called *knock-knees.* These conditions affect and are affected by stance. Refer to Figure 4.9 ■ for a comparison of these three deviations.

These conditions usually can result from any of the following:

- Arthritis (bony deformity)
- Joint or ligament instability
- Referral from the subtalar joint (varus/pronator, valgus/supinator)
- Weak quadriceps
- Impaired proprioception
- Weak gastrocnemius and soleus muscles
- Abnormal Q angle

Genu Recurvatum Muscle imbalance is clearly present in genu recurvatum (knee hyperextension). Two different patterns can be identified. In one pattern, neural or muscular disorders causing a weakened biceps femoris

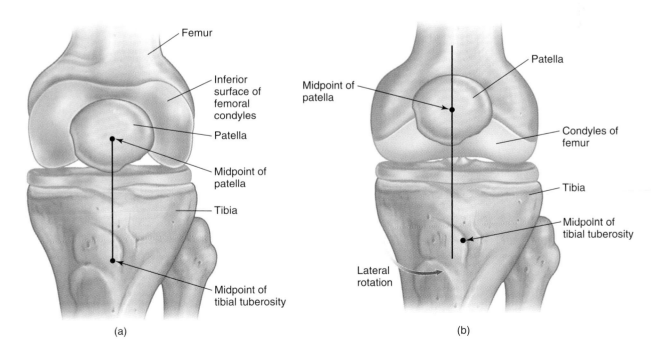

(a)   (b)

FIGURE 4.7

(a) Anterior view of the knee in a flexed position while seated. A dot on the midpoint of the patella aligns with a dot on the tibial tubercle. (b) When the knee is extended, the tubercle rotates laterally under the patella, as can be seen with the shifted position of the dot.

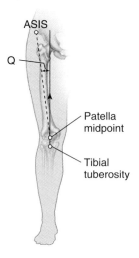

FIGURE 4.8

The quadriceps angle is measured by establishing a line from the anterior superior iliac spine (ASIS) to the midpoint of patella and along the femur from the tibial tuberosity to the midpoint of the patella.

(hamstring) facilitate hyperextension. In the second pattern, overtightening of the quadriceps femoris, which can be seen in people who habitually lock their knees, leads to hyperextension. A key difference between these two patterns is that the biceps femoris is lax in the first and hypertonic in the second.

Of all joints of the body, the knee joint has the most complex set of ligaments. Combinations of stretching and tightening opposing pairs of ligaments can be contributing factors in knee misalignment. For example, the anterior cruciate ligament (ACL) is a stabilizer that tightens upon extension to prevent hyperextension. Therefore, a person with genu recurvatum demonstrates either a weak or an overstretched ACL.

The therapist with hyperextended knees typically exhibits the following postural deviations while working:

- Trunk flexion increases tension in the back and causes low back pain. Compensation of other supporting muscles occurs as a result. (*Note:* Although back flexion is required for a variety of techniques, hyperextended knees promote back flexion when it isn't necessary.)
- Increased lordosis because of an anterior pelvic tilt changes the **lumbosacral angle** and causes shearing stresses of fifth lumbar and first sacroiliac (L5 and S1) joints.
- Flexion of the head
- Protracted chin

The therapist with genu recurvatum could develop the following problems:

- Weak or overstretched hamstrings
- Weak or overstretched calves (soleus and gastrocnemius muscles)
- Injury to posterior components of the knee joint

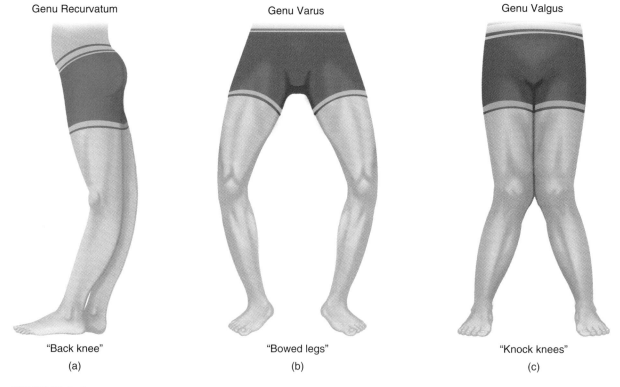

FIGURE 4.9

(a) A lateral view shows hyperextension (recurvatum). (b) An anterior view of the knees shows varus—a bowed leg effect—and (c) valgus—a knock-kneed effect or lateral angulation.

Genu Varus and Genu Valgus   When the knees appeared bowed, the distortion is genu varus, which is a lateral angulation of the knee. The distal part of the leg below the knee in Figure 4.9 is deviated inward. Most of people are born with bowed legs, a consequence of being in the uterus. However, this should self-correct in 18 months or at the latest, 3 years of age. If it hasn't corrected by this time, the condition is either genetic or caused by other medical conditions, such as infection, tumors, skeletal problems, and, in rare cases, rickets (lack of vitamin C) or Blount disease (tibial osteochondrosis).

Genu varus in adults can occur as a consequence of arthritis or postural habits as displayed by the "cowboy" or "cowgirl" who spends hours per day in the saddle.

The individual displaying genu valgus (medial angulation) of the knee whereby the distal part of the leg is deviated outward has a knock-knee appearance. As in genu varus, this condition can be inherited or acquired but is less common than genu varus. Knock-knees usually self-correct during adolescence, but corrective measures such as splints, braces, and—if necessary—surgery can be recommended.

The therapist with genu varus or genu valgus is likely to exhibit the following:

- Decreased limb stability
- Compensation proximal or distal to the knee
- Knee pain
- With valgus, weak pronators that are overstretched because of pronation at the ankles and supinators that are shortened and tightened
- In varus, weak supinators and tight pronators (opposite of valgus)

PREVENTIVE MEASURES

The first key to preventing PDs of the knee is understanding what constitutes neutral alignment of the knee and making an assessment to determine alignment. Then, depending on the contributing factors, such as muscle weakness, surgery, or poor posture, the corrective measures must be determined. For example, the bodyworker with a leg-length discrepancy because of a fused knee should have the quadratus lumborum (QL) massaged to help stretch and relax the hip hiking/elevation that occurs as a result of engaging the QL in muscle reversal. Muscle reversal occurs when a muscle's origin is pulled toward the insertion. An overall prevention plan includes being mindful of misuse and initiating corrective measures as soon as a pattern is identified. Suggested corrective measures are:

- Strength training for weak leg muscles
- Stretching and massage for overly tight leg muscles
- Maintaining range of motion within safe limits
- Using correct posture

Pelvis

The pelvis is made up of a ring of fused bones. A ring commonly represents wholeness and integration, so it seems fitting that the primary functions of the pelvis are to support and stabilize the body. It is the attachment point for the legs, and it transmits force up the spine as the body moves in all three planes. Stability is the key descriptor for the pelvis.

NEUTRAL ALIGNMENT

An anterior view of your pelvis while standing in a neutral position should show the ASIS as being level. From a lateral view, both the ASIS and the pubic symphysis should line up on a vertical plane. When they do, the angle at which the sacrum articulates with the fifth lumbar vertebra (lumbosacral angle) is 140 degrees. This position maintains a pelvic angle of 30 degrees (see Figure 4.10a ■). The spinal erectors, hip flexors, hamstrings, and abdominal muscles maintain the alignment. For the pelvis to be properly positioned on the heads of the femurs, these muscles must be strong, mobile, and balanced.

THE CAUSES AND IMPACT OF DEVIATIONS

When the pelvis tilts away from neutral as a result of an imbalance of the muscles attached to it, a corresponding opposition occurs in the joints above and below it. Three types of pelvic tilts are common: anterior, posterior, and lateral.

Anterior Tilt   An anterior tilt occurs when the pelvis tilts forward from the vertical line; that is, the ASIS moves anteriorly and the pubic symphysis moves posteriorly (refer to Figure 4.10b). The pelvic angle increases as the lumbosacral angle decreases and the hip joints flex. Hyperextension of the lumbar spine causes lumbar lordosis (swayback). The lumbosacral angle change puts excessive stress on L5 and S1.

Anterior tilt can result from a number of conditions, including:

- Congenital defects, such as congenital hip dislocation
- Neuromuscular disorders
- Skeletal disorders, such as spondylolisthesis, a partial forward dislocation of one vertebra over the one below it
- Postural compensation for kyphosis of the thoracic region
- Improper posture and muscle imbalance
- Genu recurvatum

Anterior tilt can be associated with the following conditions:

- Weak abdominal muscles
- Weak gluteus maximus
- Tight or contracted hip flexors (iliopsoas muscle, rectus femoris)
- Tight or contracted spinal extensors (erector spinae)

Obesity, pregnancy, high heels, and general, poor conditioning create an increased risk for the postural-triggered anterior tilt.

The therapist with an anterior tilt can develop:

- Herniation of the lumbar disc, commonly to the L5 disc

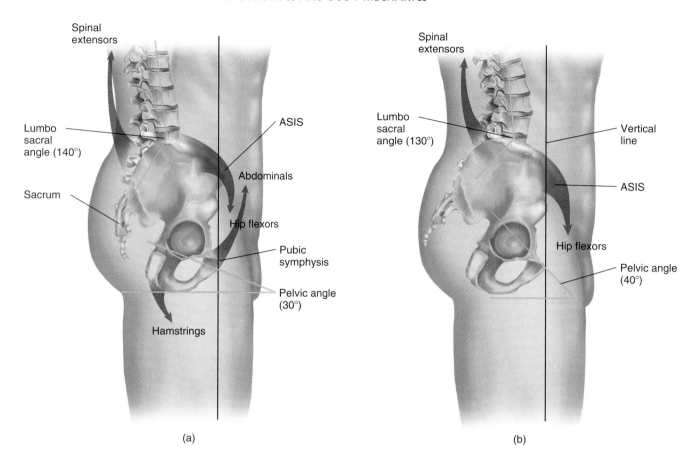

(a)   (b)

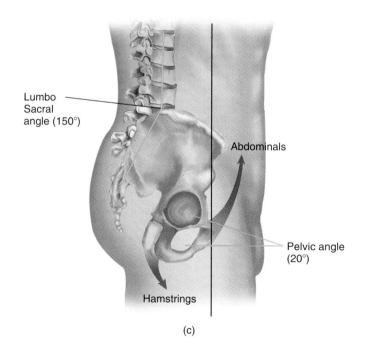

(c)

FIGURE 4.10

(a) The pelvis is in neutral alignment when the ASIS lines up vertically with the pubic symphysis in a lateral view. The pelvic angle and lumbosacral angle are also shown. (b) An anterior tilt occurs when the ASIS moves forward of the vertical line. (c) A posterior tilt is reversed, with the ASIS moving posterior to the vertical line.

- Pain radiating down the back and lateral side of the leg(s) to the sole of the foot (sciatica)
- Muscle weakness in one or both legs
- Lumbar lordosis and its complications

Posterior Tilt   A posterior tilt results in a decrease in the lumbar curve (flat back). The ASIS moves posteriorly to the pubic symphysis, causing the pubic bone to jut forward as though it is leading the person. The lumbosacral angle becomes straighter than normal and the pelvic angle decreases to 20 degrees (see Figure 4.10c).

Posterior tilt can develop as a result of:

- Compensation for abdominal or low back pain
- Compensation for weak hip flexors
- Improper posture and muscle imbalances

The muscle imbalances associated with posterior tilt are the opposite of that for anterior tilt and include:

- Weak paraspinal muscles
- Tight or contracted gluteus maximus
- Tight or contracted hamstrings
- Tight or contracted abdominals

The therapist with a posterior tilt can develop limited lumbar extension and be at higher risk for developing rounded, protracted shoulders. These changes occur as a result of altered vertebral curves.

Lateral Tilt   Some lateral tilt occurs naturally during the swing phase of walking (see Figure 4.11a ■). The **swing phase** of walking occurs when one foot leaves the ground; this lowers the pelvis on that side. The pelvis moves as one unit, so when one side is down, the other side is up. When the body is stationary, there should be no tilt (Figure 4.11b) and weight bearing should be equal across the pelvis.

Lateral tilt when the body is stationary typically results from discrepancies in leg length or muscle imbalance. The side of the tilt is determined by the weight-bearing hip (i.e., a left lateral tilt would occur when the left hip is bearing the weight and the pelvis is rotated on the head of the left femur). It can involve either (1) hip abduction, "hip hiking" (elevation of the opposite side of the pelvis) or (2) hip adduction, "hip drop" (dropping of the opposite side of the pelvis) as in Figure 4.11c. As a result of the abnormal rotation of the pelvis on the head of the femur, the position of the weight-bearing leg changes in relation to the pelvis. In hip abduction, the weight-bearing hip/leg becomes abducted and in hip adduction, the weight-bearing hip/leg becomes adducted. Lateral tilt because of muscle imbalance is based on the following typical patterns. Hip hiking can result from:

- Tight hip abductors of the opposite side
- Tight erector spinae of the opposite side, specifically the quadratus lumborum
- Lateral abdominal contracture of the opposite side
- Weak gluteus maximus on the side of the tilt

Hip drop results from:

- Tight adductors
- Tight tensor fascia lata and tight iliotibial band

The hip involved with the lateral tilt is at higher risk for injury because of the increased load placed on it. In addition, a habitual lateral tilt creates compensation as the joints above and below the tilt shift in an attempt to keep the body balanced. In a left lateral tilt, the result is a bend in the spinal column to the right. The spinal column bends to the left when the pelvis is laterally tilted to the right.

See Table 4.1 ■ for a comparison of the three pelvic tilts and their associations between the pelvis, vertebral column, and hip joints.

PREVENTIVE MEASURES

To maintain a healthy back and spine, it is extremely important to maintain neutral alignment with the pelvis. Daily habits, such as standing with weight predominately on one leg, cause the hip to hike up and out (lateral tilt). Carrying items such as a child or grocery bags on the hip also causes hip hiking. Excessive abdominal weight creates a risk for an anterior tilt, and even shoes affect the pelvic angle. Changing those patterns and conditions that can be changed is imperative for people who have a pelvic tilt. In addition, working with a body therapist or movement specialist to reeducate the movement patterns is recommended.

Head and Trunk

As with pelvic stability, spinal stability is essential for movement and support of the whole body. The vertebral column forms the longitudinal axis of the body, supports the head, and with the pectoral and pelvic girdles, acts as the anchor point for the attachment of the limbs. Muscles originating along the column stabilize the head, girdles, and the column itself and provides for movement. The curves of the vertebral column act as shock absorbers and improve flexibility. The vertebrae and vertebral discs provide a structural framework that allows spinal nerves to pass through unimpeded.

NEUTRAL ALIGNMENT

The vertebral column is considered triaxial, meaning that it allows for movement in three planes: saggital, frontal, and transverse. The motions include flexion, extension, hyperextension, lateral flexion/bending, and rotation. From the posterior view, the vertebral column is straight, but from the lateral view, it demonstrates the curves that play a role in shock absorption. The lumbar region immediately superior to the pelvis shows a convex curve; the lumbosacral angle is established by the pelvic tilt. Most flexion and extension occurs in the lumbar region of the spine. The thoracic region displays a concave curve and is the most stable, allowing the least amount of mobility because of the articulation of the ribs with the sternum. Nevertheless, most lateral flexion and rotation occur in this region. The cervical

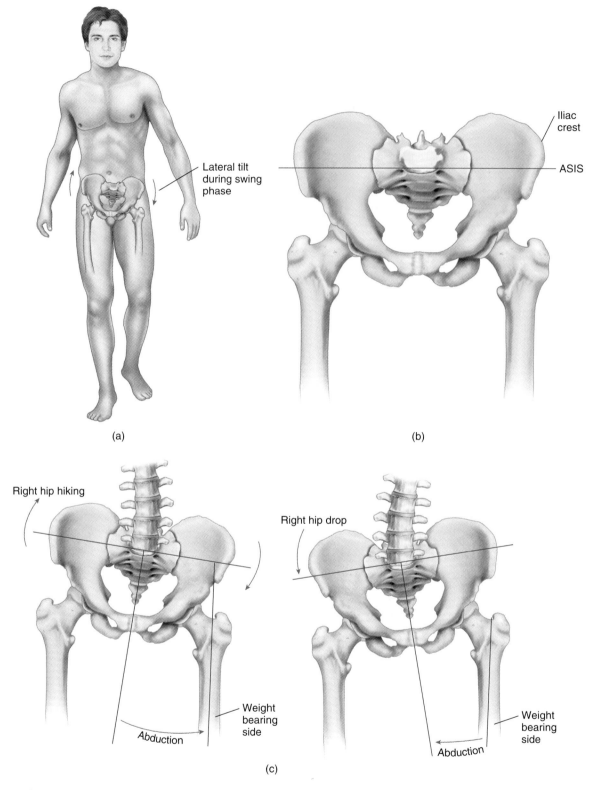

(a)

(b)

(c)

FIGURE 4.11

(a) A normal lateral tilt occurs during the swing phase of walking. (b) When standing, the iliac crests and anterior superior iliac spines should be level. (c) A lateral tilt while standing is determined by the weight-bearing hip. The illustration shows a left lateral tilt with the pelvis rotated on the left hip. The tilt may result from hip adduction or abduction of the opposite side.

TABLE 4.1	Comparison of Pelvic Tilts	
Pelvis	Vertebral Column	Hip
Anterior tilt	Hyperextension	Flexion
Posterior tilt	Flexion	Extension
Lateral tilt	Lateral tilt to opposite side	Abduction or Adduction

spine displays a convex curve. It has the greatest range of motion and provides for the head's mobility.

Intervertebral discs and ligaments play an important role in the structure of the spine. The intervertebral discs absorb shock, provide proper spacing between the vertebrae for exit of spinal nerves, and maintain flexibility of the vertebral column. In the cervical area, they contribute greatly to the normal spinal curvature. Excessive range of motion or repetitious movements in any of the planes can functionally or structurally damage the discs. The ligaments of the back prevent both excessive flexion and hyperextension.

Any exaggerated curve puts strain on the musculoskeletal system and vertebral alignment and predisposes the person to back pain and impaired movement. Abnormalities can involve either an exaggerated or reduced curve of the lumbar, thoracic, or cervical regions, or they can involve an abnormal lateral curve. Injuries occur most often in the lumbar spine because it has to absorb the bulk of body weight and anything a person carries. However, any of the areas of the spinal column can be injured with excessive movement or force. One example is the strain on the thoracic spine that occurs when lifting an object with extended arms while rotating the body.

THE CAUSES AND IMPACT OF DEVIATIONS

Several PDs of the vertebral column can occur. We discuss scoliosis, which can affect any portion of the vertebral column. When performing an assessment, bodyworkers shouldn't be surprised to find several misalignments occurring together. This commonly happens because as a change in one curve occurs, the center of gravity shifts, causing other changes.

Scoliosis   Scoliosis can be classified as either a structural or functional defect. The deformity of the vertebrae in structural scoliosis causes the vertebral bodies to rotate toward the convexity of the curve. See Figure 4.12 ■ for a right thoracic curve, where the vertebral bodies rotate to the right. When bending forward, the abnormal curve is still present. If the scoliosis is in the thoracic region, the ribs on the convex side push posteriorly, creating a rib "hump," and the thoracic cage narrows on the convex side. The deformity can interfere with breathing and the functioning of other internal organs.

Functional scoliosis of the lumbar and thoracic region result from leg length discrepancy; muscle spasms of the iliopsoas, quadraus lumborum, and/or paraspinal muscles;

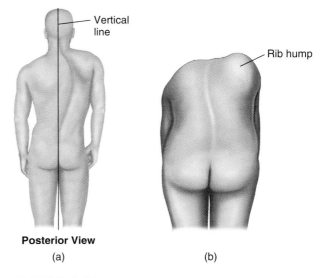

Posterior View
(a)   (b)

FIGURE 4.12

(a) A right thoracic curve has a convexity toward the right.
(b) Flexion of the torso reveals a "rib hump."

and compensation from pain, such as nerve impingement in the lumbar area; these conditions can be reversed by correcting the cause. Also, unlike structural scoliosis, the curve disappears with forward flexion because there is no vertebral rotation. Rotation of the trunk alters the plantar contact (BOS) and weight distribution and thereby affects the feet, knees, and pelvis. It also compromises the thoracic and abdominal cavities and can affect the internal organs.

Scoliosis in the cervical region, involving a lateral tilt or rotation of the head, can occur as a congenital problem or be caused by injury or habitual misuse. Examples of injury or misuse include:

- Postural compensation for other changes in the vertebral column or stance
- Weak neck muscles
- Temporalmandibular joint problem
- Compensation for hearing problems or wearing bifocal or trifocal glasses

A person with a habitual tilt or rotation doesn't necessarily display it while active, but when the person relaxes, the tilt/rotation reappears.

Other Postural Distortions of the Spine   Other changes from the neutral position of the spinal curves occur in a variety of forms and combinations (see Figure 4.13 ■).

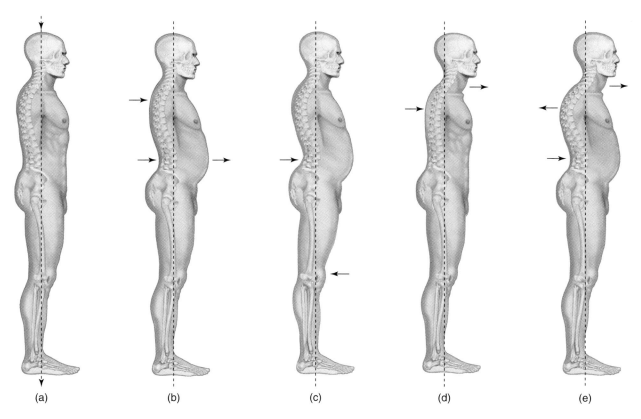

(a)   (b)   (c)   (d)   (e)

FIGURE 4.13

(a) Normal, good posture; (b) relaxed, poor posture; (c) lumbar lordosis with hyperextension of the knees; (d) kyphosis with protraction of the shoulder and head; (e) lordosis, kyphosis, with protraction of the head.

Although these misalignments can have a congenital or pathological basis, the most common problem is poor postural habit. Correct posture requires that the muscles supporting the spine be strong, flexible, and adaptable. Conditions that contribute to functional misalignment of the spinal curves include:

- Standing or sitting for long periods of time, which reduces muscle tone and balance and triggers a tendency to slouch
- Muscle tightness in the shoulder or pelvic girdle (e.g., pectoralis minor or iliopsoas)
- Muscle spasm of the paraspinal muscles
- Altered positioning to compensate for chronic pain
- Respiratory problems
- General weakness
- Loss of proprioception
- Excess weight

PDs of the lumbar region are measured using the lumbosacral (LS) angle, which is normally 140 degrees when standing. This angle depends on a pelvic angle of 30 degrees. A change in the pelvic angle (i.e., anterior or posterior tilt), in turn alters the LS angle. A posterior tilt is compensated for with a decrease in the LS angle that is commonly referred to as a *flat back.* An anterior tilt is

compensated with an increase in the LS angle and is known as *lumbar lordosis.* Of the two conditions, lordosis is more common; it develops from:

- Tight hip flexor and tensor fasciae latae
- Weak abdominal muscles
- Heavy abdomen from excess weight or pregnancy
- Weak hamstring muscles (semimembranosis)
- Compensation for other deformities such as hyperextension of the knees, or *kyphosis,* an exaggerated thoracic curve, which is the most common deformity of the thoracic spine
- Congenital problems, such as dislocation of the hip
- Pathological problems such as osteoporosis of the lumbar vertebrae

To help maintain their center of gravity, people with lordosis often develop sagging shoulders, increased thoracic curve, medial rotation of the legs, and/or protraction of the head.

Kyphosis can result from a variety of factors including:

- Congenital defects
- Tuberculosis
- Vertebral compression fractures, as seen in osteoporosis
- Compensation for lordosis
- Postural habit of slouching

When kyphosis occurs as a result of postural changes, a typical pattern of muscle imbalances occurs:

- Short upper trapezius and levator scapulae and weak middle and lower trapezius causing the shoulders to elevate and protract
- Short, tightened pectorals causing rounding of the shoulders
- Weak serratus anterior causing winging of the scapulae

In addition, the rounding of the thorax decreases thoracic cavity size, and this in turn reduces respiratory efficiency and capacity.

As stated, the cervical spine has the greatest flexibility, which allows for the necessary head movement. Two significant factors determine the head position and movement: directing the eyes and keeping the head balanced on top of the vertebral column. A dynamic relationship exists between the hands and the position of the head because of the process of keeping the eyes focused on the hands' activity. Balancing the head on top of the body is a component of overall posture control. Head movement influences the rest of the vertebral column just as distortions of lower regions trigger compensation in head position.

Therapists are prone to postural kyphosis along with rounded shoulders. Kyphosis causes the face to look downward. To be able to look forward, a person raises the head using the cervical extensor muscles. This increases the cervical curve, creating cervical lordosis, and causes the chin to become protracted. The pressure on the vertebral discs change, and impingement on cervical nerves can occur. Hypertonicity of the extensor muscles and compression of the cervical discs contribute to neck pain and headaches.

PREVENTIVE MEASURES

The functional distortions of the vertebral column are relatively easy to correct once the underlying cause has been identified. As with PDs of other regions of the body, therapy consists of strengthening weak muscles, commonly the abdominal muscles, and stretching the tight muscles, which commonly include the iliopsoas and quadratus lumborum. It is also important for people to realize it is their responsibility to maintain correct upright posture whether standing, sitting while performing daily and work activities.

Structural PDs of the spine, which most often arise from bone deformity, are more complex and commonly can be corrected only with surgery. However, instruction on proper posture can often relieve symptoms.

Shoulders

We have probably all heard the saying that "for every loss there is a gain and for every gain there is a loss." This is particularly true of the shoulder girdle and glenohumeral joint structure. The shoulder has the widest range of motion in the body, but accomplishing this sacrifices stability. This makes the region vulnerable to injury and PDs.

NEUTRAL ALIGNMENT

The shoulder girdle with which the humerus articulates comprises both the concave scapula on the posterior surface, which follows the contour of the rib cage, and the clavicle on the anterior side, which acts as a strut to tie the girdle to the sternum. From the posterior view, the medial borders of the scapulae should be parallel with each other and with the spine. From the lateral view, each acromion process should align vertically with the ear lobe and the top of the iliac crest.

Muscles originating from the vertebral column, sternum, and ribs stabilize the shoulder girdle. In turn, muscles originating from the shoulder girdle stabilize and move the humerus. The scapula is capable of elevation, depression, adduction, abduction, and rotation. This variety of motion allows for:

- The glenoid surface to be oriented for optimal contact with the maneuvering arm
- Additional range for elevating the arm
- A stable base for the controlled rolling and sliding of the head of the humerus

Stabilizing the shoulder girdle to maximize the arm motion represents dynamic stability. Contraction of the trapezius and serratus anterior muscles produces upward rotation of the scapula. Abduction without rotation of the scapula involves the serratus anterior and pectoralis minor, which are used together in most movements involving pushing with the hands.

The axilla is also an important structure of this area. This pyramid-shaped space forms the passageway for the nerves, blood vessels, and lymphatic vessels that extend from the root of the neck and pass into the upper arm. Misalignment and muscle tightness in the area can impinge on these structures and lead to impaired circulation, numbness, tingling, and pain.

THE CAUSES AND IMPACT OF DEVIATIONS

The focus of this section is two PDs that involve the scapular position: protracted (rounded) shoulders and elevated shoulders. Both of these conditions can be the cause of or caused by an increased thoracic curve.

Protracted Shoulders Protracted shoulders are quite common with bodyworkers and usually occur because of the repetitive action of pushing with the hands. Protracted shoulders occur as the scapulae roll forward and the acromion process moves anteriorly. These shifts cause chest concavity (Figure 4.14 ■). Increased use of the serratus anterior and pectoralis minor creates a muscle imbalance in the shoulder girdle. These two muscles tighten and shorten, and the trapezeus and rhomboids become weakened and stretched. A number of interrelated complications can result from this situation.

- A tight, short pectoralis minor overworks the thoracic extensor muscle and contributes to thoracic pain.

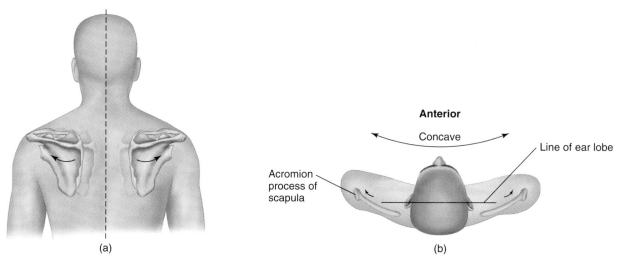

FIGURE 4.14

(a) Scapulae move lateral from the spine with protraction of the shoulders. (b) The acromion process moves anterior to the lobe of the ear and the chest becomes concave.

- The pectoralis minor can compress the brachial plexus and cause thoracic outlet syndrome involving pain, tingling, and numbness that radiates down the arm.
- Medial rotation of the humerus occurs with protraction, which affects the orientation of the lower arm. It causes the elbows to abduct and the palms of the hands, which should be facing the lateral aspect of the thighs in neutral alignment, to medially rotate and face posteriorly.
- The head is pulled forward and the thoracic curve increases. To compensate, the muscles in the back of the neck tighten to lift the face upward, which increases the cervical curve and puts more compression on the cervical discs. A long-term risk is degeneration of the discs and impingement of the cervical nerves.
- Compression of the nerves, hypertonicity of muscles, and resulting fatigue causes the practitioner to slouch. Slouching decreases lung capacity and affects breathing.

Elevated Shoulders Elevation can involve either one or both shoulders. The shoulder of the dominant side is commonly lower. However, exaggerated elevation of one shoulder can occur in response to muscle imbalance resulting from injury or improper posture, often developing as a result of the shortening and tightening of the upper trapezius and levator scapula.

Postural habits that cause these muscles to shorten include chronically holding the shoulder or shoulders in an elevated position as when cradling a phone between the shoulder and chin, supporting a shoulder bag, or working at a surface that is too high. This elevation of the shoulder(s) decreases the scapula's stability for arm movement and limits arm abduction. In addition, tightened muscles commonly cause pain. Nerve impingement because of hypertonic

muscles produces numbness and tingling sensations. Compensation occurs as a consequence, causing upper back and neck tension, which increases the potential for thoracic outlet syndrome (compression of the brachial plexus nerves.)

PREVENTIVE MEASURES

Because the scapulae are essentially held in place with muscle, maintaining a balance between all of the muscles of the shoulder girdle is the central means of preventing the PDs discussed. This can be achieved through strengthening and stretching of the shoulder muscles, as discussed later in Chapter 7, and assessing the position and movement of your arms while you are working to ensure that you are avoiding unnecessary protraction or elevation of your shoulders. This can require that you change your work surface or your method of working.

Wrist and Hand

Functions of daily living require the use of the hands often and in a variety of ways, thereby making them highly susceptible to injury. In addition, it's important to realize that the use of the hands subtly and significantly influences the entire body's posture.

The two joints of the wrist are the radiocarpal joint and the midcarpal or intercarpal joints. The radiocarpal joint allows for flexion, extension, and radial deviation (adduction), and ulnar deviation (abduction). These motions combined are circumduction. The midcarpal joints permit gliding motions that assist the wrist. The palmarcarpal ligament, transverse ligament, and extensor retinaculum ligament function to secure the tendons when the wrist flexes or extends.

The major functions of the wrist are to control the hand and provide stability. The extrinsic muscles of the hand have a role in supporting the wrist because their proximal attachment is above the wrist and their distal attachment is on the hand. The primary functions of the joints of the upper extremity are also to position the hand to carry out the many tasks required.

The hand's intrinsic muscles attach proximal or distal to the carpal bones and insert on the phalanges. These muscles are responsible for the hand's precision movement and fine motor control. The thumb, which has the greatest range of movement of all the digits, has three joints: the carpometacarpal joint, metacarpalphalangeal joint, and interphalangeal joint. They allow for extension, flexion, opposition, adduction, and abduction. The fingers have four joints, the metacarpalphalangeal joint and three interphalangeal joints. Motions of the fingers are flexion, extension, adduction, and abduction. They all serve to provide mobility and stability.

The proximal carpal, distal carpal, and longitudinal carpal muscles assist in various types of grasping tasks, and the ligaments of the hand provide support by holding the tendons close to the wrist during extension and flexion with the exception of the transverse carpal ligament, which lies deeper and arches over the carpal bones to form the carpal tunnel. This ligament is often surgically cut to alleviate the symptoms of carpal tunnel syndrome.

NEUTRAL ALIGNMENT

Neutral alignment is considered midway between flexion and extension while the hand is in a straight line with the forearm. The neutral wrist is zero degrees (or straight). The following is the approximated range of wrist movement for each of the four directions:

- Flexion (palmar) 0–90 degrees
- Extension (dorsal) 0–80 degrees
- Adduction 0–35 degrees (ulnar deviation)
- Abduction 0–25 degrees (radial deviation)

Although these are established ranges of movement of which the wrist is capable, using the full range while working is not recommended. The farther the wrist is from neutral to zero degrees in any direction, the greater the risk for injury.

THE CAUSE AND IMPACT OF DEVIATIONS

Complications that arise from overuse and deviations from neutral alignment follow:

- Carpal tunnel syndrome (CTS) is compression of the median nerve.
- Lateral epicondylitis (tennis elbow) becomes chronic after an acute phase of a tenoperiostial tear of the wrist extensors because of repetitive gripping motions.
- Medial epicondylitis (golfer's elbow) occurs with repetitive wrist flexion and pronation as in gripping when golfing or playing tennis. The medial side of the elbow is affected at the tenoperiostial junction of the pronator teres and flexor carpi radialis.
- Cubital tunnel syndrome occurs when the tunnel becomes narrow and the ulnar nerve becomes entrapped from repetitive flexion, such as hammering,

or sustained flexion as a result of sleeping with the arm flexed.

Acquired problems of the wrist and hand are due to:

- Repetitive motion
- Overuse
- Muscular tightness
- Strained ligaments
- Nerve impingement
- Tenoperiosteal tears
- Cumulative stress
- Loss of synovial fluid
- Excesses in range of motion (i.e., breaking neutral and working outside safe zones)

Also note that pain in the wrist and hand can be caused by the elbow, shoulder, or cervical areas in addition to direct wrist trauma.

How far or close an object is from the person while working—whether it is the client, the keyboard, or the knife used to chop vegetables—determines wrist alignment. Assess your own work habits to determine whether any of the following common deviations occur while you are working:

- Ulnar deviation, wrist abduction
- Radial deviation, wrist adduction
- Hyperextension
- Excessive thumb abduction

Any of these can create degenerative conditions such as arthritis and/or thickening of ligaments.

PREVENTIVE MEASURES

It is important to keep the arms and hands in neutral alignment or as close to neutral as possible while working. The position of the arms influences alignment of the hands. If the arms are too elevated or too low or if the elbows are abducted or adducted, neutral alignment of the wrist is lost.

Bodyworkers need to be attentive to minimizing repetitive motion. Altering work habits is prudent as a preventive measure and necessary once problems arise. Rather than using the hands all of the time, bodyworkers should use the ulnar surface and olecranon over large muscle groups such as quadriceps and hamstrings to rest the hands and wrists. Excessive use of any one area (i.e., thumbs, fingers, palms) leads to complications.

Having good body mechanics is especially important when a person lifts and carries objects. The location of the object and its weight in relation to the body influences the position of bodyworkers' hands and overall posture. Many bodyworkers make house calls and must carry and maneuver their tables in and out of vehicles and through tight spaces. Following prescribed safe zones while lifting and moving an object as in Figure 4.1 reduces the risk for injury to the wrists as well as other areas.

The habit of sleeping with an overflexed wrist and elbow can trigger problems such as cubital tunnel syndrome defined earlier. Use a pillow to prop the arms and

CASE FOR STUDY 4.1
Implications of Lifting

Elena is a very talented massage therapist whose practice picked up markedly when she began to make house calls and travel to businesses. She is 32 years old, stands 5'7" and is slightly overweight at 155 pounds. Although she does not eat an excessive amount, she admits that her physical exercise is limited due to her busy work schedule and care of a family. She has been complaining of low back and right shoulder pain since her business began to expand and recently began to notice stiffness in her wrists and occasionally pain in her knees.

Although a number of factors can contribute to Elena's complaints, the challenges of moving her table to the various sites should be considered. Her table is 45 pounds, and she carries it in the trunk of her mid-size car, which is fairly deep. To lift the table out, she has to bend forward with her knees locked in position. The table bag has a shoulder sling that she uses to help position and lift the table, but nevertheless, it is still quite awkward.

Elena tried to use a cart to move the table once it was out of the trunk but having to move it on stairs and through narrow hallways with corners caused it to be of limited use. As a result, she usually carries the table using the shoulder strap but in tighter corners, she needs to slide the unit around on its edge.

1. Considering the position Elena has to be in to lift the table, what is the maximum weight she should be lifting based on the safe zone depicted in Figure 4.1?
2. Identify the various times when Elena is moving her table that she is likely working outside the recommended safe zones.
3. Explain an improper body mechanic that Elena is doing that attributes to each of the following: low back pain, right shoulder pain, wrist stiffness, and knee pain.
4. What recommendations and guidelines would you have Elena follow?

---

discourage elbow flexion. Stretching, massage, ice/heat therapy, and splinting the wrist or elbow are recommended to treat wrist and shoulder syndromes when indicated by pain or swelling. Health care professionals should be consulted for the best treatment protocol.

In conclusion, this chapter has addressed how PDs can involve the entire body. The challenges of working safely

and effectively are multifaceted and involve maintaining neutral alignment, staying within the safe zones, and minimizing repetitive motions.

See Case Study 4.1 for an example of how a simple task can impact multiple regions of the body.

CHAPTER SUMMARY

- Postural distortions can occur as genetic, congenital, or acquired conditions and can be classified as structural or functional.
- Postural habits and improper ergonomics often cause PDs, but when recognized, posture modification and work methods can correct the conditions.
- PDs involving vertical misalignment of the foot include calcaneovalgus, calcaneovarus, forefoot valgus, and forefoot varus. These conditions create unequal weight bearing on the foot, which leads to injury. PDs involving the arches of the feet reduce the shock absorption ability.
- The three common PDs of the knee are genu recurvatum, genu valrus, and genu valgus; they are associated with changes in the feet and pelvis as well as muscle imbalances of the leg.
- PDs of the pelvis include anterior and posterior tilt, which can affect the lumbar region and the knees, and lateral tilt, which can affect the torso and cause an unequal weight distribution to the feet.

- Scoliosis is an abnormal vertical curve of the spine that can result from a variety of factors. Other PDs of the vertebral column involve either an exaggeration or a reduction of the normal curves. The two most common forms are lordosis, the exaggeration of the lumbar and/or cervical curves, and kyphosis, the exaggeration of the thoracic curve. All PDs of the vertebral column compromise the musculoskeletal system and predispose the person to back pain and impaired movement.
- Muscle imbalance is the major factor for the two shoulder PDs: protraction and elevation. These conditions lead to pain and impaired movement.
- Common deviations when using the hands include ulnar deviation of the hand, radial deviation of the hand, hyperextension of the wrist, and excessive thumb abduction. Deviation of the hands while working, repetitive motion, overuse, and working outside the safe zones are the major risk factors for injury and pain of the hands, wrists, and forearm.

REVIEW QUESTIONS

1. Three PDs of the spinal column are
   _____, _____, and
   _____.
2. The three general causes of PDs are
   _____, _____, and
   _____.
3. Postural habits facilitate _____ PDs.
4. Acquired PDs can result from _____,
   _____, and _____.
5. The most common PDs of the shoulder are
   _____ and _____.
6. The general pathological basis for PDs is (are):
   a. skeletal misalignment or malformation
   b. muscle imbalance
   c. loss of stability of joints
   d. a and b
   e. a, b, and c
7. PDs affect the body in which of the following ways?
   a. increased risk for injury
   b. reduced range of motion
   c. change in muscle tone
   d. pain
   e. all of the above

8. Deviations of the foot include:
   a. genu varus and genu valgus
   b. pes planus and pes cavus
   c. genu recurvatum and calcaneovarus
   d. scoliosis and lordosis
   e. a and b
9. What is the ideal position for the knee when standing?
10. What angle relates to knee distortions?
11. Give the clinical term for knee hyperextension.
12. Describe the neutral position of the pelvis from the anterior and lateral views.
13. True or false? The vertebral column is triaxial.
14. True or false? A structural defect that causes a PD can be corrected without surgery.
15. True or false? The shoulder has the widest range of motion and the least stability of any joint.
16. True or false? Safe zones address only the maximum weight of objects.

REFERENCES

Magee, D. (2006). *Orthopedic physical assessment* (4th ed.). Philadelphia: W.B. Saunders.

Porter, R. (2005). *Musculoskeletal disorders and ergonomics.* Atlanta: Back School of Atlanta.

SUGGESTED READINGS

Hendrikson, T. (2003). *Massage for orthopedic conditions.* Baltimore: Lippincott Williams & Wilkins.
Lippert, L. S. (2000). *Clinical kinesiology for physical therapist assistants* (4th ed.). Philadelphia: F. A. Davis.

Norkin, C. C., & Lavangie, P. K. (1992). *Joint structure and function: A comprehensive analysis* (2nd ed.). Philadelphia: F.A. Davis.

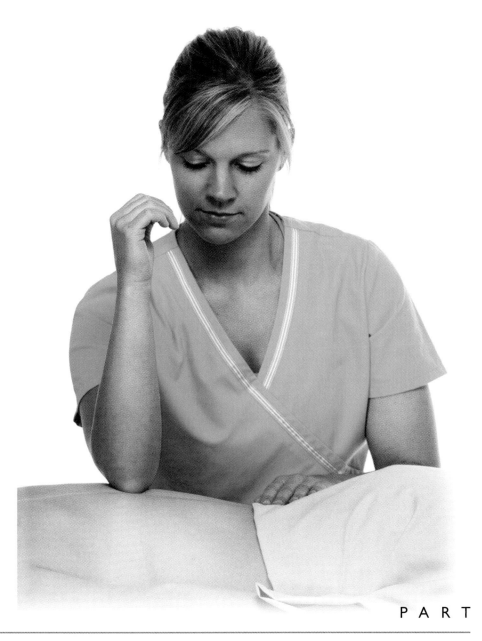

PART

2

Principles into Practice: Techniques, Environment, and Self-Care

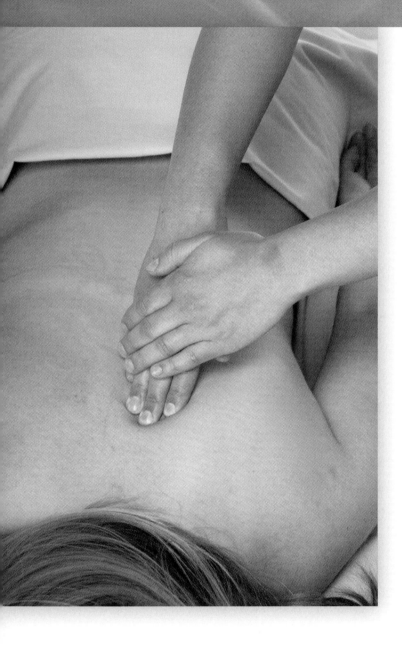

5 Ergonomic Techniques for the Bodyworker

 CHAPTER OUTLINE

LEARNING OBJECTIVES

Upon successful completion of the chapter, you will be able to:

1. Identify the neutral checkpoints of the body.

2. Determine the correct biomechanical positions of the bodyworker's body while applying therapeutic techniques.

3. Determine how to modify the client's position on the table to enhance the therapist's ergonomics.

4. Identify props used to aid therapists in their work.

5. Utilize the triangle of power when working.

KEY TERMS

Diagonal stance 86

Direct stance 85

Martial stance 84

Negative space 83

Triangle of power 80

Bodyworkers and massage therapists can become so involved in delivering treatment that they can fail to be mindful of their own body mechanics. The previous chapters have set the foundation for knowing what is ergonomically neutral whether stationary or moving. This chapter is the practical application of the foundations. Its emphasis is on safe and effective body mechanics while working and to teach therapists to observe and reflect on the best practice in different scenarios.

This chapter addresses ergonomics for working on each region of the client's body. Although this is not a book about therapeutic technique, it does briefly discuss some as a point of reference for the correct body mechanics. Description of ergonomic techniques continually refers to ways to maintain neutral alignment and recommends how to reduce repetitive action and impact on high-risk body areas. For example, this chapter includes working while seated as an alternative to the common standing position. Imbedded throughout the chapter are lists of checkpoints bodyworkers should watch for to assess proper ergonomics. Always be mindful of the breath and use it to aid not only providing depth of pressure but also to stay focused on the client and the work being performed. Bodyworkers who have worked in the field very long, could have found that physical aches and pains motivate change, but we recommend taking a proactive approach by critiquing yourself via video to identify poor work habits before you compromise your body's health and well-being. The values of having a peer make a video as you work are incomparable, and the video feedback call attention to flaws in your approach. Worksheet 5.1 is a guide for critiquing your work.

OVERVIEW OF ERGONOMIC TECHNIQUES

Key ergonomic principles apply to the individual regardless of the area being worked or the position used while working. These principles relate to neutral alignment and ways to improve stability.

Neutral Alignment

Maintaining neutral alignment prevents and alleviates repetitive motion injuries and reduces the risk of joint injuries. Identifying neutral checkpoints and recognizing when the bodyworker moves out of neutral while working is the starting point for achieving proper ergonomics. The foundation is basically the same for all techniques, whether energy work or Swedish or a neuromuscular technique. Consciously practicing proper body mechanics in sessions with peers, in the classroom, and when working on a client establishes muscle memory, over time helping the therapist to become unconsciously competent. "Variety is the spice of life" and in ergonomics relates to the advantage of varying the way the therapist works to minimize the effects of repetitive movement. Varying the techniques used to avoid overuse syndromes is best for bodyworkers.

Spinal and head alignments should be checked constantly while working whether seated or standing. The eyes are a major proponent in determining head position and posture. Bodyworkers have a natural tendency to look at what they are doing and where they are working. A common risk factor in bodywork is flexing the neck to be able to look down at the body being worked on. Being mindful of this can help to correct this bad habit. Closing the eyes or working blindfolded can help to train bodyworkers to rely less on their eyes and become more aware of their posture. Creating verbal or written cues are also beneficial.

Bodyworkers often overuse the upper extremities. Awareness of correct arm width and distance from the body can be lost during the course of the treatment. Whether the technique is static as in some energy work or moving, checking for neutral alignment is important. These following checkpoints are further discussed following the list.

- Keep arms as close to the body as possible.
- Do not abduct brachium more than 45 degrees.
- Do not adduct brachium past normal resting position (causes ulnar deviation).
- Avoid radial and ulnar deviation of the wrists.
- Keep fingers adducted.
- Keep thumb adducted when it is used.
- Relax the thumbs.
- Stack joints as much as possible.
- When using the fist, keep the thumb relaxed, not tucked into the palm.
- When using the ulnar surface, adjust the body to minimize torso torque (rotation).
- Focus on the breath and flow of energy.

Bodyworkers most often use and abuse their thumbs and fingers. Unfortunately, they are not designed to withstand what is asked of them. As a saddle joint, the thumb has a wide range of motion but not as much stability. Its design is for opposition to the fingers for grasping but not for applying compressive force, which is the tendency in bodywork. Instead, bodyworkers need to minimize the use of their thumbs and maximize working with their fists, ulnar surface, olecranon (elbow), and fingers. However, when deliberately using the thumb, it should be supported by keeping it close to the fingers. Likewise, fingers need to be adducted to support one another. Abduction and single-digit work cause undue stress.

Avoiding compressive force of the joints is virtually impossible when practicing modalities that require force such as Swedish and neuromuscular techniques. However, bodyworkers can align or stack the joints to minimize the effects. Remember that neutral alignment is always the best alignment. The finger joints ideally are stacked in alignment with one another and with the wrist, elbow, and shoulder (Figure 5.1 ■). When circumstance and technique prevent joint alignment of the limb from the shoulder to the finger, bodyworkers should maintain as much joint alignment as possible.

WORKSHEET 5.1

Assessment for Neutrality

Instructions: Use an outside observer and/or a video of your work to assess your work habits. Repeating this exercise periodically provides continued improvement. Comments in addition to the key will guide you on areas for improvement in ergonomic techniques.

Assessment for Neutrality

Body Area Worked	Head	Spinal Curves	Shoulders	Brachium	Wrists	Fingers and Thumbs	Triangle of Power	Stance	Weight Shift	Knee	Use of Props	Self-Awareness of Misalignment
Head/Neck												
Feet												
Upper extremity												
Lower extremity												
Back												
Gluteal area												
Chest												
Abdomen												

KEY

ab = abducted	↑ = elevated	Rt/L = right lateral tilt	r = rotated	re = retracted
ad = adducted	↓ = depressed	Lt/L = left lateral tilt	pro = protracted	N = neutral
at = anterior tilt	kp = kyphosis	h = hyperextend	ud = ulnar deviation	
pt = posterior tilt	ld = lordosis	f = flexed	rd = radial deviation	

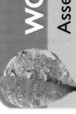

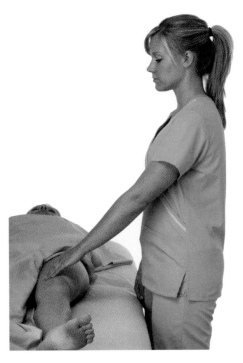

FIGURE 5.1

Joints are stacked from the fingers to the shoulder demonstrating ideal joint alignment.

Application of a stroke involves four body parts: fingertips, fists, palm, and elbow (olecranon process). Joints need to be stacked between the shoulder and the point of contact. The following list of checkpoints need to be followed when working in a seated or standing position.

- When using the fingertips, maintain a stacked alignment from shoulder to elbow to wrist and through the finger joints as in Figure 5.1. Note that there is no ulnar or radial deviation of the wrist.
- Use of the fist should follow the same neutral wrist alignment with the exception of the fingers being in a relaxed, flexed position (see Figure 5.2 ■). Use the dorsal side of the fist from the metacarpal phalangeal joint to the proximal interphalangeal joint. Don't tuck the thumbs into the fist; doing so compresses the thumb joints and alters the flat surface used to deliver the stroke.
- Use of the palmar surface increases the risk for hyperextension and radial deviation. Using the palms requires the bodyworker to continually adjust her or his stance to keep neutral alignment. Note the hyperextension of the wrist when standing straight (Figure 5.3a ■). By adjusting the stance (Figure 5.3b), the wrist alignment can be maintained. Delivering the stroke requires lengthening and deepening the stance that lowers the elbow and keeps neutral alignment.
- When using the olecranon, there are no joints to stack; however, the wrist, hand, and fingers remain relaxed but neutral (see Figure 5.4 ■).

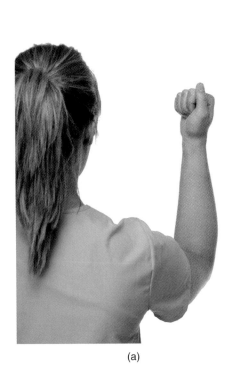

(a)

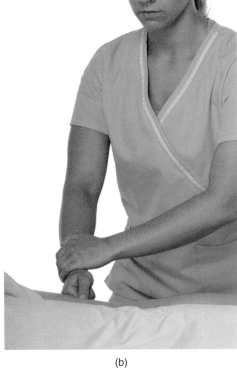

FIGURE 5.2

Use the dorsal side of the fist with relaxed fingers and thumb. (a) Note the fingers are cupped, relaxed and the thumb rests alongside the fist. (b) Applying the stroke using the fist.

(b)

FIGURE 5.3

(a) The wrist is shown in hyperextension when using the palmar surface. (b) Adjusting the wrist alignment by lengthening and deepening the stance.

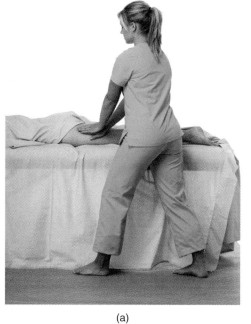

(a)

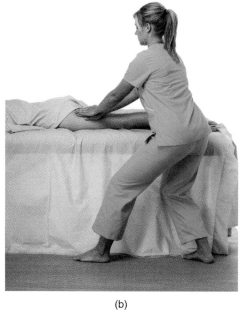

(b)

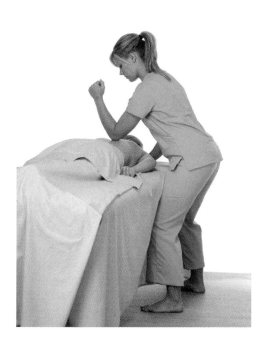

FIGURE 5.4

Proper alignment of the wrist, hand, and fingers is demonstrated when using the olecranon. Keep the torso and head in neutral alignment also.

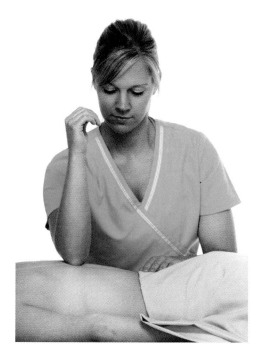

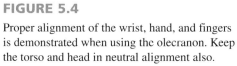

FIGURE 5.5

Correct olecranon alignment when applying a neuromuscular stroke to the back along the erector spine.

The elbow (olecranon) is a wonderful tool for applying depth when needed. Important alignment when using it is first to have the elbow as close to the body as possible. Pay attention to the shoulder and brachium. From an anterior or posterior view, keep the brachium in alignment with the side of the body to avoid adduction, abduction, or rotation of the brachium, which will be felt in the deltoid. See

Figure 5.5 ■ for the alignment of the arm when using the olecranon to apply a neuromuscular stroke to the erector spinae. Two positions are used to vary the depth of the stroke (Figure 5.6 ■). Using the body correctly and focusing on breathing allow for the application of more depth with less effort. Being mindful of the internal approach while practicing enhances the bodyworker's performance and

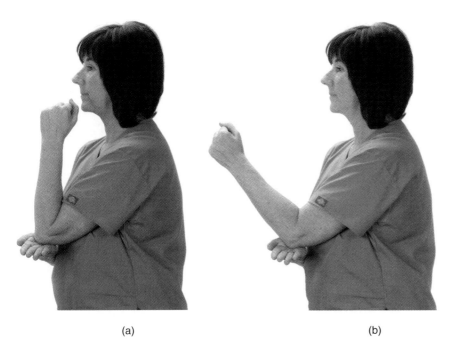

(a)   (b)

FIGURE 5.6

Two positions are used to vary the depth of stroke when using the olecranon: (a) forearm perpendicular to palm; (b) extending the forearm increases pressure on the palm.

provides career longevity. Practice these positions using the palmar surface of the opposite hand to feel the change in depth after adjusting the olecranon from position 1 to position 2. Helpful Hint 5.1 details the instructions.

Stability While Working

Stability is important for holding position, such as in trigger point and energy work and while delivering strokes. Stability can be achieved by using conscious body mechanics and persistent self-awareness.

A concept that we use in teaching ergonomics is the **triangle of power**, also referred to as the *tripod*. When performing a stroke, a bodyworker should create a triangle whether with the hands, fingers, elbow, fist, and so on. Regardless of the body part being used, forming a triangle provides support and stability while applying the technique. This sense of stability facilitates confidence, which is conveyed to the client and allows the bodyworker to relax into the stroke, trigger point, and so forth. In addition, this approach can deliver more depth with less effort when

needed. See Figure 5.7a ■, b, and c for an illustration of the triangle of power in a variety of positions. See Helpful Hint 5.2 for an activity for increasing awareness of the effects of the triangle of power.

We have a good friend and professional engineer Betsy Pearson, who says that the triangle is probably the most important shape in engineering. Each triangle side is supported by the other two when the triangle is under stress. Unlike a rectangle or any other polygon, a triangle cannot be deformed unless a side or junction breaks. In fact, one of the simplest ways to strengthen a rectangle is to add supports that form triangles at the corners or across its diagonal length. A single support between two diagonal corners greatly strengthens the rectangle by turning it into two triangles. Bridge trusses and geodesic domes have numerous triangles that make them stable.

Breath work and self-awareness (internal approach) are also fundamental to ergonomics for bodywork. Bodyworkers should be mindful of getting set, sinking (initiating movement), and completing the movement. Whenever they work on the body regardless of the technique to be used,

HELPFUL HINT 5.1
Adjusting the Olecranon for Depth

Place your left palm facing up and position your right elbow in the center of the palm.

Place the arm in position 1 as in Figure 5.6a with the forearm straight up perpendicular to the palm and fingers relaxed. Extend

the forearm until the olecranon can be felt (Figure 5.6b). Observe the change in depth that the position creates as the point of the olecranon is balanced on the palm. Overextension reduces the contact and depth.

FIGURE 5.7

The triangle of power can be used regardless of which body part you are using to employ the technique: (a) hands, (b) fists, (c) elbow/olecranon. The other arm is used to stabilize the olecranon.

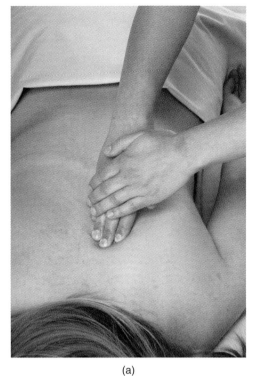

(a)

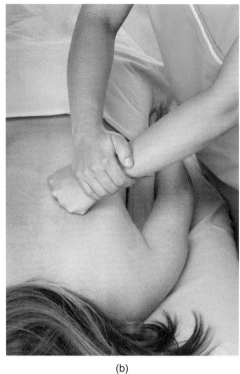

(b)

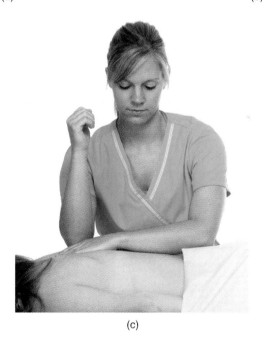

(c)

they should first set their intention, next sink into the stance, and then initiate and complete the movement. The therapists will have a sense of being centered and balanced as well as the feeling of moving into the fascia in such a way that conveys confidence and expertise to the client. We repeat the words "set, sink, move" like a mantra to our students. Its deliberateness provides a focus that slows the student/practitioner down and gives him or her the opportunity to feel the fascia from the beginning of the contact to the end. This concept can be employed with energy work as well.

Another important consideration for stability is aligning the body with the direction of movement or intention. The saying "energy follows intention" has significant validity in the field of bodywork.

WORKING WHILE SEATED

As teachers, we believe it is very important to demonstrate to our students several approaches to a situation. The field of bodywork has many modalities and many approaches to

HELPFUL HINT 5.2
Activities Increasing Awareness of the Effects of the Triangle of Power

Practicing the positions in Figure 5.7 in addition to seeking feedback from a peer or client will help you to develop an increased awareness of the benefits and effects of forming a triangle when you are working.

Begin by standing at the head of the table with the client in a prone position. Place your right hand on the left side of the client's back and your left hand on his or her right side. Apply a long gliding stroke such as effleurage with little or no lubricant. Repeat several times. Next, place your hands together so your thumbs are overlapped or linked as in the figure and then repeat the stroke several times. Do you feel the difference? Does your client?

When using the olecranon for deep tissue or neuromuscular technique, which is ideally suited for the erector spinae, begin with a wide stance at the side of the table facing your client's back. This is the exception to the toes lined up with the direction of the movement. You can try this in two ways: (1) the feet facing the client's body and (2) the foot closest to the client's head with your toes pointed toward the head (direction of movement) and the foot closest to the lumbar region with your toes pointed diagonal to the client's body. This is also the exception to splitting the energy. If you are on the right side of the table, your right olecranon is used, placing your body energetically behind the stroke for pushing through the stroke instead of pulling.

When using your fist remember to keep your thumb relaxed, not tucked into the fist; decide which fist is more appropriate and feels right for the area being worked on. Your side, location, and stance will determine this and the triangle of power that is used.

If you do trigger point work, we recommend using the olecranon as your primary tool and the knuckles as your secondary tool. Avoid using the fingers and thumbs because of the contact stress placed on these weaker more vulnerable areas. Stance and body alignment are critical to establishing an effective BOS from which to administer trigger point technique. Contact stress occurs regardless of the body part being used, but the negative impact can be alleviated by mindfulness of posture, leverage, movement (set, sink, move), and the techniques and tools being used.

---

them. Ergonomically, using both seated and standing positions makes sense. Areas of the client conducive to work on while seated are the head, neck, and feet. Other areas can be adapted to seated massage if the situation warrants it, such as an injury that prevents the bodyworker from standing for a prolonged period of time. Practitioners who travel and work with professional athletes or dancers most likely have experienced cramped conditions that are not favorable for moving around a table. An option is to adapt a seated position on the table while working. We discuss some ergonomically safe ways to practice bodywork in these conditions.

Following General Guidelines

One of the greatest challenges of working while seated is to become accustomed to the position after having been trained to perform the techniques while standing. Practitioners can feel that working in a seated position limits range of motion. Height becomes a factor that is easily remedied by adjusting the stool. When seated, the ischial tuberosities (sit bones) create the foundation or base of support (BOS). When resting on the ischial tuberosities, practitioners should find the center point and then gently rock back and forth to ascertain the range of motion and observe the subtleties of the core muscles, specifically the abdominal and the lumbar muscles. This is a good exercise to determine where practitioners feel comfortable and a good place to use the internal approach of centering through breath and visualization. Are the ischial tuberosities centered (i.e., neutrally balanced) or tilted anteriorly or posteriorly? Residing on the anterior portion hyperextends the lumbar spine causing lordosis. Residing on the posterior region of the ischial tuberosities cause the lumbar spine to be kyphotic. Refer to Chapter 4 regarding postural distortions related to an anterior or posterior tilt.

At times a deliberate shift from the center is effective in deepening a stroke. This allows the practitioner to use the energy from her or his body core. Applying traction requires a shift from the center of the ischial tuberosity to the posterior. Applying pressure requires an anterior shift that should both be done while keeping normal spinal curves and head position.

While seated, the practitioner's feet should be firmly planted approximately hip distance apart and parallel or staggered. The lower leg forms a 90-degree angle, and the seat can be either passive (resting against a seat back) or active (requiring the use of the core muscles) because either there is no back or the bodyworker is positioned away from the seat back (see Figure 5.8 ■). We use backless stools with a pneumatic lever for ease of adjusting to the correct height while working. The upper body is neutral (i.e., has normal spinal curves); the head is aligned to the torso with no protraction, flexion, or extension. The optimum position for flexion of the brachium is 0–45 degrees and the forearm at 90–130 degrees. The brachium should rest against the bodyworker's side or be abducted approximately 20 degrees.

Working on the Head and Neck

Preparation for seated head and neck work is the same regardless of the style of bodywork. Begin by establishing the neutral checkpoints. The worker will need an adjustable

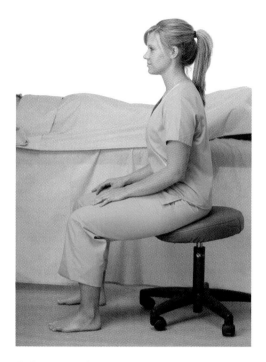

FIGURE 5.8

Use core muscles to maintain neutral alignment while seated without using a chair back.

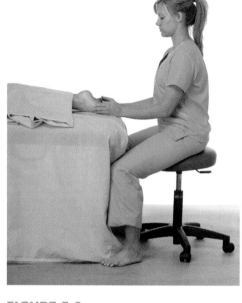

FIGURE 5.9

stool with or without a back with a minimum of five legs for stability and caster wheels for maneuverability. Make sure the surface around the treatment table is not too slippery as a linoleum surface would be, for example. If it is slippery, purchase appropriate floor mats for safety.

A checklist for remaining neutral while working on the head and neck follows:

- Feet flat on the floor, hip distance apart, and parallel or staggered
- Lower leg at 90 degrees
- Balance on the ishial tuberosities
- Spinal curves neutral and head neutral
- Upper arms 0–45 degrees and forearms at 90–130 degrees
- Focus on the breath and flow of energy

Stool height should be adjusted to keep the forearms in the correct position while working on the face or feet (see Figure 5.9 ■). The stool needs to be lower for working on the cervical area than it does on the face; otherwise, the forearm is not in neutral alignment. The stool itself should be repositioned as needed to have better access to the specific area of the head or neck and to create neutral wrist alignment. Shifting to a right diagonal position to work on the right side of the head or neck naturally corrects hyperextended wrists (Figure 5.10 ■). The seated position generally is not used for working on the cervical area while the client is in the side-lying position, but it can be used for the patient in the prone position.

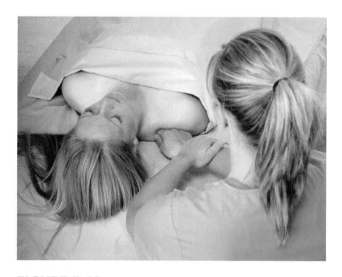

FIGURE 5.10

Hyperextension of the wrist can be prevented by adjusting the seated position to the diagonal.

Energy work lends itself to working while seated. The addition of props supports a static position. Use props to fill **negative space** such as between the forearm and the table (see Figure 5.11 ■). The prop's position should provide maximum support and maintain neutral alignment. Aligning the prop lengthwise rather than perpendicular with the forearm provides more support. Breathing, settling into the seat/stance, and using the internal approach enable

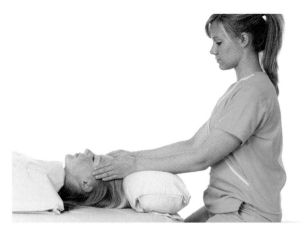

FIGURE 5.11

Use a prop (bolster) to fill negative space between the forearm and the table when doing energy work.

the bodyworker to stay connected to the client and to maintain awareness of his or her own body.

Working on the Feet

The same neutral checkpoints previously stated for the head apply when working on the feet in a seated position. A therapist who notices the wrist breaking neutral should slide the stool to the diagonal. The therapist can apply several modalities to the feet when the client is in the supine or prone position with some ergonomic modifications between the positions. Some tips for working on the feet include working on the plantar side of the foot when the client is in the prone position and using a bolster propped under the anterior portion of the ankle (Figure 5.12 ■). The therapist should elevate the stool to the appropriate height so his or her arms are at the correct angle before administering the techniques. It is challenging to avoid radial and ulnar deviation of the wrists when working on feet. One way to keep neutral wrists while applying a petrissage stroke is for the therapist to position the stool beside the client's lower leg with his or her back to the client (Figure 5.13 ■). The therapist should remember to use the

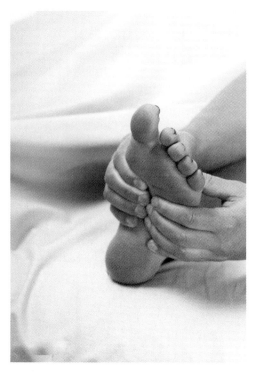

FIGURE 5.13

Positioning your body to face the client's feet while administering a petrissage stroke to the plantar surface of the foot.

knuckles and fists as alternatives to the fingers when providing foot massage. Refer to Figure 5.14 ■ for some examples of these techniques. We know a reflexologist who uses the eraser end of a pencil as his favored tool when applying pressure, but remember that the tools that often make a particular technique easier to apply can present a greater challenge to good body mechanics. When performing energy work on the feet, working from the side supports neutral alignment. Align the prop perpendicular to the forearms (Figure 5.15 ■). A checklist for remaining neutral while working on the feet is the same as that for working on the head and neck with the addition of the use of props used as needed.

WORKING WHILE STANDING

Standing is the most common position while working. It is optimal for working on the torso and the limbs because of the advantage of leverage and depth on the larger muscles. The BOS depends on the feet and their position, referred to as *stance*. Knowing when to shift weight and maintain balance are important factors to working safely and effectively. We teach *tai chi* as part of our program because it provides a good foundation to learn how to have a stable, balanced BOS and how to use a shift in weight to administer a firm or deep stroke. Work is more effortless when using the principles of tai chi. We refer to this as the **martial stance:** ready, poised, and centered with knees slightly bent while standing. Whether the therapist is

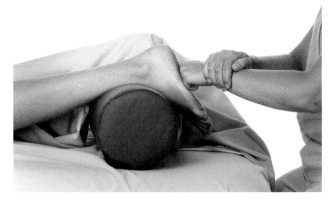

FIGURE 5.12

Use a prop (bolster) to support the anterior ankle while working on the plantar side of the foot.

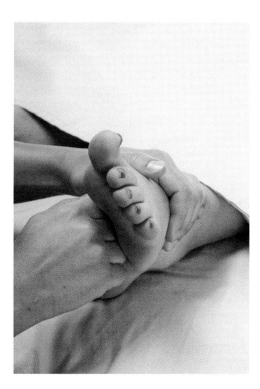

FIGURE 5.14

Use knuckles or the fist to work on the plantar surface of the foot.

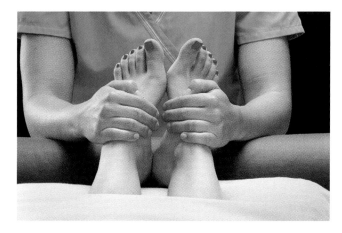

FIGURE 5.15

Align the prop perpendicular to the forearms when doing energy work on the feet.

applying a stroke, traction, or stretches, her or his stance determines the degree of effort.

General Guidelines

The triangle of power mentioned earlier also applies to how the therapist stands. The foot's BOS is the calcaneus and the first and fifth metatarsals. The position of the feet creates the stance and effects how weight is shifted from one foot to the other. Proper position helps to deliver a deeper, more fluid stroke; conserve energy; and be more ergonomically sound. The following is a list of checkpoints pertaining to neutral stance.

- Feet at shoulder or hip width apart, parallel, or staggered
- Staggered back foot at 30–45 degrees
- Knees not locked (hyperextended)
- Knees possibly in martial arts position softly flexed or in the knee-screw home position (15 degrees of extension)
- Hips level
- Neutral spinal curves (the upper torso in flexion during stroke applications)
- Head aligned with the spine
- Arm joints aligned as much as possible
- Shoulders relaxed (not elevated or depressed)
- Feet pointed in the direction of movement
- Focus on breath and flow of energy

Some common problems that occur when standing are protracting and flexing the head, collapsing the spine, hyperextending the knees, and having the feet too close together. These can be corrected by being mindful of them and by reeducation. Awareness of the center of gravity will help to maintain neutral alignment. Core muscles maintain balance, so the therapist should be mindful of engaging these muscles when seated or standing to maintain an upright posture. Refer to the core strengthening exercises in Chapter 6.

Two stances are recommended for position in relation to the client—direct and diagonal. In **direct stance**, (Figure 5.16 ■) the therapist faces the body area being worked on. The feet are usually parallel, and the preceding list of checkpoints for stance applies. This stance places the therapist directly above the working area and makes stacking

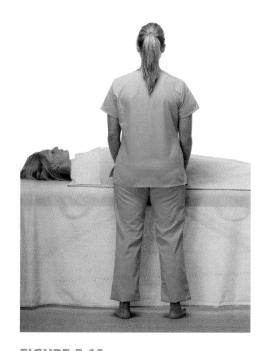

FIGURE 5.16

Feet are usually parallel and shoulder or hip width apart for the direct stance.

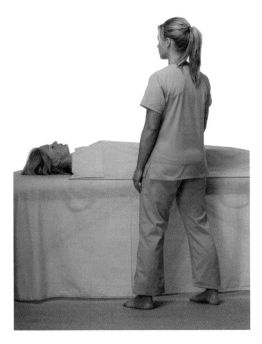

FIGURE 5.17

Feet are shoulder/hip width apart and staggered. The diagonal can be facing either the head or the feet.

the arm joints easier. In the **diagonal stance** (Figure 5.17 ■), the therapist is at an angle to the body area being worked on. The feet are staggered and approximately shoulder wide. The leg closest to the table should be the back foot and the one farthest should be the lead foot. The length of stance should be adjusted for the stroke length. More weight is initially on the back foot and then shifted to the front as the stroke is delivered. The front knee never extends past the toes, and the back foot should remain on the floor during the transfer of weight. This stance facilitates delivery of longer strokes and so is suggested for the back and legs.

If staying within these parameters cannot cover the area, the bodyworker can slide the back foot forward during the stroke and adjust the front foot accordingly to finish the length of the stroke. Placing the back foot in front of the lead foot should be avoided because it creates a twist in the torso.

In both direct and diagonal stances, the feet should generally be pointed in the direction of the movement with exception of the back foot in the staggered martial stance, which is slightly on the diagonal. This ensures better pelvic alignment. A bodyworker positioned beside the table with one foot facing it and the other turned out forming a 90-degree angle creates undo stress in the hip joint and energetic splitting, going in two directions. To best understand what we mean by this notion of energetic splitting, the exercise in Helpful Hint 5.3 should be performed while viewing Figure 5.18 ■. These splits happen often throughout the day without being noticed until the bodyworker becomes tuned into the nuances and energetics of his or her posture and movement. The bodyworker should feel the difference between the alignments of the feet pointing in the direction of the intention of movement versus split and observe the difference viscerally, energetically/internally. An exception to the rule occurs when the therapist uses the olecranon to apply a deep stroke to the back. In this case, his or her feet can face the client (Figure 5.19 ■). The direction of the movement is at a right angle to the feet. The front foot can also be positioned diagonally, which somewhat modifies the split.

Working on the Upper Extremity

When the client is in a supine position, the bodyworker should adjust her or his stance and the level of the squat to maintain the appropriate posture. Experience has shown that working this area has a high risk for flexion of the head, so the bodyworker should be very aware of maintaining neutral alignment of the torso and head. Electric tables

HELPFUL HINT 5.3
Energetic Splitting

Exercise 1

To build a deeper awareness of this concept, begin by sitting in a chair with a back support. Sit with your feet flat on the floor, parallel or staggered, with your lumbar area against the seat back for support and your body upright. Close your eyes and observe the sensations and become aware of the different parts of your body as they make contact with the chair. Slowly begin to flex your forearms and brachium in front of your body approximately 6 inches away. Observe the sensations. What do you feel?

Once you have noted the sensations, begin to slouch. Your lumbar area is no longer making contact with the seat back and your feet are on the chair legs; the slouch causes protraction of the head. Next, flex your forearms again and extend them about 6 inches from your body. Feel the difference? You will notice a

pulling sensation especially at the posterior side of your neck and upper back. It is as though part of your energy is going to the posterior and the rest of the action through the arms is going to the anterior. This splitting of the energy can be depleting. Sitting upright and with your energy moving forward is a more dynamic position.

Exercise 2

Stand beside your treatment table using a direct stance facing the client's body. Observe and make a mental note of your sensations. Next, turn one foot out 45 degrees or more and observe the difference. This affects the gluteal muscles on the side turned out as well as the abductor muscles. When you add applying a stroke to this equation, you will feel as though you are being split directionally.

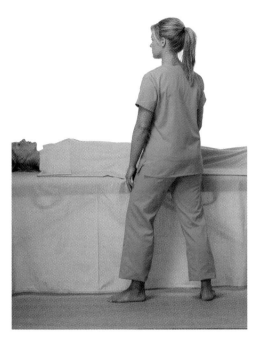

FIGURE 5.18

The feet placed in opposition to one another (90-degree angle) splits the energy and disrupts pelvic alignment.

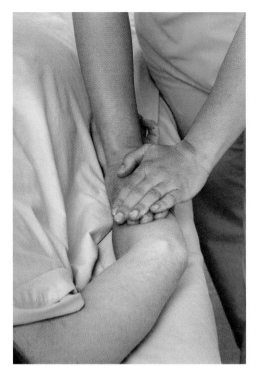

FIGURE 5.20

There is a greater risk for hyperextension of the wrist when not using props.

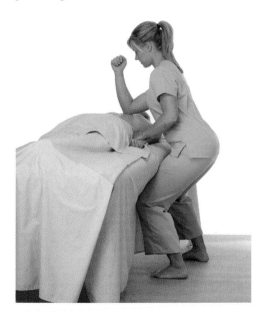

FIGURE 5.19

When using the olecranon on the back along the erector spinae, take a direct stance at the side of the client even though the direction of movement is toward the head.

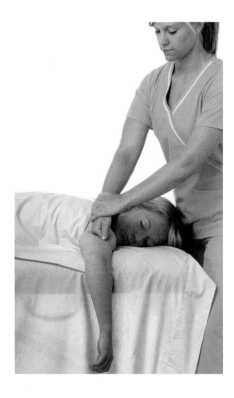

FIGURE 5.21

Work on the triceps while the client is in the prone position for greater ease and depth.

can be adjusted to the appropriate height to reduce the tendency for flexion. We endorse the use of bolsters and pillows to prop the arm in a variety of ways and positions to complete different strokes because leaving the arm on the table typically causes hyperextension of the wrists while the therapist is working as in Figure 5.20 ■.

Working on the triceps when the client is prone and the arm is flexed at the elbow with the forearm hanging off of the table makes the arm easily accessible and allows the therapist to apply more depth to the stroke with increased ease (Figure 5.21 ■).

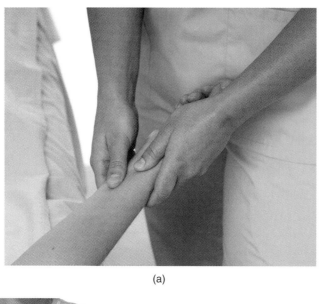

(a)

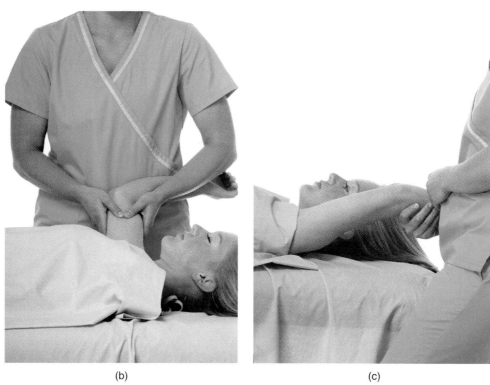

(b)   (c)

FIGURE 5.22

(a) Petrissage on the ventral side of the forearm. (b) Simultaneously working on the biceps/triceps
while propped. (c) Triceps in the propped position for increased ease and depth.

Another way to make working on the client's arm
easier is for the therapist to prop it on his or her body.
Refer to Figure 5.22a ■, b, and c for three variations for
propping the arm. Figure 5.22a illustrates the ventral side
of the forearm propped while the therapist applies a
petrissage or cross fiber stroke, Figure 5.22b shows the
arm propped to allow for working on the biceps/triceps
simultaneously, and 5.22c depicts the triceps propped in a
stretched position during the administration of a deeper
stroke.

The following are checkpoints for working on the
upper extremity:

● Feet hip or shoulder distance apart
● Feet either direct or diagonal (stance)
● Knees screw-home position or slightly flexed

- Neutral spine
- Neutral head
- Shoulders relaxed
- Brachium 0–45 degrees
- Wrists neutral
- Props used
- Focus on the breath and flow of energy

Working on the Lower Extremity

Work on the leg is done predominately while the practitioner is standing, and developing and maintaining good postural habits is essential. These include a solid base of support, proper stance, and good knee alignment. The practitioner should remember this whether she or he is a proponent of the knee-screw home position or the martial stance with the knees softly flexed. He or she should not twist at the knee or squat so far that the patella extends beyond the toes.

When the practitioner is working on the anterior side of the lower extremity, we recommend a direct stance, facing the side of the client for most of the strokes and techniques to better align the body. After the initial effleurage strokes to the leg, which are usually applied from the foot of the table, the practitioner should move to the side of the table to apply direct alignment to the body area. The joints are in better alignment and allow for achieving significant leverage if needed.

Many clients need a bolster under their knees when they are in the supine position to prevent low back discomfort. The practitioner needs to make some adjustments and modifications to his or her posture and technique depending upon the size of the bolster. It often raises the leg especially around the knee area to a height that increases the odds for postural distortions especially to the shoulder and wrist areas. An electric table comes in handy here because it can be easily lowered to keep the leg at the best working height. However, few practitioners have an electric table and having the client get off the table while it is being lowered is not practical, so other options are available: The practitioner can set the table lower to begin with and deepen the stance, being mindful of his or her knees in this position, or keep the table at the recommended height and sit on it or use a solid wide-based stepping block to stand on.

Working on a client's posterior leg when she or he is in the prone position also often requires using a prop under the anterior side of the ankle. Use the same guidelines for the posterior leg as for the anterior leg. Remember that anytime a body area is elevated with props, the practitioner must adjust the table or his or her own body accordingly. Adjusting the table to a lower position to accommodate the intended use of several props and a neuromuscular technique is best.

Incorporating diverse approaches to work on a body area enables the practitioner to work his or her own muscles differently, decreases boredom from repetition, and

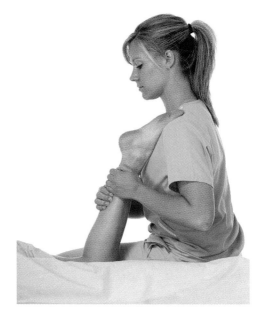

FIGURE 5.23

Several stroke variations while the client is prone and the lower leg is flexed.

minimizes the negative effects of working the same way every day on his or her body. Clients will also appreciate this approach. A practitioner who always works on the posterior leg when it is extended should try flexing the lower leg and applying a variety of strokes with his or her hands, fingers, and ulnar surface (see Figure 5.23 ■).

Checkpoints for working on the lower extremity follow:

- Feet hip or shoulder distance apart
- Feet either direct or diagonal (stance)
- Knees screw-home position or slightly flexed
- Neutral spine
- Neutral head
- Shoulders relaxed
- Brachium 0–45 degrees
- Wrists neutral
- Props used
- Focus on the breath and flow of energy

Working on the Back and Gluteal Areas

According to an osteopathic publication in Great Britain, 66% of people treated seek help for occupation-caused back pain (http://rheumatology.oxfordjournals.org/cgi/content/abstract/20/4/239, accessed 7/15/08). The back is the most requested area of the body for treatment in the authors' clinic. Because of its proximity and involvement with the gluteal muscles, we believe incorporating techniques for the gluteal area in the treatment protocol is very important. This area is significantly overworked in the activities of daily living, which are exacerbated by other activities such as, running, cycling, and so on.

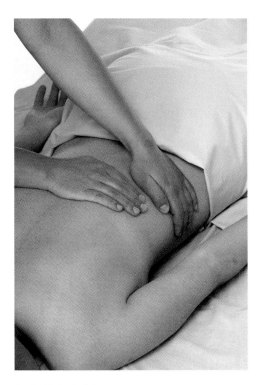

FIGURE 5.24

Neutral alignment is shown while applying a wringing stroke to the back.

Self-critiquing the way they work on the back is important for bodyworkers. They should investigate whether they move from one side of the table to the other side or often reach across the back. We recommend that bodyworkers stay on the same side of the body area being treated rather than reaching across the client with the exception of applying the wringing stroke; this is better for joint alignment and leverage. When the therapist uses a wringing stroke, we recommend standing against the table with a direct stance and squatting with the quadriceps touching the table to shorten the reach distance. The spine and head should be aligned with slight flexion, and reaching to the opposite side to initiate the wringing stroke. The stroke should be stopped before the wrist breaks neutral, which usually occurs just past the midline (spine) (Figure 5.24 ■).

Minimize working above the head of the table to reduce reaching except when applying strokes to the upper back. The bodyworker should not twist the torso but should stay aligned, squat sufficiently to keep his or her body upright as much as possible. Some forward flexion is unavoidable; however, the head should be kept aligned with the spine; protraction or flexion of the head should be avoided. A diagonal stance is useful when giving extra attention to an area such as the quadratus lumborum. This approach allows the bodyworker to be closer to the area without compromising her or his body mechanics. Using the triangle of power for strength, depth, and overall

power is a great asset to work. Apply the set, sink and move approach.

Two positions—prone and side lying—for working on the gluteal area are preferred regardless of the technique/modalities used. In both positions, the therapist should be sure to work while standing adjacent to the area to avoid overreaching or twisting.

The prone position provides an easy transition from the back or the legs. Many of the same checkpoints regarding the back apply to the gluteal area. Depending on the client's gluteal mass, working this area can cause the therapist to elevate the shoulders, but he or she can avoid this by taking a diagonal stance. Selecting the direction of stance depends on the specific work and the direction of the muscle fibers. Adjusting the stance can maintain optimum ergonomic position and improve efficiency. For example, when a therapist works the piriformis, a direct stance best serves working the length of the muscle fiber, and either a front or rear diagonal stance could be used for working cross fiber. See Figure 5.25a ■ and b.

As when working with any area of the body, the therapist should avoid abduction of the brachium as mentioned earlier. We commonly see abduction beyond the recommended 20 degrees because of the change in mass (height) of this area when the student/practitioner does not correct for the transition from the back or posterior leg to the gluteal area. Two ways to correct this when it occurs are to change the stance from a direct to a diagonal and/or to lower the elbow to reduce the angle. This rotates the palmar surface from a palm-down to the palm-lateral position while keeping neutral alignment of the wrist (see Figure 5.26a ■ and b).

The side-lying position has three considerations to take into account. First, when the client goes from a prone or supine position to side lying, the area being worked on is elevated. The two ways to compensate for the transition from prone or supine to side lying are to lower an electric table or to modify the posture and stance, making sure to keep the head and torso in neutral alignment. The second consideration of side lying is that it causes the gluteal muscles to stretch, making them tauter, which requires less pressure for deep work, hence, less contact stress to the body. A third consideration of side lying is that because the surface area of the muscles changes, the orientation for working on them shifts. A key checkpoint is elevation of the shoulders (Figure 5.27a ■ and b), which can be avoided by using a diagonal stance and approach facing the head or the feet with the fists, ulnar surface, or olecranon:

- Form a triangle with the fists (Figure 5.28a ■). The supporting hand is the hand closest to the client.
- Use the ulnar surface that is the one closest to the client. Support the active arm by forming a triangle (Figure 5.28b).
- Form a triangle for the olecranon with a supporting hand (Figure 5.28c). The active olecranon is again the one closest to the client.

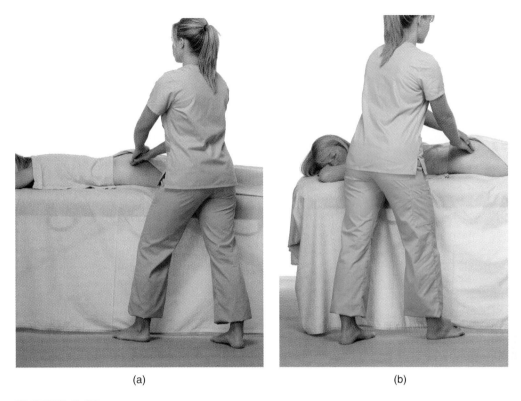

(a)   (b)

FIGURE 5.25

(a) A diagonal stance facing toward the front of the client facilitates working the length of fibers.
(b) A diagonal stance facing toward the foot of the client facilitates working cross fiber.

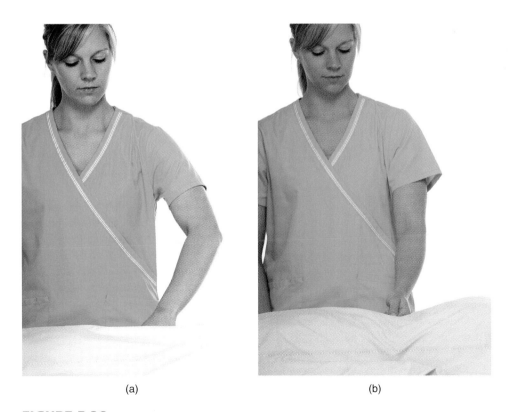

(a)   (b)

FIGURE 5.26

(a) Abduction of the brachium and elbow. (b) Adjust abduction of the elbow by lowering it. This rotates the palm from facing down to lateral while maintaining neutral alignment of the wrist.

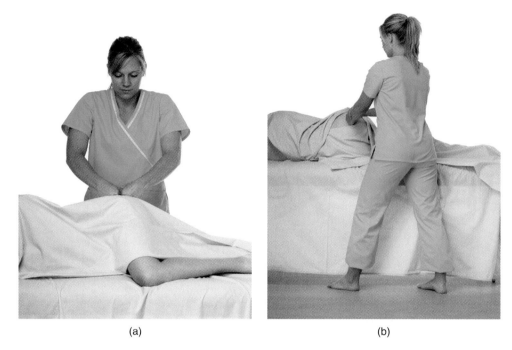

(a) (b)

FIGURE 5.27

By adjusting stance and technique you can maintain neutral alignment while working the gluteus in a side-lying position. (a) Direct stance increases risk for elevated shoulders. (b) Diagonal stance allows the shoulder to drop to a neutral position.

Checkpoints for working on the back and gluteal area are the same as for the lower extremities.

- Feet hip or shoulder distance apart
- Feet either direct or diagonal (stance)
- Knees screw-home position or slightly flexed
- Neutral spine with no twisting
- Neutral head
- Shoulders relaxed
- Brachium 0–45 degrees
- Wrists neutral
- Props used
- Focus on the breath and flow of energy

Working on the Chest and Abdomen

The chest and abdomen are often overlooked during a treatment unless the client requests it or a site-specific injury necessitates treatment. A student/practitioner who is uncomfortable working on these vital areas most likely do not practice the techniques learned after their training. However, good skills and the proper body mechanics make the techniques more comfortable for the practitioner to apply. Use of the fingers, thumbs, and palmar surfaces are best suited for these areas because of the sensitivity of these vital organs.

We recommend working on the chest from the head of the table. The area from the clavicle to the middle of the sternum can easily be accessed from this position without compromising body mechanics. Points to be mindful of with this position are to:

- Assume a direct stance (feet shoulder width)
- Use the knee-screw home position or softly flex the knee as in a martial stance
- Maintain head and spine alignment

One alternative method is to use a diagonal stance on the left side of the client's body while treating the right side of her or his upper chest and vice versa. Another is to use a direct stance facing the client on the side that will be worked on.

We recommend that when therapists work on the abdominal area, they use the same approach as the one employed on the back. Use a direct stance for side-to-side work and for a wringing stroke. A common pitfall to the wringing stroke is hyperextension of the wrists. The diagonal approach is effective for getting closer to an area and getting deeper as when working on the psoas.

MAKING SPECIAL ACCOMMODATIONS

As bodyworkers, we are sometimes asked to work in situations or conditions that are far from ideal for our body mechanics. One of the authors was the massage therapist for a ballet company and frequently toured with it and was periodically called to work on a dancer backstage in what is

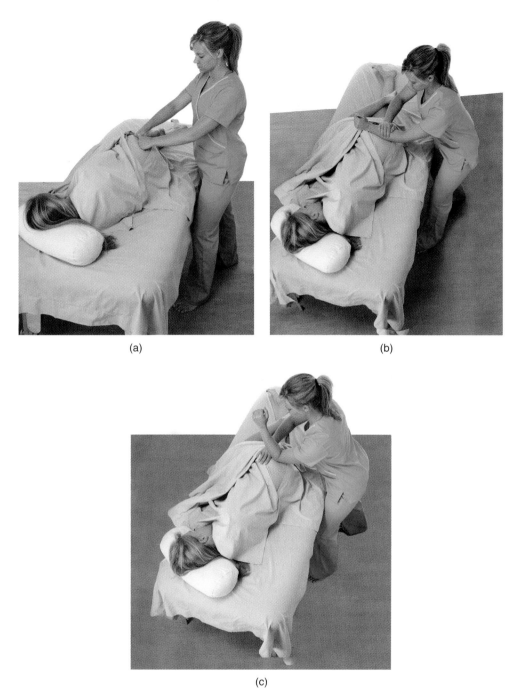

(a)   (b)

(c)

FIGURE 5.28

(a) Using the fist. (b) Using the ulnar surface. (c) Using the olecranon.

referred to as the *wings,* an offstage area to the left or right of the performance space that the audience does not see. The wings are used as a warm-up area for the dancers, a set storage area, and a work area for stagehands. Wings also hide technical equipment, such as lights and pyrotechnics that project from the side of the stage. Due to these factors, the author often has had very limited space—approximately a foot—around the table, which required being creative to prevent undue body strain.

The following sections offer some helpful tips for working in tight spaces, giving a chair massage, accommodating wheelchairs, working on someone who is hospitalized, and using draping techniques.

Tight Spaces

Therapists who must work in a small space without much room to move around the table (less than 3 feet in circumference) can work some areas of the body while seated on

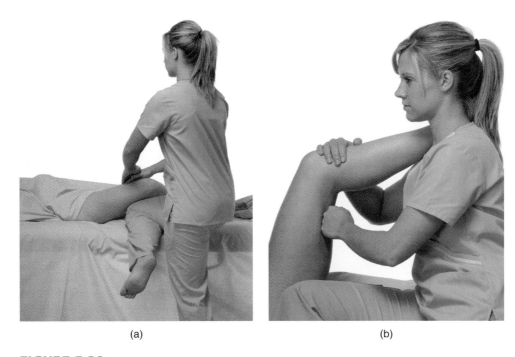

(a)   (b)

FIGURE 5.29

(a) Client leg propped on bodyworker leg for better access to adductors. (b) Client leg propped on bodyworker shoulder for posterior leg work.

the massage table. Key points to remember when working in tight spaces are:

- Work seated if it assists proper body mechanics
- Be mindful of breath and internal awareness
- Prop the extremities
- Use props in general to help maintain good body mechanics
- Maintain neutral alignment of the wrists
- Do not compromise the body for the client

Figure 5.29 ■ shows the practitioner seated on the table (after asking the client's permission) with the lower leg propped on the practitioner's upper trapezium while the practitioner applies an effleurage or fascia release stroke to the hamstrings.

Chair Massage

Chair massage can be physically demanding. Our program provides students many opportunities to practice chair massage, especially during their clinical component. Several of them say that this form of practice is too hard on their bodies. One of the complaints refers to working over clothing, which abrades the skin after giving several chair massages. We recommend purchasing or making satin or silk hand savers (Figure 5.30 ■).

Other helpful tips for chair massage include:

- Use of ulnar surface to save the hands from fatigue
- Use of the olecranon process for deep work
- Use of a stool (we recommend carrying a small one, preferably with wheels) (Figure 5.31 ■)

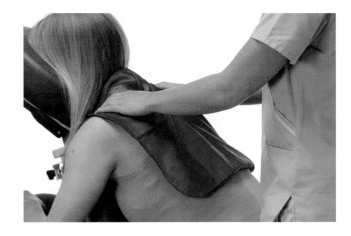

FIGURE 5.30

Satin or silk hand savers reduce abrasion when working over clothing.

While working on the back during a chair massage, the practitioner should transition from a standing position (for the upper back) to a seated position (for the low back).

Wheelchair

A client in a wheelchair presents several ergonomic challenges. We recommend working on the client while she or he is seated in the wheelchair. This prevents risks to both client and practitioner while the latter attempts to assist the client out of the wheelchair and onto the table. Safe lifting training videos are available for the certified nursing assistant (CNA) and nursing professions; however,

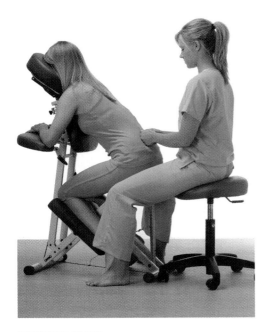

FIGURE 5.31

Sitting for lower back work helps maintain neutral alignment.

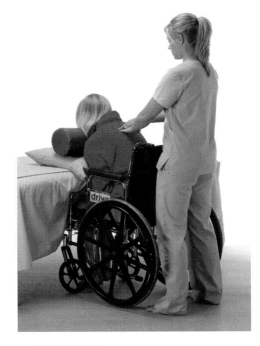

FIGURE 5.32

A wheelchair-bound client can be made comfortable for back and shoulder work by having them lean forward onto a table and supporting them with props.

most of them demonstrate the use of lifting aids such as a board, a Hoyer Lift™, or other device. If the place of practice requires moving clients, lifting videos can be found at www.medfilms.com and www.osha.org.

To work on a client in a wheelchair, position the chair alongside the massage table with the client facing the table. Use props such as pillows to support the client while he or she rests his or her head and upper chest on the massage table (Figure 5.32 ■). Massage techniques can be administered to the scalp, shoulders, back, and arms in this position. However, this position requires more bending over than usual, so be careful:

- Not to hyperextend the knees
- Keep the head and neck aligned with the back
- Bend at the hips
- Use diagonals

Hospital Bed

Modalities best suited to practicing safe ergonomics for the client in the hospital are reflexology and energy work. We recommend limiting massage because of the ergonomic challenges of working on a nonambulatory client. Lower the bed rails and position yourself beside the client. Apply Swedish modalities using a wide stance and flexed knees to support the body as you bend forward. The client's hands and feet can be worked on while the practitioner is seated. Use the same guidelines as for the client in a wheelchair. If they are acceptable to the client and the hospital, use some of the propped techniques while sitting on the bed as recommended for working in tight spaces.

Draping Technique

Specific draping techniques can compromise good ergonomic habits. We often see good body mechanics go out the window when a student is draping the client. Multiply the number of clients assisted per day by the number of times each client must be draped to calculate body stress and tension. Key points to using good body mechanics while draping are to:

- Minimize reaching while draping
- Maintain neutral alignment
- Avoid awkward postures

Ergonomic Demands

In summary, learning to be correct ergonomically demands that practitioners be mindful of body position and movement. Doing so requires a conscious approach. At first they should separately focus on each area of their own body (arm, hands, feet, knees, hips, torso and head) for alignment. They can do this with the help of a peer or by watching a video of their work and following Worksheet 5.1 to document what they are doing correctly and where corrections need to be made. Adjustments should be made while the practitioners notice the change in the sense of balance and feel. Repeat this while moving from one area of the client to the next to begin to see a pattern of not maintaining neutrality, such as perpetually having elevated shoulders. As the bodyworkers move to each area, they should check their BOS and neutral alignment. Developing proper ergonomic habits takes time and commitment but will pay off in the long run.

CHAPTER SUMMARY

- Spinal and head neutral alignment is required whether seated or standing. Flexion of the head to look at the work area is a common ergonomic error.
- Ergonomic checkpoints for the arm and hands include keeping the arms close to the body with no more than a 45-degree abduction of the brachium and stacking the joints from shoulder to point of contact to keep neutral alignment.
- Fingers and thumbs are at high risk for injury in body-work. Keeping them adducted when using them minimizes the risk. Use the fist, palm, ulnar surface, and olecranon as alternative techniques to reduce the use of the digits. Each technique requires always maintaining neutral alignment of joints. This can require altering the stance.
- Use of both hands, one as the active hand and the other as the supporting hand, creates a triangle of power and improves stability and support when applying a technique.
- The seated position for work provides an alternative to standing to reduce impact on the legs and feet and can readily be applied to work on the client's head, neck, and feet. Being seated requires maintaining proper neutral alignment of the spine and head while one is balanced on the ischial tuberosities. Keep the feet flat on the floor at hip width and knees flexed at 90 degrees. Adjust stool height so that the shoulders are not elevated and the arms are in alignment with the work.
- Adjust between direct or diagonal alignment with the client to maintain neutral alignment of the arms, wrist, and hands and to reduce the risk of shoulder elevation or protraction. This applies to both seated and standing work.
- Use props to fill negative space between the arm and table when doing static work.
- Proper stance while standing maintains neutral alignment of the legs, spine, and head and allows for shifting weight in a balanced fashion while applying a stroke. The feet should be hip width apart and can be either parallel or staggered and pointed in the direction of movement. The knees should not be locked.
- Work on the arm and hands can be done on the table or in several propped positions. Maintaining neutral alignment applies as always, and the high risk for flexing the neck when working this area should be noted.
- A direct stance is favored for working on the anterior surface of the leg to be directly positioned above the area. Propping the knee elevates the work height and requires either lowering the table or adjusting the position to prevent shoulder elevation.
- Work the posterior leg with the patient in a prone position and adjust table height or position to maintain neutral position. Working the lower leg in a flexed position provides an alternate technique.
- Most work on the back is from the side of the client. Adjust between a direct and diagonal stance based on the technique used and area being accessed.
- The gluteal area can be worked in either a prone or side-lying position. When a risk is possible, avoid elevating the shoulder by using a diagonal stance. Use of the fist, olecranon, or ulnar surface is an option to be able to increase pressure to this area that commonly has more mass.
- Fingers, thumbs, and palmar surface are appropriate to use for treatment of the chest and abdomen. Special attention needs to be paid to keep the fingers and thumbs adducted and to prevent deviation of the wrist. Direct stance with knee-screw home position or slight flex and proper head and spine alignment also apply.
- Even if they are brief, routine actions such as draping require conscious performance with proper ergonomics in mind.

REVIEW QUESTIONS

1. Identify a benefit of critiquing one's ergonomics via video.
2. How do neutral checkpoints help practitioners work more efficiently?
3. True or False? The head and spine should remain neutral whether seated or standing.
4. True or False? The eyes play a major role in determining our posture.
5. True or False? The thumb is not designed for compressive force.
6. Stacking the _____ minimizes the effects of compression.
7. It is important not to _____ the thumb when using the fist.
8. The _____ is aligned with the side of the body when using the olecranon.

9. Using triangles when working will:
   a. facilitate application of the stroke
   b. increase stability and power
   c. require more effort to deliver the stroke
   d. decrease the pressure of the stroke
10. The ishial tuberosities provides:
    a. a base of support when seated
    b. the ability to deepen a stroke
    c. a way to rock to and fro
    d. all of the above
11. The stance is determined by each of the following except:
    a. the direction of movement
    b. the client's position
    c. the area being worked
    d. the lead foot

6 The Workplace Environment

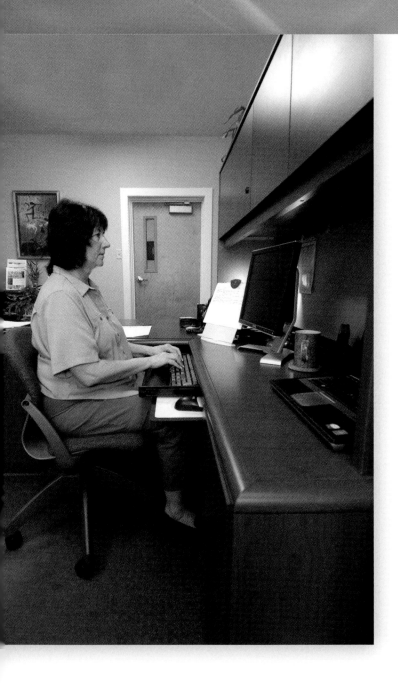

 CHAPTER OUTLINE

LEARNING OBJECTIVES

Upon successful completion of the chapter, you will be able to:

1. Discuss the purpose and significance of the governmental regulations that address ergonomics and the workplace.

2. Categorize and list factors that contribute to indoor air quality that are attributed to sick building syndrome and building-related illnesses.

3. Explain the benefits and challenges of heating, ventilation, and air conditioning systems.

4. Describe the effects of the quantity of light, contrast, and glare on vision, and explain how to create proper lighting in both the office and treatment room.

5. Design an office space, including the setup of the computer and selection of furniture, for optimal ergonomic considerations. Follow best work practices to avoid the risk of computer vision syndrome and musculoskeletal disorders.

6. Design and set up a treatment room with a comfortable and aesthetically pleasing feel that is also efficient and ergonomically sound.

7. Assess office and treatment room work spaces.

KEY TERMS

Building-related illnesses (BRI) 101

Computer vision syndrome (CVS) 104

National Institute for Occupational Safety and Health (NIOSH) 107

Sick building syndrome (SDS) 100

Video display terminal (VDT) 104

Volatile organic compounds (VOC) 101

An important part of ergonomics is the examination of the working environment to meet the worker's needs. This aspect encompasses a broad area, which includes the practitioner's physical abilities and limitations, anthropometrics, equipment design, and other indoor environmental factors such as temperature, ventilation, and lighting. Attention to these details can help to prevent injuries, assist with functional limitations, and help maintain the bodyworker's health and well-being. The importance of being proactive to reduce workplace injuries and illnesses is reflected by established federal and state regulations. Implementing an ergonomic safety program whether for oneself or a business and its employees is not only wise but also prudent. Maintaining neutral postures is fundamental in avoiding musculoskeletal injury. Proper design of the workplace and proper technique can achieve this. In addition, proper ventilation and building maintenance play a critical role in preventing **sick building syndrome (SBS),** a condition where workers complain of symptoms during working hours that disappear outside the workplace. This chapter addresses the physical features of the bodyworker's office and treatment space that complement and/or support safe ergonomic techniques.

U.S. OCCUPATIONAL SAFETY AND HEALTH ADMINISTRATION (OSHA)

A discussion of ergonomics is not complete without an introduction to the Occupational Safety and Health Administration (OSHA) and its role in the workplace whether it is an office, classroom, or clinic. Demographics show that a significant number of massage school graduates choose to be employed by spas, clinics, salons, and fitness centers rather than self-employment. Therefore, it is beneficial to have a basic understanding of OSHA's role (American Massage Therapy Association, 2004).

The U.S. government established the Occupation Safety and Health Administration in the early 1970s for the purpose of providing safe and healthy working conditions for the American people. Prior to this, approximately 15,000 work-related deaths and more than 2 million work-related injuries were reported annually. Before OSHA, states were solely responsible for creating safety guidelines and laws. Currently, states have the option to establish their own plan as long as it is equal to or more stringent than the federal plan. Since 2004, OSHA guidelines and recommendations have applied to 6.5 million employers and 100 million workers. In its first three decades, workplace deaths have been cut in half, and the number of injuries and illnesses have dropped by 40%. OSHA states that "nearly every working man and woman in the nation comes under OSHA's jurisdiction" (OSHA's Role, http://osha.gov/oshinfo/mission.html).

It is commonly thought that OSHA's main function is to prevent major trauma and death in the workplace. However, according to OSHA, work-related musculoskeletal disorders (MSDs) are the cause of more than one-quarter of all occupational injuries reported to the Bureau of Labor Statistics (BLS) every year. MSDs represent the largest job-related injury problem in the United States today (Bureau of Labor Statistics, 2007). The U.S. Department of Labor defines MSD as an injury or disorder of the muscles, nerves, tendons, joints, cartilage, and spinal discs but stipulates that it excludes disorders caused by slips, trips, falls, motor vehicle and/or similar accidents.

OSHA expects employers to follow the general duty clause of the OSH Act of 1970, which states that "a place of employment must be free from recognized hazards that are causing or likely to cause death or serious physical harm to employees." Sprains and strains were the leading nature of injury in every major industry with the service industry reporting the highest rate at 29% (Loy & Greer, 2007).

The high rate of musculoskeletal disorders and their impact on the economy through loss of production, loss of wages, medical expenses, and disability claims, set the stage for the development of the Final Ergonomics Program Standard in 2000. The purpose of this program, which applies to all employers, is to reduce risk for injury and medical costs. OSHA had estimated that the program would save employers $9 billion over ten years (Occupational Safety and Health Administration, 1999).

The Department of Labor followed in 2002 with a four-pronged strategy to address the continuing musculoskeletal disorder issue. The plan addressed both industry-specific and task-specific strategies. It encompasses guidelines, enforcement, outreach, and assistance, and it established a national advisory committee on ergonomics whose focus includes research. OSHA's emphasis on identifying specific needs of individual work groups in addition to supporting enforcement, training, and research is ongoing. OSHA's efforts reflect sincere interest in communicating the value of ergonomics. The four-pronged strategy is important because the number of workers' compensation claims filed per year is in the billions of dollars, and the highest number of claims falls under the category of musculoskeletal disorders, many of which can be prevented (Anshel, 2008).

The American with Disabilities Act (ADA) requires employers to accommodate employees with disabilities. Business and institutions such as schools need to comply with this act. Any adjustment or change to a job, work, or school environment that allows the individual, employee, or student, to perform the necessary tasks is considered an *accommodation*. If an employee or a student has an identified need, the employer has an obligation to make accommodations to meet that need. More information about this is available at http://www.jan.wvu.edu/links/adalinks.htm.

INDOOR ENVIRONMENT

Most bodyworkers practice indoors. This environment can affect them and their clients. Factors to be aware of include indoor air quality (pollutants, particulates, humidity, and temperature), noise and vibrations, and lighting.

Indoor Air Quality

The potential impact of the indoor workplace environment on health is highlighted by the recognition of two conditions: sick building syndrome (SBS) and building-related illnesses (BRI). The World Health Organization coined the term SBS for the situation in which 25–30% of the workers complain of symptoms during working hours that diminish over the weekend and during holidays. Symptoms include:

- Eye irritation
- Skin irritation
- Headache
- Throat irritation
- Recurrent fatigue
- Chest burning
- Cough
- Wheezing
- Nasal congestion
- Problems with concentration or short-term memory

Causes of SBS are nonspecific but have been attributed to tobacco smoke, microbes including fungi associated with water damage or collection areas, **volatile organic compounds (VOC)**, particulates, and psychosocial factors. It has been suggested that the psychosocial component occurs because of a "mismatch between environmental demands and individual abilities" (Lahtinen, Huuhtanen, & Reijula, 1998). SBS may be associated with a single room, region of a building, or the entire building.

Building-related illnesses (BRI) have some of the same symptoms as SBS such as cough and chest tightness. Its symptoms can also include fever, chills, and muscle aches. In contrast, however, BRI is a diagnosable illness that can be specifically linked to an indoor contaminate. Often specific antibody production correlates with airborne contaminates in the building. Recovery after leaving the building is more prolonged.

Contributing factors to SBS and BRI include:

- Inadequate ventilation
- Chemical contaminants from indoor sources
- Chemical contaminants from outdoor sources
- Biological contaminants
- Particulates

Addressing both potential sources of contaminants and the way to dilute or eliminate them need to be considered for all buildings. See Table 6.1 ■ for a short list of chemical pollutants, their potential sources, and effects.

Indoor chemical pollutants are abundant. Formaldehyde was identified as a contaminate in particle board more than 30 years ago. Since then, studies conducted by the Environmental Protection Agency (EPA) have identified significant levels of more than 107 known carcinogen in modern offices (Arnold, 2001). These and other VOCs are especially prevalent in new and refurbished buildings. High levels of some VOCs can cause chronic or acute disorders, and even moderate to low levels of a mix of compounds can trigger acute reactions. Sources of these contaminants come from items such as:

- Upholstered and manufactured wood furniture
- Carpets and adhesives used to lay carpets and tiles
- Copy machines
- Pesticides
- Cleaning agents

Tobacco smoke is a source not only for VOCs but also particulate matter. The increase in smokeless buildings has taken great steps toward reducing this hazard. Perfumes, scented oils, and any room scents—for example, candles or potpourri—add to VOC levels and can cause problems especially for those with allergies or with a sensitivity to scents.

Air vents and open door/windows can draw outdoor pollutants into the building. Exhausts (from traffic, nearby

TABLE 6.1	Chemical Pollutants Associated with SBS and BRI	
Chemical	**Potential Sources**	**Health Hazard**
Formaldehyde	Pressed wood products including furniture and cabinets; paints and coating products; upholstery and drapes; tobacco smoke	Eye, nose, and throat irritation; wheezing and coughing; nausea; fatigue; skin rash
Carbon dioxide	Metabolism of occupants and pets within the building	Reduction of the ability to concentrate
Carbon monoxide	Back drafts from furnace and heaters; automotive exhaust from adjacent garages, roadways, and parking lots; tobacco smoke	*Low concentration:* fatigue *Moderate concentrations:* impaired vision and coordination, headaches, confusion, nausea, and flulike symptoms that disappear after leaving the building; *High concentration:* Death
Ozone	Certain air cleaners	Throat irritation and cough; lung inflammation and reduced function; aggravation of asthma
Radon	Decay of uranium that percolates from underlying soils through cracks and holes into the building where it accumulates; less often from building materials or well water	Lung cancer in nonsmokers

garages, and heating units of adjacent buildings), pollens, pesticides, herbicides, and industrial chemicals can all be introduced depending on the building's location. Proper placement of ducts and vents and proper filtering units reduce or remove the contaminants. Business should avoid opening windows if there is a risk for drawing in contaminants.

Biological contaminants can include pollen, mold and mildew, bacteria, viruses, dust mites, and bird and rodent droppings. Water damage, whether in the walls, carpeting or ceilings, is noted for its high risk for mold and mildew problems. However, another source can be stagnant water in humidifiers or ducts and drain pans of ventilation systems. Microbes are able to proliferate and be disseminated through the ventilation systems. Awareness of this contaminant source peaked when an outbreak of pneumonia, which came to be known as *Legionnaires' disease*, occurred following an American Legion convention. The bacterium, later named *legionella*, was isolated in the convention center's air conditioning system. Infectious agents can also be spread among building occupants by means of droplets and contaminated dust particles in the air.

Particulate sources include dust, dust mites, tobacco smoke, and pollens. The size and composition of the particles determine the health impact. Small particulates can stay airborne longer and when breathed in can reach deeper regions of the lungs. The risk of lung cancer from asbestos particles is well known, and regulations are strict for renovations of buildings that have asbestos. Fortunately, unless disturbed during remodeling and construction, for example, asbestos is not a threat.

Dust particles can also carry infectious microbes. A room's cleanliness and the air currents influence the amount of dust in the air. Frequent cleaning surfaces, ideally when the room is unoccupied, can effectively reduce particulates. Use of vacuum cleaners with a micropore filter system or central vacuums that exhaust outdoors will more efficiently remove the small particles. For the sake of the housekeeper's health, adequate ventilation should be provided during cleaning. Air cleaners and filter systems in ventilation systems can also assist in reducing particulates although small particles are more difficult to remove. Electric air cleaners have been found to be more effective for small particles; however, they have the potential to produce ozone.

Although each person has her or his own personal preference in regard to thermal comfort, studies have shown that high room air temperature (above 25 degrees C) is correlated with an increase in SBS and affects work performance and productivity (European Collaborative Action, 2003). Setting thermostats lower in the winter months in temperate climates and using proper ventilation throughout the year can help achieve optimal temperature.

Ventilation should deliver sufficient outside air to dilute and remove body odors and chemical contaminants and effectively distribute the air to the occupants. Ventilation also assists in temperature control by distributing heat or cool air. Three types of ventilation are recognized: natural (windows/doors), mechanical (duct work with fans often associated with heating systems), and heating, ventilation, and air conditioning (HVAC) systems. Interestingly, natural ventilation shows the lowest incidence of SBS symptoms, even though the mechanical and HVAC systems can filter the air. In addition, HVAC systems can regulate air temperature and humidity. A study examining HVAC systems determined that poor maintenance of the systems, intermittent use, lack of moisture control, and the likelihood that systems can directly emit pollutants contributed to SBS (Seppaanen & Frisk, 2004). Although occupants of a building likely do not have immediate control over its maintenance, being able to recognize characteristics of SBS to alert the building supervisor of possible concerns is important.

Vibration and Sound

Vibration is wave energy with a specific amplitude and frequency. When the frequency is within the range that human ears can detect, we refer to it as *sound*. Vibration is produced by equipment and can be an ergonomic factor for handheld equipment.

Bodyworkers often use handheld equipment such as vibrators. Excessive use of these tools presents an additional ergonomic challenge. Prolonged use of a vibrator can cause spasms in the small blood vessels, which reduce blood flow to the hands/fingers. Sensory receptor feedback can be interrupted, which leads to an increase in handgrip on the device. A stronger grip magnifies the impact of the vibration on the vasculature. This situation is one cause of Reynaud's phenomenon or white finger syndrome. The hands will have increased sensitivity to cold and severe conditions can cause the skin of the fingers to peel.

The frequency/pitch of sound is measured in hertz (Hz), and the amplitude/loudness of sound is measured in decibels (dB). The dosemeter, or sound level meter, measures the decibels of sound. Loud sound can damage hearing. Loss is usually gradual but permanent, so we have to take every caution to prevent it. According to OSHA, safe levels of sound should be no greater than 80 dB, and levels of more than 100 dB can cause headaches and increase blood pressure. OSHA regulates the maximum hours of exposure to decibels higher than 80 even with the use of personal protective equipment (PPE) (i.e., ear protection).

Unlike those who work in construction or industry, bodyworkers are much less likely to need to protect themselves from sound. However, location of an office near an airport, high traffic location, or industrial area can result in high levels of background noise. Normally, bodyworkers would avoid these locations because these environments would not be relaxing for the client.

Exposure to loud sounds during personal activities such as listening to music and attending concerts or games are a more likely cause of hearing loss. The sounds can result in temporary and permanent hearing loss, create stress, and cause missed or misunderstood communication.

LIGHTING AND VISUAL CONSIDERATIONS

Vision affects virtually everything we do, and proper lighting is necessary for each situation. "Over 80% of our learning is mediated through the eyes, indicating the important role vision plays in our daily activities" (U.S. Census Bureau, 2008). Lighting requirements vary according to the individual and the activity. Improper lighting can lead to eye strain and fatigue. Computers at work and at home bring new challenges for eye strain.

The eye is profound, intricate, and complex. Structures including the conjunctiva, lids, lacrimal system, and vasculature are responsible for protecting, lubricating, and nourishing the eye.

A sufficient amount of light entering the eye is required for sight. The cornea is the front window of the eye that initially bends or refracts light rays that then pass through the pupil, which acts like a shutter. It controls the amount of light entering the back portion of the eye. The iris is the colored area surrounding the pupil. Light rays next pass through the lens, which can change its shape to bend and focus the rays on the retina. These "windows" into the eye can change because of aging, cataracts, and other damage, causing the need for more light. The light-sensitive retina, which is a thin layer of tissue that contains millions of nerve cells referred to as *rods and cones,* reacts to the light and sends a record of it to the brain via the optic nerve (Figure 6.1 ■). Rods are responsible for peripheral vision and motion detection and respond to dim light, providing night vision. Cones require bright light and detect color. Their high concentration at the fovea centralis, the central focus point on the retina, allow for detailed vision.

Environmental factors can trigger dry or irritated eyes that impact vision, an example of SBS symptoms. Three basic factors that optimize vision and reduce eye strain are:

1. Quantity of light
2. Contrast (the difference in brightness between two areas)
3. Glare

Light that is too dim first causes loss of the ability to detect color and detail. It also causes eye strain. On the other hand, light that is too bright floods the retina, causing eye strain and squinting. The amount of light is measured in lumens by a light meter. A lumen is a 1-foot candle that illuminates a space of 1 square foot (*Handbook of Building Contractors,* 1929). Detail work requires direct, brighter light. Adding a desk or work lamp to the overhead indirect light can supply the necessary light. Lighting standards dictate that office lighting should measure between 100–200 feet per candle (fc), depending on intensity, angle, luminance, and proximity of the source to the line of sight. When they are not doing detailed work, most people find indirect lighting in general to be more pleasant. The two sources of indoor light are incandescent and luminescent (including fluorescent). Incandescent light burns "hot," does not last as long as luminescent light, and uses more energy. Use of luminescent or fluorescent lighting diminishes our carbon footprint.

The difference in brightness between two areas determines contrast. Increased brightness of the immediate work area is desirable for detailed work. Also, the use of contrasting color on printed material or computer screens is easier on the eye and improves vision.

Glare is an annoying distraction and causes eyestrain and headaches. Extraneous light coming from a window, an

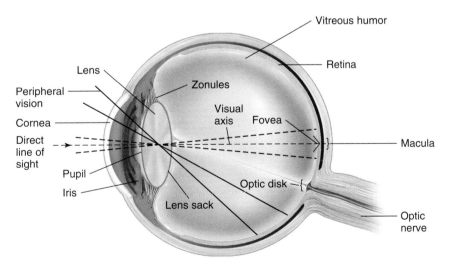

FIGURE 6.1

The dashed line represents the pathway of light for images we are directly focused on. The light passes through the cornea, pupil, and lens before it hits the fovea, where there is a high concentration of cone cells. Peripheral vision involves light coming in at an angle to the cornea and ultimately stimulating rod cells located in the peripheral regions of the retina.

overhead light, reflective surfaces, and direct light can produce glare. All light sources in an office should be evaluated and any that cause glare should be blocked or turned off.

The human eye has not evolved in more than 40,000 years, but the way humans use their eyes has changed significantly. Although at one time humans used predominately distant vision, the development of printed material and the advent of **video display terminals (VDTs),** have significantly increased the amount of close vision needed. According to the Census Bureau, more than half of all households in the United States own computers. Of all children between 3 and 17 years of age, 65% have a computer (Anshel, 2008). The gaming and the monitor-viewing population is getting younger and the full effect of gaming and looking at a VDT is yet to be determined. As a rule, the eyes must work harder when viewing a VDT. The contrast between the letters and the background, glare, reflections, and distance and angles from the VDT impacts vision. The eyes must continually adjust and refocus causing stress and strain. Maintaining one position during extended times while sitting in front of a VDT affects posture and can contribute to MSDs.

Computer vision syndrome (CVS) is the set of eye and vision problems that occur with prolonged VDT use. The symptoms associated with CVS can range from headaches because of eyestrain, dry eyes, blurred vision, and neck and shoulder pain.

According to an article in *Review of Ophthalmology* (Lee, 2003), 75% of computer users experience eyestrain, and 143 million Americans use computers daily. A study by the University of Alabama-Birmingham indicates that having correct lens prescription improves the users' productivity (American Optometric Association, 2008).

Tips and guidelines avoiding physical problems while working at a computer are:

- Rest your eyes for at least 20 seconds every 20 minutes by closing them or gazing at something in the distance.
- Blink often to lubricate the eye.
- Focus on the breath to relax.
- Clean your screen and filter if you use one.
- Eliminate or reduce overhead lighting to reduce glare.
- Use low glare lenses and louvers on overhead lighting.
- Eliminate or cover reflective surfaces such as windows.
- Use a high-quality monitor, at least 70 Hz and a resolution of 800 by 600.
- Increase the computer font size.
- Keep work within easy viewing distance.
- Keep the screen perpendicular to your line of sight.
- Use glasses if necessary; those with a slight tint to help to cut glare.

CVS occurs in part from poor lighting, screen glare, improper positioning, and use of materials that are difficult to read because of font size, lighting conditions, and/or physical position. Most users report a decline in symptoms after ending the computer session. If reduced or discontinued usage is not an option and/or you have any of the aforementioned symptoms, consulting an ophthalmologist for screening and testing for CVS and/or prescribing corrective lenses to use when you work on the computer is important. Additional recommendations on computer use are provided later.

A last point regarding vision is the relationship between it and the movement of the rest of the body. Vision is required for most tasks. The body follows the line of vision. As we move our head to focus the eyes on our target, a ripple effect moves through the body. When a person riding a horse moves their head, the shoulders, trunk, hips, and legs shift and the horse can feel that movement. In the office setting, simply taking a book from a shelf is a chain reaction of head, neck, torso, shoulder, hands, and so on. This relationship is important to consider when designing and setting up a workplace. Notice as you work when you need to search visually for an item to the reach for it. Having items frequently used properly positioned can reduce repetitive motion. Also, notice whether you have a proper line of sight when you are in the favored neutral position. If not, adjust the works space so that the two "match up." Otherwise, you will find that you move out of neutrality while you work, which will result in muscle fatigue.

DESIGN ELEMENTS OF THE OFFICE

The amount of time that bodyworkers spend in the office varies. However, they need to spend some time recording information and maintaining their practices. Therefore, the office and desk should be organized to efficiently complete tasks. The environment—lighting, temperature, colors, and other environmental factors such as odors—should provide a pleasant working environment.

Office Organization

A good office floor plan is the result of considering several factors when it is created. One is making an assessment of the layout, design, and equipment for ease of use, efficiency, and safety. The workspace should be organized in a manner that supports the tasks to be performed there. Constantly having to twist to reach for the phone or other item, cradling the phone between the ear and the shoulder while working create tension, pain, and musculoskeletal problems. Another task analysis is to sequence tasks that are currently being performed to be more effective and efficient. Look for ways to best support neutral alignment, minimize movement, and optimize the movements required to fulfill the tasks.

The overall effect of environment and the placement of office furniture and accessories are important in designing office space. One principle of feng shui is that a room free of clutter frees the mind. Harmonious placement of furniture and items is important to the flow of chi (energy) in the

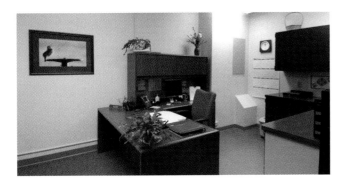

FIGURE 6.2

Office space should be organized, clutter-free, clean, with sufficient lighting, a comfortable temperature, and a quiet workplace.

office environment. See Figure 6.2 ■ for an office with an efficient and pleasing design.

This being said, make sure the office is comfortable for its employees. It should express the owner's individuality. The colors in the room should be pleasing, and the accessories, whether pictures or a fountain, should enhance the work environment. The features of the room including desk and chair should support the work done there. An L-shaped desk, for example, would overpower a small room. Windows are wonderful for letting in natural light, but they need to be considered when planning where to place the desk and computer to prevent reflective and glare effects.

Chair and Desk

The quality of equipment and accessories should be as high as the budget allows. The adage "you get what you pay for" is most often true. Various types and models for almost all office equipment are available, and it usually pays to do some research before selecting an item whether it is a glare reduction filter for the computer monitor, a document holder, a riser for a computer, or a chair. We recommend trying the furniture for fit and feel before purchasing it. Helpful Hint 6.1 provides several sources for equipment and accessories.

A chair should be fully adjustable and ergonomically rated; it should be checked and adjusted to ensure that the seat pan, back, and armrest fit: The hips should be slightly higher than the knees. It is beneficial to have a footrest available in the event that the chair needs to be raised to a level so that the feet do not touch the floor. Footrests maintain good alignment of the lower leg and feet and thereby aid blood circulation of the lower extremities. If the chair causes undue pressure in the posterior thigh, using a footrest will be helpful. Select a chair with five legs for stability; one with fewer than five can easily tip over, presenting a safety hazard. The back of the knees (popliteal fossa) should never be impinged or restricted and the knees should

HELPFUL HINT 6.1
Equipment and Accessories

We recommend the following suppliers from the many sources for equipment and accessories for the office.

- AOA Commission on Ophthalmic Standards
  - 243 N. Lindbergh Blvd., St. Louis, MO 63141
  - http://www.aoa.org
- Air Technologies Corporation
  - 27130 Paseo Espada, Ste. 1405-A, San Juan Capistrano, CA 92675
  - 800-759-5060
  - http://www.airtech.net
- Ergonomic Products, Inc.
  - 1817 S. Home, Mesa, AZ 8520
  - 800-476-9868
  - http://www.cybertrails.com/ergonomic
- AliMed
  - 297 High St., PO Box 9135, Dedham, MA 02026
  - 800-225-2610
  - http://www.alimed.com
- ARV Computer and Office Accessories
  - 33800 Curtis Blvd., No. 110, Willoughby, OH 44095
  - 800-729-7200
  - http://www.arv.com/arv.html

- Ergonomic Sciences Corporation
  - 2672 Bayshore Parkway, Ste. 520, Mountain View, CA 94043
  - 650-964-313
  - http://www.ergosci.com
- Ergopro.com
  - PO Box 25914, No. 225, Houston, TX 77265
  - 800-ERGO-PRO
  - http://www.ergopro.com
- Ergo Systems
  - 1347 Spring St., Atlanta, GA 30309
  - 800-700-9141
  - http://www.ergosystems.com
- Ergoview
  - 11 East 26th St., 8th Floor, New York, NY 10010
  - 800-888-3537
  - http://www.ergoview.com

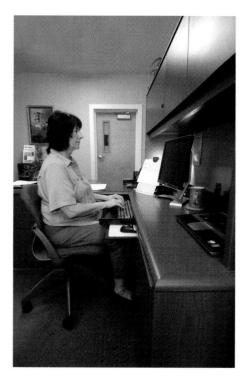

FIGURE 6.3

Proper ergonomic alignment when working at a desk or computer keeps the body in neutral alignment and maintains the proper alignment and distance from the computer screen.

extend a few inches beyond the chair seat pan (Figure 6.3 ■). Props can be purchased to accommodate for a chair back that does not fit either the thoracic or lumbar areas. One recommendation is the Medicair$_x$^{R} Back Pillo, an air pillow made by Corflex. Some additional details necessary in a chair are:

- Padded seat pan
- Minimum 18.2-inch wide seat pan
- Seat pan adjustable in height and depth
- Seat back's angle and height adjustable

The desk size and shape is best determined by the size of the room and tasks performed at it. Virtually all desks today are equipped to accommodate a computer. Depending on the amount of additional equipment (e.g., phone, fax, printer, books), an L-shaped desk could best meet these needs.

Office desks are made at standard heights; unfortunately, people are not. Standard sizes are determined on anthropometric data in Helpful Hint 6.2. When a person is seated three points at which the body should make contact with a surface are the desk or keyboard, the seat, and the floor. Adjustable chairs take care of the second two, but the standard desk size causes the first to be fixed. Someday adjustable desks will be the norm, but until such time, accommodations must be made to fit a person to his or her desk. Short individuals need to raise their chair so their arm position and line of vision are correct and to have a footstool to properly position their feet. Taller people need to adjust their chair for proper alignment and, if needed, place their computer on a riser for proper visual alignment. In all cases, the space under the desk should be ample for the legs to move freely.

The standard anthropometric criteria for desks are for writing rather than typing. When writing, a person's desktop should be approximately 50 millimeters above the elbow; when typing, the home row of the keyboard should be approximately level with the elbow, as shown in Figure 6.3.

HELPFUL HINT 6.2
Anthropometrics Explained

Anthropometry is the study of the range of human physical dimensions. Height, width, and distance between anatomical points such as, shoulders, hips, and arms are factored into the equation of fitting the worker to the task. Anthropometry follows a set of guidelines that are quantitative in determining the absolute and relative variables of the shape and size of the human body that are universally applicable. Tools for assessing these measurements can include:

- Weight scales
- Skin fold calipers
- Bioelectric impedance analyzers to measure body size and composition
- Body volume tanks for underwater measurements
- Anthropometer, a calibrated instrument used to measure the trunk and limbs

Anthropometric data is based on the norm and uses the 5th to 95th percentile. This means that data of the smallest and the largest are sizes are not included; therefore, it reflects the average for 90% of the sizes (Anshel, 2008). You may find it interesting to know that the shortest people in the world are pygmies living in Africa and the largest are in Sudan. The data do not factor in gender difference (e.g., the average height of males is 64.96 inches and of females is 60.5 inches). Two general rules apply to variation in physical aspects among ethnic groups. Bergman's rule states that the body size varieties increase with the mean temperature of the habitat. Allen's rule states that the relative size of exposed portions of the body (i.e., nose, ears, toes), decrease with decreasing temperature, and extremities will be proportionately smaller (Pheasant, 1991).

(Loy & Greer, 2007). An adjustable keyboard tray allows a person to adjust to her or his needs.

Computers and VDTs

VDTs are revolutionizing workplaces. As usage continues to increase, so will concomitant stressors. VDTs, including their position, angle, size, type, and distance must be assessed as part of office design.

Individuals are at high risk for fatigue and MSDs when they spend extended time in front of a computer. The small movements and fixed positions lead to fatigue, which eventually leads to tension, muscle pain, and injury. Poor work habits and/or design of the computer work space most affect the eyes, neck, back, shoulders, wrists, and hands. Selecting proper computer equipment can prevent or reduce fatigue and injury. Laptops should not be the primary computer because they are less adjustable, making it harder to maintain neutral postures. However, docking stations for this type of computer can help, as can a separate, larger monitor and separate keyboard. Keep in mind that wrist pads on the keyboard are intended as a brief resting pad from typing. Do not use them while typing to avoid hyperextension of the wrists.

A document holder is important for people who spend a significant amount of time on the computer working from other documents. This helps to keep the head/neck in a neutral position. Many models to choose from are available, but we personally prefer the type that clips or adheres to the monitor in order to keep the eyes, head, and neck in alignment with it. Fortunately, eyestrain does not seem to be of concern when the document holder and the monitor are at different distances.

The type of mouse used is a personal preference; more important is to position the mouse to keep neutral alignment with the wrists. One benefit to an external wireless mouse is its maneuverability and the ease of changing hands. The built-in laptop mouse and small keyboard surface are the worst choice for maintaining proper hand position. Wrist problems develop as a result of overuse, and repetitive radial and ulna deviation (Figure 6.4 ■). Wrist supports can be helpful; however, it is better keep the wrists neutral, change hands, and take breaks to avoid problems.

Conventional practice recommends that the viewing distance from a person to a monitor should be anywhere from 18 to 30 inches from the eyes, but current recommendations extend the distance as far as 40 inches to take advantage of eye relaxation that occurs when the eyes are focused on a more distant point. The screen should be at least 4 to 5 inches below eye level. Others recommend the center of the screen to be 7 to 10 inches lower than the horizontal line of sight to prevent eyestrain, fatigue, and headaches (U.S. Department of Labor & OSHA, 1997). These measurements should be made from the center of the screen. The monitor should be placed directly in front of the person and centered over the desk's knee well; refer to Figure 6.3.

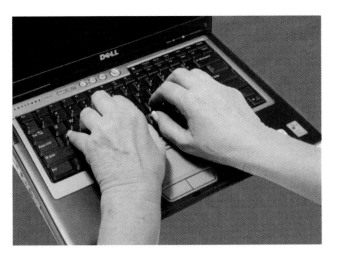

FIGURE 6.4

The laptop computer presents ergonomic challenges. The central station position of the built-in mouse and small keyboard surface increases the risk for ulnar deviation.

Even several hours a day of looking at a computer screen can be stressful to the eyes. Ease stress by reducing surrounding light to increase contrast. Adjust background and font color to give optimum contrast. If the monitor flickers, reduce the brightness of the screen. Individuals should experiment by adjusting the brightness of the screen to determine the level that works best for them. Another contributing factor to eye strain is glare, which a monitor glare guard can help reduce. Glare reduction filters recommended by the American Optometric Association (AOA) are best. Its specifications include filter construction, quality, image degradation, and environmental testing. The filter should not degrade the quality of the image but should withstand humidity, resist abrasion, and varying temperatures. See Table 6.2 ■ for some AOA accepted filter models and the companies that sell them. Ideally, the monitor should be placed at a right angle to a window to reduce glare. Cover windows and turn off light sources that create the glare.

Some VDT users are concerned that electromagnetic field emitted from VDTs could be harmful. No conclusive evidence that the low levels of radiation emitted pose a health threat, but because of the possibility, the **National Institute for Occupational Safety and Health (NIOSH)** has a published resource about VDTs (Lee, 2003).

In conclusion, some general tips to keep in mind when for working at a personal computer are:

- Break up repetitive and static postures with breaks
- Keep the head and neck neutral; no flexion or extension
- Adjust keyboard to elbow height
- Keep the wrists neutral while keyboarding; no flexion or extension
- Use an external mouse on a laptop to avoid excessive radial and ulnar deviation caused by built-in mouse

TABLE 6.2	Ergonomic Supply Company Sources for Screen Filters	
Company	Contact Information	Acceptable Filters
Fellowes Manufacturing Company	1789 Norwood Ave. Itasca, IL 60143 http://www.fellowes.com	○ Premium glass antiglare/some tint ○ Premium glass antistatic/radiation/some tint ○ Premium glass antistatic/radiation/traditional tint ○ Picture perfect antiglare/static/radiation
Kantek, Inc.	3067 Hampton Rd. Oceanside, NY 11572 http://www.kantek.com	○ Spectrum Universal ○ Spectrum Universal Contour
Kensington Technology Group Division ACCO Brands, Inc.	200 Alameda de las Pulgas San Mateo, CA 94403 http://www.kensington.com	○ Kensington high contrast ○ Kensington true color ○ GlareMaster premium ○ Contour and flat frame ○ GlareMaster premium antiradiation contour
3M Corporation Optical Systems Division	260-5N-10/3M Center St. Paul, MN 55144-1000 http://www.3m.com	○ AF-100 ○ EF-200 ○ EF-250 ○ BF-10

DESIGN ELEMENTS OF THE TREATMENT ROOM

The treatment room should be set up to include comfort, aesthetics, efficiency, and sound ergonomics.

Room Design

The dimensions of the treatment room should be of sufficient size for the practitioner to move comfortably around the table when working. A room with a minimum of 8 x 12 square feet will work for the standard table size. The clearance around the table should have at least 2.5 feet. The room should have no obstacles, such as electrical cords or area rugs that are a hazard for tripping or protruding furniture to bump into. The room needs to have adequate storage for the supplies and equipment needed while working or the space under the table must have an area for storage. The room in Figure 6.5 ■ is one example of a warm, inviting, aesthetically pleasing yet functional treatment room.

Equipment

An adjustable table and stool are imperative for the practitioner. The preference is for an electric table that allows the bodyworker to adjust for each client and during treatment. If an electric table is not available, adjustments for the client must be made before she or he arrives and appropriate props available to allow work to be performed ergonomically correctly.

We recommend varying techniques and using a seated position when possible. An adjustable stool on casters is the optimum for this. The choice between a backless seat or one with a back is a personal preference. However, a backless seat requires the core muscles to be engaged, which is considered an active seat.

Recommended props to have available in the treatment room include a bolster, which is not only beneficial in aiding client comfort (e.g., under the knees when the client is supine) but also can be used to support the bodyworker's lower arms during energy work so the shoulders can relax. This posture can be maintained for a more extended period

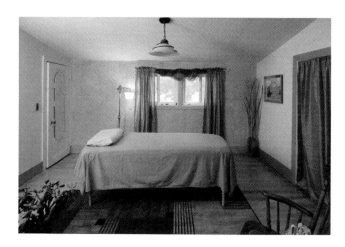

FIGURE 6.5

The treatment room should be aesthetically pleasing and spacious enough to allow at least two and a half feet of clear space around the table.

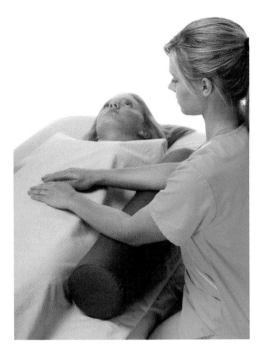

FIGURE 6.6

The same bolster used to support the client legs
can be used to support the lower arms when
holding a position for a long period. This
reduces the stress on the shoulders.

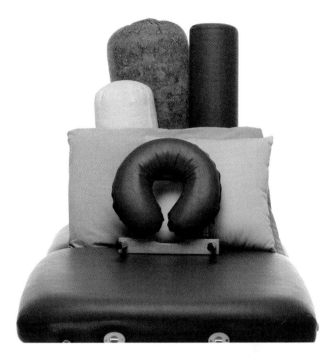

FIGURE 6.7

An adjustable face cradle and a variety of pillows and bolsters
are essential for a well-equipped treatment room.

with support (see Figure 6.6 ■). Other standard props used
to position the client include pillows, adjustable face cradle,
and different sizes of bolsters (Figure 6.7 ■).

Floors and Mats

Flooring needs to be level and any factor that could cause
unsteady footing or could be a tripping hazard needs to be
eliminated. Carpet or a mat under the table improves stability. Carpet pile should not be deeper than 0.5 inch.

Because they have multiple clients during the workday
and each treatment can last over an hour, many bodyworkers spend much of their time standing. This can cause blood
to pool in the legs and feet, increasing the risk for varicose
veins and associated vascular problems and general fatigue
of the legs and feet. Antifatigue mats can increase productivity by reducing fatigue and the risk for plantar fasciitis,
varicose veins, and low back pain. Research shows they
encourage subtle contracting and relaxing movements of
the lower leg muscles, thereby decreasing blood pooling
(O'Dell, 2008). Having antifatigue mats around the massage table is especially important when the treatment room
has a concrete or hardwood floor. Many types of mats are
available; they are made from a variety of substances such
as vinyl, rubber, and/or polyvinyl chloride (PVC). We recommend those that meet ergonomic standards. Refer to
Helpful Hint 6.1 for mat sources.

ERGONOMIC ASSESSMENT OF THE WORKPLACE

A full ergonomic assessment addresses both the physical
workplace and the practitioners' techniques. Obviously, the
two are not mutually exclusive, however; because this chapter has focused on the workplace, we end it by providing
assessment guidelines and a worksheet for an assessment
of your own office and treatment area. We also use three
case studies to demonstrate how to spot problems and find
solutions.

Few practitioners likely have had their work analyzed for
ergonomic factors. To identify elements that cause the workplace or techniques not to be ergonomic, they can start by
considering past and any current injuries. Refer to Table 6.3 ■
for symptoms that point to ergonomic issues for the arms,
hands, legs, and feet. If any of these symptoms exists, practitioners should seek professional assistance to determine the
underlying cause. They should also identify their tasks that
require twisting, bending, using forceful exertion, assisting
clients physically, and taking positions for prolonged periods and consider how often they occur. After these factors
have been identified, the practitioners can reflect on how to
modify the work space to reduce the occurrence of these
risks. While sitting at the desk and while standing and/or
sitting at the massage table, bodyworkers should determine

TABLE 6.3	Warning Signs for Ergonomic Problems
Hands and Arms	Back and Legs
Tingling	Back pain
Numbness	Muscle spasms
Sore muscles	Cramps
Shoulder and arm fatigue	Circulatory problems
Stiffness	Inflammation
Loss of dexterity and grip	Sore joints, stiffness, and swelling

whether the heights and alignments for each are correct and have sufficient space surrounding them. Based on these observations, practitioners can make initial adjustments. Ultimately, they should have someone else analyze their work, either while they are working or by watching a videotape of their work. The job assessment should address both the physical space and techniques.

Refer to Case Studies 6.1, 6.2, and 6.3 for methods to use to identify poor ergonomic conditions. Worksheet 6.1 is a checklist regarding air quality, lighting, tools, and potential hazards in a workplace setting. Completing the worksheet and becoming more aware of your work space will help you make adjustments to improve ergonomics.

CASE FOR STUDY 6.1
Office Space Basics

Aaron found the only available space to set up an office in his home. From friends, family, and a yard sale, he outfitted his office, but for some reason, he could not stick with his office tasks long enough to get things done. He also left the office feeling fatigued. Review the diagram of his office space in Figure 6.8 ■. What problems can you identify, and how can they be corrected?

Did you notice the inadequate chair? The seat back is too short, the lack of armrests is problematic, and the glare from the window can wreak havoc with his vision. The notebook computer is not ideal and can contribute to loss of neutral position.

Solutions:

- New adjustable chair with higher seat back and arm rests
- Window coverings to reduce/eliminate glare
- External keyboard for the notebook (laptop) computer
- Riser for the notebook to elevate it for proper viewing height or a separate, larger monitor
- Ergonomic training for proper use of equipment and posture

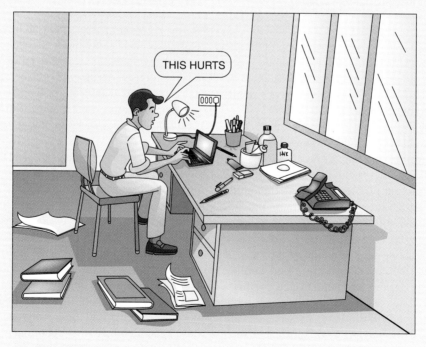

FIGURE 6.8

An office area with poor ergonomic conditions.

CASE FOR STUDY 6.2
Further Improvement of the Office Space

Aaron recognized that his space needed revamping and began to make some changes with window covering and a new light, chair, desk, and computer (Figure 6.9 ■). How is he faring now?

The space is beginning to look more like an office, but did you notice that the chair does not have the recommended five-leg base for stability and that this particular design tilts his upper body forward? The forward tilt and lack of armrests will cause shoulder and neck problems. Resting his arms on the desk edge can impinge the ulnar nerve. The light in the room is reflected toward the ceiling instead of lighting the work area.

Solutions:

- Chair needs armrests and five legs
- Proper lighting for the task and overall room
- Training for proper body mechanics while working

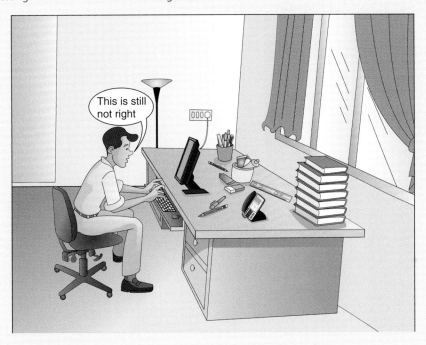

FIGURE 6.9

The ergonomics of the office are improved, but not perfect.

CASE FOR STUDY 6.3
The Treatment Room

Alice is a new graduate and has started her own practice. She notices that by the end of the day, her shoulders and wrist hurt. What problem do you see in Figure 6.10 ■ that could be causing her symptoms?

This is a classic example of poor body mechanics while working. Her head is protracted, her shoulders are slightly elevated, and her wrists are hyperextended. Posture and technique are part of the problem, but what is the equipment's role in this? The table needs to be adjusted, but in which direction? Raising it

would be appropriate for Swedish technique; this would reduce the shoulder protraction and hyperextension of the wrists. Lowering the table would be appropriate for neuromuscular techniques. A clue in the figure is the elevated shoulders, indicating the need to lower the table. Alice was practicing neuromuscular techniques.

As this case history illustrates, a full job analysis addresses both the workplace and the tasks being performed.

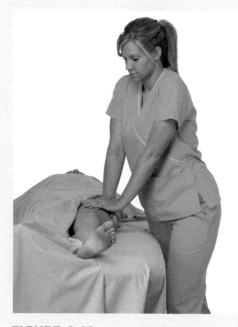

FIGURE 6.10

WORKSHEET 6.1
Ergonomic Assessment of the Physical Workspace

Indoor Environment

Do you consistently experience symptoms associated with SBD while working? _____ yes _____ no   Circle any that apply.

- Eye irritation
- Skin irritation
- Headache
- Throat irritation
- Recurrent fatigue
- Chest burning
- Cough
- Wheezing
- Nasal congestion
- Problems with concentration or short-term memory

Office and Computer Area Assessment

Desk

Room for legs _____ yes _____ no

Adequate room for tasks _____ yes _____ no

Items within easy reach without twisting _____ yes _____ no

Chair Fit

Seat pan

Padded _____ yes _____ no

When seated with your back against seat back, is the back of the knee (popliteal fossa) resting on front of seat pan? _____ yes _____ no

Height

Adjusted so the elbow is 90 degrees to desktop (writing) or keyboard _____ yes _____ no

Feet flat on the floor or on footrest _____ yes _____ no

Seat back

Lumbar support comfortable _____ yes _____ no

Thoracic support comfortable _____ yes _____ no

Monitor

Height is 4–10 inches below horizontal line of sight _____ yes _____ no

Distance of at least 18 inches to you _____ yes _____no

Lighting

Any glare _____ yes _____ no

Position at right angle to window _____ yes _____ no

Keyboard

Height is at elbow level with home row _____ yes _____ no

Treatment Room Assessment

Layout

Space

Minimum of 2.5 feet around table _____ yes _____ no

Free of obstacles _____ yes _____ no

Accessories and supplies readily available _____ yes _____ no

Table

Adjusts in height _____ yes _____ no

Wide enough to accommodate average person _____ yes _____ no

Stool

Adjustable _____ yes _____ no

Minimum of 5 legs with casters _____ yes _____ no

Flooring

Nonskid surface under table _____ yes _____ no

Antifatigue mats _____ yes _____ no

CHAPTER SUMMARY

- Federal and state regulations have been established to improve the safety of the workplace and reduce the cost of work-related injury or death. OSHA's efforts are ongoing in the areas of enforcement, training, and research, and since its inception in 1970, workplace death and injuries have dramatically declined.
- Chemical, biological, and particulate contaminants can reduce indoor air quality to the point of causing sick building syndrome and/or building-related illnesses. Sufficient ventilation, moisture control, and effective air filtering systems are necessary to reduce such hazards. Temperature, sound, and lighting are other key factors of the indoor environment to assess.
- Lighting needs to be appropriate for each specific task. The amount of light as well as contrast and reduction of glare need to be considered.

- Computers and VDTs have created a new health challenge. Computer vision syndrome, which can occur with prolonged monitor use, includes a range of symptoms from headaches to eye irritation, blurred vision, and neck and shoulder pain.
- Offices should be organized to be efficient and safe. Proper selection of a chair for fit is critical, and suitable setup of the computer, including the keyboard, mouse, and VDT can reduce the stress of desk and/or computer work.
- Treatment rooms need to be esthetically pleasing and comfortable for the client and be an organized, safe environment for the bodyworker. An adjustable table, stool for seated work, and props are necessary, and an antifatigue mat is highly recommended.
- A job assessment starts with a critique of the physical space and includes a full assessment of techniques.

REVIEW QUESTIONS

1. The role(s) of the Occupation Safety and Health Administration is(are) to provide:
   a. guidelines and regulations to reduce workplace accidents
   b. safety training
   c. ongoing research on safety
   d. all the above
2. True or False? Sick building syndrome is a diagnosable disorder.
3. Name three contributing factors for SBS and/or BRI.
4. True or False? Overuse of vibrating tools can damage small blood vessels in the hands, leading to a condition known as Reynaud's phenomenon.
5. Name four ways to reduce eyestrain when working at a computer.
6. Which of the following is correct for the selection of or fit of the office chair?
   a. It should have three legs for stability.
   b. The back of the knees should rest right at the edge of the seat pan.
   c. Chairs with armrests are preferred over those without.
   d. The use of footrests should always be avoided.

7. In regard to working at a computer:
   a. the monitor should be directly at or above eye level
   b. the internal laptop mouse is preferred over an external mouse
   c. the monitor should be within 18 inches of the eyes
   d. a document holder helps to keep the head and neck in neutral alignment
8. The number of minimum feet around the massage table should be
   a. 1
   b. 2.5
   c. 4
   d. 6
9. True or False? Antifatigue mats improve blood flow in the legs when a person is standing and working for extended periods of time.
10. A job assessment critiques both _____ and _____.

REFERENCES

American Massage Therapy Association. (2008). Retrieved January 25, 2008, from http://www.amtamassage.org/

American Optometric Association. (2008). Retrieved January 15, 2008, from http://www.aoa.org/x6024.xml?prt

Anshel, J. (2008). Visual ergonomics in the workplace: Improving eyecare and vision can enhance productivity. Retrieved January 13, 2008, and January 29, 2008, from http://www.tifaq.org/article/vision_health_management-may99-dr_anshel.html

Arnold, K. (2001, June). Sick building syndrome solutions. *Professional Safety*, 46(6).

Bureau of Labor Statistics. (2007). Nonfatal occupational injuries and illnesses requiring days away from work, 2007 (USDL 08-1716). Retrieved January 22, 2008, from http://stats.bls.gov/

European Collaborative Action (ECA). (2003). Urban air, indoor environment and human exposure, ventilation, good indoor air quality and rational use of energy. Report 23. Retrieved January 30, 2008, from http://www.buildingecology.com/publications/ECA_Report23.pdf

Herman, A., and Watchman, G., U.S. Department of Labor, & OSHA. (1997). Working safely with video display terminals. http://www.osha.gov/Publications/videoDisplay/videoDisplay.html

Lahtinen, M., Huuhtanen, P., & Reijula, K. (1998). Sick building syndrome and psychosocial factors—A literature review. *Indoor Air*, 8(Supplement 4).

Lee, J. (2007). *Handbook of Building Contractors*. Retrieved January 20, 2008, from http://books.google.com/books

Lee, J. (2003, September). Screen for struggling computer users. *Review of Ophthalmology*, 88–89.

Loy, B., & Greer, J. (2007). Ergonomics in the workplace: A resource guide. Retrieved January 30, 2008, from http://www.jan.wvu.edu/media/ergo.html

Occupational Safety and Health Administration (1999). Ergonomics program. Retrieved September 10, 2010, from http://www.osha.gov/pls/oshaweb/owadisp.show_document?p_table=FEDERAL_REGISTER&p_id=16305

O'Dell, L. (2008). Anti-fatigue mats for the standing worker. Retrieved August 1, 2008, from http://www.americanfloormats.com

Pheasant, S. (1991). *Ergonomics, work and health*. Gaithersburg, MD: Aspen.

Seppaanen, O., & Frisk, W. (2004). Summary of human responses to ventilation. *Indoor Air*, 4(Supplement 7).

U.S. Census Bureau. (2001). Retrieved January 1, 2008, from http://www.informationweek.com/story/IWK20010906S0010

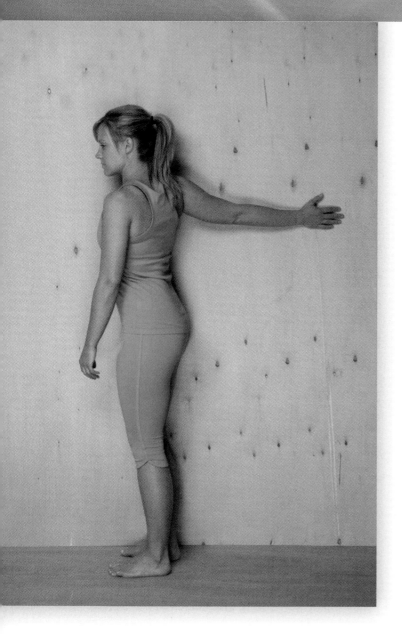

CHAPTER

7 Self-Care: Exercise

 CHAPTER OUTLINE

Engaging in Strength Training

Promoting Cardiorespiratory Fitness

Stretching

Using Suggested Strengthening and Stretching
  Exercises by Body Area

Summary

Review Questions

LEARNING OBJECTIVES

Upon successful completion of this chapter, you will be able to:

1. Differentiate between stretching and strengthening and identify the role of each in an exercise program.
2. Differentiate the three different types of muscular contractions and how they are used in exercise programs.
3. Discuss the benefits of strengthening, endurance, and stretching to bodyworkers.
4. Define cardiorespiratory fitness.
5. Calculate your target heart rate (THR).
6. Identify the different modes of stretching and uses of each.
7. Design and implement an exercise program the meets your needs.

KEY TERMS

Bodyworkers who want to enjoy a long career need to take care of themselves. This chapter describes exercises that will help achieve muscle fitness to better maintain neutral positions, avoid postural distortion, and work more efficiently. Professional athletes achieve great performance day in and day out by maintaining a good balance of strength and flexibility. Although practitioners aren't professional athletes, bodywork is physically demanding, and an exercise routine that improves practitioners' strength and flexibility will increase their vitality, efficiency, and improve overall well-being. Bodyworkers need their muscles to perform a wide variety of sometimes strenuous tasks on a daily basis. The best way to avoid injury and fatigue is to have a thorough and consistent stretching and strengthening program and to use proper body mechanics. Muscles must be strong enough to handle the demand placed on them or they will quickly fatigue. Fatigue will lead to less effective work, misalignment, and personal injury. Additionally, if the surrounding muscles are inflexible, a joint will not be able to work through its complete range of motion (ROM). When it is limited, the muscles are forced to work in a shortened state, which will lead to a number of physical problems ranging from headaches and soreness to overuse syndromes.

Physical fitness is important for all people to reduce chronic diseases, address obesity, and slow the aging process. In addition, fitness programs can be tailored to meet individual needs. Although this chapter provides general fitness recommendations that can apply to the entire population, much of it addresses fitness training to prevent or combat the development of postural distortions that are common for bodyworkers. Use the assessment you completed as Worksheet 4.1 as a tool to help you begin to identify your individual fitness needs.

Health screening is important prior to initiating a fitness program to determine whether any special medical considerations exist. A general guideline is for people older than 35 or if they have a history of:

- Heart problems or high blood pressure
- Family history of early stroke or heart attacks
- Dizziness
- Fatigue with mild exercise
- Lung disorders including asthma
- Joint problems or severe muscle or tendon problems
- Metabolic disorder including diabetes mellititus, thyroid disorders, kidney disease, or liver disease

A life of inactivity and obesity increases an individual's risk for chronic disease and early death, so a medical condition shouldn't keep him or her from exercising. Instead, the individual should consult a physician and follow his or her recommendations. Also, hiring a personal trainer to help assess the physical condition and to act as a guide for starting a program is wise. Certified personal trainers, athletic trainers, and exercise physiologists should be available at local YMCAs, rehabilitation centers, and sports medicine facilities, or contact American College of Sports Medicine

(ACSM) or the National Council on Strength and Fitness (NCSF) for a qualified instructor. Trainers are reliable sources for information and know how to individualize a program for specific needs. If it is not possible to hire a personal trainer, suggestions for designing a program of activities that are varied and fun are available from a number of publications and websites that focus on fitness. Some suggested websites are listed in the Suggested Readings and Websites section at the end of this chapter.

Fitness requires a permanent lifestyle change but provides life-long benefits including:

- Reduced risk for cardiovascular disease
- Reduced high blood pressure or the risk of developing it
- Reduced risk of colon and breast cancer
- Reduced body fat and increased lean body mass
- Reduced anxiety and depression
- Increased energy level to enjoy leisure activities and meet daily demands
- Improved performance
- Improved cardiorespiratory (heart and lungs) function
- Increased blood supply to muscles
- Increased HDL (good) cholesterol

Physical fitness incorporates four basic components: muscular strength, muscular endurance, cardiorespiratory endurance, and flexibility. Before beginning an exercise program, it is useful for individuals to understand what each component includes so they can better recognize how to keep a balanced program.

Muscular strength refers to the muscle's ability to produce force at a given velocity (i.e., how much weight and how quickly a person can pick it up). Not all muscle cells (or myofibers) are the same. Some muscle cells known as *fast twitch fibers* can provide an explosive, fast, and powerful contraction. They are able to do so because they have more contractile filaments and a faster contractile rate. When we perform a movement against resistance that requires a forceful contraction, these are the muscle cells recruited for the work. Muscle strength develops as the muscle fibers increase their contractile components allowing them to contract with more force. The muscle cell also hypertrophies (i.e., enlarges) and contributes to the increased muscle mass seen in weight training. Although fast twitch fibers provide significant force of contraction, they fatigue easily. This is so because the fibers need to rely on anaerobic metabolism to provide the rapid supply of adenosine triphosphate (ATP) that is necessary for the quick contractions. Anaerobic metabolism does not use fuel efficiently, so it depletes the glycogen stores in the muscle cell quickly and fatigue occurs.

In contrast, muscular endurance is the ability of muscle to continue repeated contractions without fatigue. A second muscle cell type known as the *slow twitch fiber* is recruited in endurance activities that occur for extended periods of time because they are resistant to fatigue. The availability of myoglobin, which stores oxygen within the cell, a better capillary network around the cells, and the use of aerobic respiration that efficiently produces ATP allows the slow twitch fiber cells to function much longer before depleting their fuel supply and causing fatigue. With improved muscle endurance, the myoglobin supplies and the mitochondria (the "powerhouse" of the cell) increase for improved ATP production; however, the number of contractile filaments does not, so the muscle cells do not increase in their contractile strength or hypertrophy. Muscle endurance also develops in strength training and relates to being able to do more repetitions with a given weight without fatigue. The fast twitch fibers become more efficient at storing glycogen and using the fuel to produce ATP; however, the ATP production is still by means of anaerobic metabolism, so fatigue still occurs relatively soon.

Cardiorespiratory endurance, or fitness, is the body's ability to maintain sufficient blood flow to the muscle to provide it the necessary nutrients and oxygen and to remove waste products. Cardiorespiratory endurance is closely tied to muscle endurance, but the two can most easily be distinguished by noting that cardiovascular endurance relates to the body's ability to supply muscles with oxygen and fuel, and muscle endurance is the muscle's ability to continue contractions because of available fuel. Cardiorespiratory endurance depends on the health of the heart, vasculature (arteries and veins), and lungs to pump a sufficient volume of blood through the body, properly distribute the blood to the tissues, and provide for adequate oxygen and carbon dioxide exchange. Endurance training increases the demand placed on the cardiorespiratory systems and in turn the heart, vessels, and lungs adapt for improved circulation and gas exchange.

Flexibility is defined as the ability to move through the full range of motions. The health of the joint structures and muscle's ability to relax and yield to the forces being placed on them determine flexibility. Stretching extends the length of muscles by relaxing more muscle cells and increasing elasticity of the connective tissue scaffolding within muscles and, thus, improves flexibility. Strengthening exercises result in muscle shortening, and stretching results in muscle lengthening. Both are important to incorporate into exercise routines to maintain muscle balance.

ENGAGING IN STRENGTH TRAINING

Strength training uses resistance to develop muscle strength and bone density. Proper strength training focuses on the core/stabilizer muscles and major muscle groups and ensures that there is a balance of training of angonist/antagonists pairs to maintain proper neutral alignment.

Strength training is important for bodyworkers because it supports proper body mechanics. A body that has good tone and muscle balance is able to perform the physically demanding tasks of bodywork with increased power and proper body alignment. This results in a decreased risk of repetitive motion disorders, postural distortions, and musculoskeletal disorders (MSDs). As a result, the body can remain pain free and work in a more energized state.

Failure to maintain muscle strength has lifelong implications including:

- Gait and balance problems
- Risk for falls and fractures
- Risk for chronic disease including osteoporosis and diabetes
- Lethargy
- Immobility

Strength training offsets these risks by increasing physical strength and body tone, which in turn improves the ability to maneuver and prevent falls because of poor balance. Strength training helps to maintain or increase muscle mass depending on the intensity of a workout. Increased muscle mass improves muscle response to insulin, which reduces the risk for diabetes. Muscle mass also directly influences metabolic rate. More muscle relates to a higher metabolic rate and more energy, and weight control becomes easier.

A significant benefit of strength training is to maintain bone mass. This is especially important to women of all ages who are at higher risk for osteoporosis. The benefits are achieved in at least two ways. First, resistance placed on a bone during its development from birth through the twenties determines the total amount of bone mass. Strength training with proper nutrition during the teens and twenties allow for achieving a greater peak bone mass. A higher peak bone mass reduces the risk for osteoporosis. The second way strength training maintains bone mass relates to the fact that bones are continually remodeling throughout life: older bone is removed and new bone is laid down. The organization and density of the rebuilt bone is based on the physical demands that are placed on it. As muscles increase in strength, they can work with more force. This increased force places more resistance on the bones, and remodeling in those areas will improve the bone strength and reduce the overall rate at which total bone mass diminishes.

When beginning to develop a strength training program, select one for the particular muscle or muscle group that is needed for daily and occupational tasks and always include the core muscles, the fixator muscles of the torso. Strength and stability of these muscles maintains the stability of the spine for posture and provides the foundation for movement of the extremities by stabilizing the pelvis and scapulae. In addition to the group of abdominal muscles (rectus abdominis, transverse abdominis, and internal/external obliques), the core muscles include those that lie deep in the torso and attach to the spine and pelvis, including the erector spinae, multifidus, and quadratus lumborum.

The approach to strength training of major muscle groups and the core muscles is slightly different. For a major muscle group, one or two specific joints are isolated, and the muscles are worked under resistance in relationship to the joint(s), for example, the working of the biceps and triceps brachii at the elbow joint. On the other hand, working the core muscles involves stability exercises that work the entire torso at once. Abdominal bracing, which is an isometric contraction of the abdominal muscles, is a major technique during this training. Properly bracing involves an attempt to pull the umbilicus toward the spine, an action that involves the rectus abdominis, and keeps the spine in neutral alignment with a slight pelvic tilt by increasing tone of the obliques and transverse abominis. Leaving these other abdominal muscles relaxed is counterproductive to strengthening the core and only contributes to the distention of the abs. This is the reason that people complain about all of the sit-ups and crunches that they are doing but their belly seems to protrude. Equally important to proper muscle engagement is maintaining breath awareness. People should not hold their breath while doing core exercises. Crunches and push-ups can be the start of a simple core strengthening program. Specific programs that involve core training are yoga and Pilates, martial arts, and ballet. Some of the equipment used in core training is:

- Stability ball
- Medicine ball (weighted)
- Resistance bands
- Wobble boards

All strength training, regardless of whether it is for major muscle groups or the core, must ensure a balance in the training of the agonist and antagonists to ensure that neither becomes hypertonic. This means that both sides of the body (e.g., the front and the back) or both "sides" of a joint (e.g., the extensors and the flexors) should be worked. Increased strength and tone of one over the other muscle or muscle group pulls the body out of neutral alignment. For a person who already has a postural distortion because of this type of muscle imbalance, strengthening the weaker muscle should be the focus, but only to the point of bringing the body back to neutrality.

For a muscle to become stronger, it should be subjected to increasing levels of resistance. Strengthening and increased muscle mass result from a sequence of events: Motor control improves with strength remaining the same followed by an increase in strength. This increased strength is thought to be due to an increased synchronization/recruitment of muscle fibers, or increased density of contractile filaments. Ultimately, true hypertrophy of muscle occurs as the muscle fibers increase in diameter and strength. This last change starts after 10–12 weeks of proper training and is thought to occur as a result of a cycle of "tear-down and recovery."

The load or stress applied to the muscle causes minute tears in muscle tissue. These tears are rebuilt with more contractile filaments in the muscle cell, which ultimately increases the muscle's contractile force. The minute tears and inflammation they trigger is what causes the pain experienced several hours or the day following strenuous exertion known as *delayed onset muscle soreness*. It is important for the muscle(s) to rest for repair to occur and as it does, the pain diminishes. A safe and effective weight training program should consider intensity and frequency to balance the stress load used during training and the repair time made available between trainings.

The intensity of your workouts will be based on the amount of weight lifted and the number of repetitions performed. As the amount of weight is increased, the number of repetitions that you can perform will decrease. The amount of weight used is referred to as a given **repetition maximum (RM)**. One repetition maximum (1 RM) is the amount of weight that can be lifted with proper technique for only one repetition—not two. A 10 RM is the weight that could be lifted for 10 repetitions, but not 11, and so on. Increased muscle strength is gained by using low RM loads and more muscle endurance is gained using high RM loads. The American College of Sports Medicine recommends RM loads of 8–12 to best develop both strength and endurance (American College of Sports Medicine, 2000). A personal trainer can help to determine what a person's starting RM load should be, or it can be determined through trial and error. The main caution is to not attempt too high a load that could cause injury.

Types of Contractions

Various types of isometric or isotonic muscle contraction can help to achieve strengthening. Recall that during an isometric contraction, the muscle contracts without changing length. Because the muscle maintains in a static position, no change occurs in the angle of the joint. As an example, an isometric (static) contraction occurs when a person places a hand against a wall and pushes on it (Figure 7.1 ■). The wall cannot be moved, but the muscle is still contracting. As noted earlier isometric contractions of the abdominal

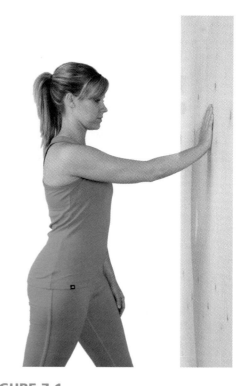

FIGURE 7.1

Pushing against a wall generates an isometric contraction in the triceps since its force cannot exceed the resistance of the wall.

muscles are a part of the strength training program for the core. Other than that, the use of isometric contraction in routine strength training programs is relatively limited, although physical therapists can use it for localized rehabilitation of selected muscles following trauma, such as torn rotator cuff muscles, or for prevention of muscle atrophy of a limb immobilized in a cast. Isometrics are also used in sport specific training, such as gymnastics.

Isotonic contractions result in a change in the muscle's length and in the angle of the joint. The contraction can be further separated into the concentric and eccentric phases. At the start of a motion, such as a bicep curl (Figure 7.2 ■), there is first a positive contraction known as **concentric contraction** or miometric contraction (*mio* meaning "less") in which a muscle shortens while contracting against resistance through the joint's range of motion. Second, there is a negative contraction known as **eccentric contraction** or pliometric muscular contraction (*plio* meaning "more") in which the muscle lengthens while contracting against resistance through the joint's range of motion. This returns the bicep curl to its starting position. For strength training to be effective, these contractions must be slow and controlled. To achieve slow, controlled contractions, it is helpful for the person to count while doing the exercise: during the concentric phase of the movement, she or he should make two counts (one, two), and during the eccentric movement, four counts (one, two, three, four) to ensure that she or he doesn't perform the movements too quickly.

A variety of methods is available for doing isotonic exercise, including body weight exercises, free weights,

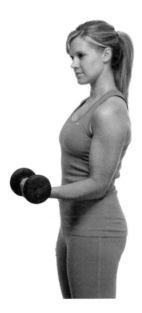

FIGURE 7.2

As the arm is flexed under resistance, the muscle is in a state of concentric contraction; then as the arm returns to its original position, the biceps is lengthening while force is still being applied, which is the eccentric contraction.

and exercises with equipment. The choice should be based on what is available and what is most comfortable. A summary of the pros and cons and tips for the different techniques and common equipment available follow.

Body weight exercises are the oldest means of strength training and offer a variety of exercises without the use of equipment. However, the body weight cannot readily be adjusted to meet the load needs for training. In the beginning, exercisers could find that their strength level prevents even one repetition (or rep) of a push-up or pull-up, which could prevent them from starting a full program. As strength develops, a limit for easily increasing load also develops. The maximum load that can be expected using purely body weight for exercise is 50% of the body's weight. Some exercises can accommodate increased load by using exercise bands, resistance bands, or wrist and/or ankle weights.

Use of free weights, which include barbells and dumbbells, is an effective training method for all ages and fitness levels. Barbells are long bars 4–6 feet in length with weights attached at each end; dumbbells are smaller, handheld weights. Instruction from an exercise professional in the use of free weights is necessary for those who have never used them to prevent injury. The use of free weights requires more muscle coordination than a weight machine. Because their use does not restrict movement, the risk for injury increases. General precautions when working with free weights include maintaining a good grip, which in part depends on using the correct size bars or handles, maintaining a stable seated or standing position, using appropriate forms, and not attempting to lift too much weight.

Weight machines come in a variety of forms from those that work a specific muscle group to multistation units that can provide workout for multiple muscle groups. The key issue for selecting the use of weight machines is their availability. Virtually all health clubs have them, and joining a club is one option. See Helpful Hint 7.1 for some guidelines for selecting a health club. On the other hand, although purchasing a home weight machine has an upfront cost, the convenience of having one often keeps people on their fitness program and is well worth the price. A multistation unit provides the widest range of exercise with minimal space and is more cost efficient. These units are constructed in a variety of ways with advantages and disadvantages for each:

- Weight stack uses a number of weights and a system of cables and pulleys. Resistance is changed simply by varying the number of weights until it feels natural and is constant through the full range of motion. The disadvantage of such machines is that they are heavy, bulky, can be difficult to assemble, and are difficult to move once assembled. When choosing this option, plan to have a permanent area for the equipment.
- Hydraulic pistons operate like shock absorbers, creating resistance with fluid within the piston. Adjustment of valves changes the resistance. The machines are much lighter in construction and easier to move than

HELPFUL HINT 7.1
How to Select a Health/Fitness Club

A health or fitness club should provide a safe environment with properly trained personnel and the programs to meet your needs at a price you can afford. Before seeking a facility, establish your exercise/fitness goals. Prepare for your visit to the facilities by formulating a set of questions that address safety and your personal needs. Recommended questions adapted from the ACSM include:

1. Is the facility conveniently located for you?
2. Is it a physically safe facility?
   - Does the facility have adequate parking during the times you would use it?
   - Does it have proper lighting outside and inside?
   - Is it clean and well maintained?
   - Does it have adequate heating, cooling, and ventilation?
   - Does it have posted emergency response and evacuation plans?
3. Does the facility provide the services and programs you need?
   - Does it provide preactivity screening to check for medical conditions or risks?
   - Are fitness screenings available for the types of activities you want to do, and are personalized exercise programs developed for the patrons?
   - Are fitness assessments available during a program to help you plot progress?
   - Are the types of exercises or programs that you are interested in available (aerobics, personal training, Pilates, martial arts, etc.)?
   - Are programs developed by qualified personnel?
   - Are staff members willing to modify programs to meet your needs?
   - If you need a rehabilitation program, is it available?
4. Is the facility properly staffed?
   - Do professional staff members have the appropriate education and training for the duties they perform? Degrees in health-related areas, including sports

medicine, physical education, exercise physiology, and kinesiology are most appropriate.
   - Do staff members, including personal trainers, managers, and supervisors, hold exercise certifications from nationally recognized organizations?
   - Do staff members receive ongoing training?
   - Are staff members properly trained in CPR and first aid?
   - Are staff members professional, friendly, and helpful?
   - Are staff members knowledgeable about your health conditions and able to help you set realistic goals?
   - Are there enough staff members to meet patrons' demands?
5. Is the facility a respected business that treats its patrons fairly? Read the membership contract thoroughly and make sure that you completely understand it before signing. Do not allow yourself to be pressured into purchasing a membership.
   - Is there a trial period that will give you an opportunity to try out the equipment and programs before you make a full commitment?
   - Are there different membership options and are all fees for services made clear?
   - Does the membership fee fit your budget?
   - Is a grace period available after joining that allows you to drop your membership and receive a refund?
   - Is there a written set of rules that establish the responsibilities of the members as well as the facility?
   - Is there a procedure for the facility to inform members of changes in charges, services, or policies?

Asking questions allow you to make an informed decision. Selecting a facility requires many considerations. There is never a guarantee that a facility will be entirely risk free or that you will be satisfied with what it offers. On the other hand, doing your homework, visiting all the facilities in your area, and selecting one that does meet your needs can be a major step toward reaching your fitness goals.

---

the weight stack. The disadvantage is that the resistance varies with pace and effort, so it becomes more difficult to stay on a program and chart progress.
- Flexible rods or bands used in conjunction with a lever and cable system are another option. Resistance is changed by varying the number of rods or bands used. Like the hydraulic systems, the machines are lighter and easier to move than the weight stack. The disadvantage is that the resistance varies through the range of motion and can become quite difficult to control toward the end of the range of motion. These machines should be tried before purchasing one to be certain that it offers a natural feel to movement.

Be sure to use any weight machine safely. Don't use defective equipment, stay away from moving parts, and protect the back from improper positions and use proper lifting techniques and perform the exercises through their full range of motion. Weight machines need to be adjusted to meet each individual's body size.

Suggestions for Strength Training

Strength training can target specific muscle(s), be individualized, and be adjusted based on the rate of progress. Strength training improves occupational performance for bodyworkers when the training is specific for the muscle groups used and the movement patterns performed in their work. A strength training program should focus on the muscles that maintain

WORKSHEET 7.1

Individualizing Your Fitness Plan

Worksheet 4.1 in Chapter 4 helped you identify PD(s) and the muscle condition (weakened or hypertonic) behind a PD. As you develop your plan for the upper body and lower body, focus on those areas in your plan as you also work to achieve overall strengthening and flexibility.

Identified PD	Muscle(s) to Strengthen	Muscle(s) to Stretch

neutral postural alignment. If a person has identified a postural distortion, strengthening the weaker muscles underlying the distortion is important. Worksheet 7.1 matches the common postural distortions discussed in Chapter 4 with muscle(s) needing strengthening or stretching. Exercises should be developed to alleviate and/or change the impact of these distortions on performance.

Individuals should be sure to warm up before and cool down after exercising. They should take one day off between strength training sessions to allow the muscles time to rest and repair. They can complete a training session that involves both upper and lower extremities in one day but should schedule alternating days for strength training or workouts every day by alternating the body area they train each day. For example, they can train the upper body Monday, Wednesday, and Friday and the lower body Tuesday, Thursday, and Saturday.

Strength training requires varying the body area being trained and identifying the amount of weight to use for each area and the number of reps performed. "Bulking up" involves using heavy weight and doing a lower number of reps, somewhere from 6 to 10. The last rep should fatigue the muscle being used. If bulking up is not a goal, a light weight and a high number of reps, ranging from 15 to 30, is appropriate, and the muscle should be fatigued at the completion of all reps. This low weight/high rep combination should result in increased muscular endurance, which is a muscle's ability to perform over a long period of time.

To continue gaining muscular strength and endurance, the amount of weight and number of reps should be adjusted as the muscle gets stronger and adapts to the stress put on it. Helpful Hint 7.2 is a guideline for determining the number of reps. When the muscle is no longer fatiguing, the number of reps with the same load can be increased. After the number of reps recommended for the result wanted (anywhere from 6 to 20) is achieved, it is time to increase the weight. Increasing the weight should be accompanied by decreasing the reps and repeating the process. The amount of weight needed to begin an exercise for a certain muscle or group of muscles varies. An individual muscle (bicep) generally requires a lighter load than a large muscle group (quadriceps). Experimenting with different amounts of weight with each new exercise is important but should be stopped when pain at the joint occurs, which is an indicator of improper body mechanics.

Guidelines for proper body mechanics while lifting are:

- Keep the neck neutral.
- Keep spine neutral.
- Keep weight-bearing joints in neutral alignment with one another, i.e., feet with the knees.

HELPFUL HINT 7.2

Guidelines for the Number of Repetitions

- 15–20 to increase muscle endurance and decrease fatigue
- 10–12 to increase muscle size (hypertrophy)
- 8–10 for basic strengthening
- 5–8 for strengthening—recruits fast twitch muscle fibers
- 1–5 to increase in power—used for preparing for an event (e.g., competition)

- Perform extension in a smooth movement.
- Perform flexion in a smooth movement.
- Breathe in when lowering a weight and out when lifting it.

For best results, record the exercise and the number of reps performed as well as the amount of weight used. This helps to track progress, adjust the weight/rep combination when needed, and change exercises regularly. See Table 7.1 ■, which includes recommendation for a cardiovascular workout discussed next. Photocopy and use Worksheet 7.2 for tracking your own program.

PROMOTING CARDIORESPIRATORY FITNESS

Aerobic/endurance training goes hand in hand with achieving cardiorespiratory fitness. During endurance training, the muscle demand for increased oxygenated blood triggers a response to increase circulation and respiration. This activity promotes a healthy heart, lungs, and vascular system. Being cardiorespiratory fit means having the ability to deliver blood and oxygen to tissues during periods of sustained physical activity. Those individuals who are cardiorespiratory fit do not fatigue as quickly as those who aren't and have a quicker recovery following physical exertion.

Society continues to become more sedentary, obesity is increasing in all age groups, and cardiovascular disease is the leading cause of death and morbidity. Perhaps these conditions resulted in the emphasis for all people to engage in aerobic activity rather than strength training. Endurance training has many benefits including these:

- The heart becomes a more efficient pump. The strength of the heart's contraction increases, pumping more blood per contraction. As a result, the heart rate decreases, giving the heart a longer rest period between contractions.
- The muscle becomes more efficient in using fat, causing the body mass to become leaner.
- Levels of HDL (good cholesterol) increase and of LDL (bad cholesterol) decrease, reducing the risk for developing atherosclerosis, a major contributor to cardiovascular disease.

Bodyworkers have a relatively sedentary job compared to those of our forefathers. Practitioners' work does not put a direct demand on their cardiorespiratory systems, so like others in society, they are at risk for cardiovascular disease. In addition, they often stand for prolonged periods of time. Regular endurance training helps to maintain good venous flow and decreases the risk for various veins and thrombophlebitis. Aerobic activities are also excellent ways to reduce stress and gain an overall sense of well-being; many of these activities help strengthen and tone the core muscles.

The same precautions for exercise and recommendations for consulting a physician discussed earlier also apply to preparing for endurance training. In particular, individuals who have hypertension, asthma, or emphysema and who are on certain types of medication, especially hypertensive medications, need to visit with their physician prior to starting an endurance training program.

TABLE 7.1	**Sample Exercise Tracking Log**								
Exercise	Date	Sun	Mon	Tues	Wed	Thur	Fri	Sat
Cardiobike/treadmill (TM)		15′ TM 20′bike	20′ TM 15′bike	15′ TM 20′bike	20′ TM 15′bike	15′ TM 20′bike	20′ TM 15′bike	15′ TM 20′bike
Bicep curl		10#15R		10#20R		10#30R		15#15R
Tricep curl		10#15R		10#20R		10#30R		15#15R
Upright row		12#15R		12#20R		12#30R		15#15R
Bench press		20#15R		20#20R		20#30R		25#15R
Shoulder press		25#15R		25#20R		25#30R		30#15R
Hamstring curl			15#15R		15#30R		20#15R	
Knee extension			30#15R		30#30R		35#15R	
Hip adduction			15#15R		15#30R		20#15R	
Hip abduction			15#15R		15#30R		20#15R	
Hip extension			20#15R		20#30R		25#15R	
Calf raise			15#15R		15#30R		20#15R	

TM = treadmill; # = amount of weight; R = repetitions; ′ = minutes

WORKSHEET 7.2
One-Week Exercise Log

The following exercise log can be copied to plan and track your fitness program one week at a time. Following is a checklist of items to include and information to consider:

- Check with your physician if you are over 35 years of age or have health problems or family history of health problems that could be negatively impacted by vigorous exercise.
- Regularity is critical. Balance your workout through the week to gain and maintain the desired level of fitness.
- Workouts should begin with 5–10 minutes of warm-up and end with 5–10 minutes of cool down.
- Include a cardiovascular exercise three to five times a week for a period of 20–60 minutes.
  - ○ Target heart rate should be maintained during the exercise.
  - ○ Calculate your THR range.

$$\text{(THR} = (220 - \text{age}) \times 55\% - 90\%$$

$$\text{THR} = \underline{\quad} \text{ bpm} - \underline{\quad} \text{ bpm}$$

- Schedule both upper body and lower body strength training and provide one day of rest between training for a given area.
  - ○ Incorporate appropriate strengthening for PDs identified.
  - ○ Incorporate appropriate strengthening for prevention of PDs common to therapists.
- Do stretches daily for at least 10–12 minutes.
  - ○ Stretching can be incorporated into the warm-up and cool-down periods of your cardiovascular workouts and strength training.
  - ○ List muscles/areas that need attention because of PDs.
  - ○ Stretching can be incorporated through the day, such as during work breaks.
- Increase intensity, frequency, and/or duration of activity over time to improve.

Cardiovascular Workout	Date						
	T/D	T/D	T/D	T/D	T/D	T/D	T/D

T = type, D = duration

(continued)

WORKSHEET 7.2 (CONTINUED)

Muscle Group Strengthened or Stretched	Exercise Name	Date						
		Rep/lbs	Rep/lbs	Rep/lbs	Rep/lbs	Rep/lbs	Rep/lbs	Rep/lbs
Abdominals								
Arms								
Upper back & neck								
Lower back & hips								
Shoulders								
Chest								
Legs								

Rep = repetition; lbs = pounds

Information for Performing Aerobic Exercise

According to the American College of Sports Medicine (ACSM), a person should perform vigorous **aerobic exercise** three to five days per week for 20–60 minutes per session. During that time, the heart should be achieving the individual's **target heart rate (THR),** measured in beats per minute (bpm). Monitor your heart rate by checking your carotid pulse as shown in Figure 7.3 ▪. The THR ranges from 55–90% of maximal heart rate. People who are just beginning an exercise program should work out at the low end, from 55–75%. The high end, 75–90%, is appropriate for those who have been exercising for long periods of time. Working within this range ensures that the heart is being exercised appropriately and is not being overstressed. See Helpful Hint 7.3 for information on how to calculate the THR.

The length of time a person needs to exercise should be adjusted according to intensity of the workout. Low-intensity workout should extend over a longer period of time. At the beginning of a program, low intensity for long periods of time is a good option. As it does in strength training, the body adapts to the stresses placed on it. As the program progresses, the exercise intensity, duration, or a combination of the two should increase. The most dramatic changes generally occur in the first 6–8 weeks of a program.

Aerobic activities that promote cardiorespiratory fitness include any that use large muscle groups (principally the muscles of the arms and legs) and can be maintained at submaximal intensity for a rhythmic, continuous period. Activities that meet this description include walking, jogging, running, bicycling, swimming, aerobic dancing, rowing, and cross-country skiing. For the beginner, walking, jogging, and cycling are excellent choices. People who

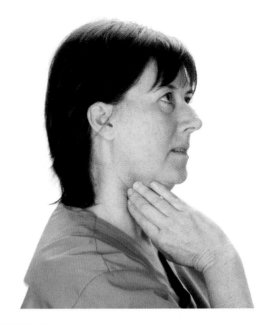

FIGURE 7.3

Palpate the carotid artery, which runs alongside the trachea. Find the position by first placing your fingertips lightly alongside the trachea and then sliding your fingers laterally. You will notice a slight groove and should be able to palpate the pulse. Be careful not to push too hard.

have joint problems or are at risk for them should select low-impact exercise options such as walking, swimming, or cross-country skiing.

A number of exercise machines on the market allow indoor exercise when weather, air pollution, or location prevents going outdoors. As with weight machines, individuals have the option to join a fitness club to have access to the

HELPFUL HINT 7.3
How to Calculate Your Target Heart Rate (THR)

First, calculate your maximum heart rate (MHR):

MHR = 220 − Your age

Perform aerobic exercise at a pace that keeps your heart *below* your MHR. The ideal range is known as the target heart rate (THR). It ranges from 55% to 90% of your maximum heart rate. Calculate your THR as follows:

Low end of THR = MHR × .55
High end of THR = MHR × .9

Here is an example based on a 25 year old:

MHR = 220 − 25 = 195
Low end of THR = 195 × .55 = 107 beats per minute
High end of THR = 195 × .9 = 176 beats per minute

Thus, during aerobic exercise, a 25 year old should reach a THR between 107 and 176 beats per minute.

- How do you check your heart rate to see whether or not you are working in your THR range? While you are exercising vigorously, pause for a moment and take your pulse. It is easiest to feel the pulse at the radial side of your wrist or over a carotid artery beneath your jaw and to the side of the trachea. Count for 15 seconds, and then multiply by 4 to calculate beats per minute.
- When beginning an exercise program, it is wise to work out at the lower end of your THR range. When you gain more experience and feel more fit, you can experiment with working out at a higher THR.

equipment or can purchase one. Purchasing the equipment is a major investment, but buying low-cost models can result in having a piece of equipment that does not meet expectations and/or requires frequent repair. Before purchasing any equipment, try a variety of types and compare various models. The following is a brief comparison of some of the more common pieces of equipment.

- A treadmill is the most popular of all exercise equipment and a logical choice for walkers and runners. A treadmill should have at least a 2.0 horsepower motor and should be rated as a continuous duty motor to constantly provide maximum power. A prospective customer is encouraged to try treadmills to be sure that their width and length accommodates customer's stride. A tall person should select a longer model. Buyers should make sure that the deck of the treadmill gives them adequate cushion to minimize the impact on the feet, ankles, and knees.
- In addition to aerobic training, stair steppers provide low body strength training and allow for both upper and lower body strength training. Before purchasing this type of equipment, the customer should make sure that the ceiling height where the equipment will be used is adequate and the floor can support the weight. Models of steppers/climbers can be costly and vary greatly as to the options they offer, such as the stepping rate and height. Customers should choose a model that provides a stepping height that is comfortable for the knees and ankles. Posture should be kept upright with hands resting lightly on the stationary rails if they are present. Make sure that the legs do the work. Select a rate of workout that slightly raises the pulse rate.
- The elliptical trainer is becoming a very popular machine for cardiorespiratory exercise. These machines provide a low-impact workout that combines the motion of stair stepping with cross-country skiing. Some devices also include poles for moving the arms. Proper fit is extremely important for maintaining a relaxed stride through the individual's normal range of motion. Make sure that the pedals accommodate foot size, that the stride length allows for leg ROM, and that the overall fit is comfortable when the user is in an upright position. When using an elliptical trainer, maintain good posture, don't lean forward, and make sure that the lower body is supporting the majority of the weight.
- Stationary bicycles provide low-impact exercise and come with several options. The upright style is most common, but people who have low back pain should choose the semirecumbent style. The bicycle's adjustment is important; poor adjustment causes discomfort, which is the most common reason that people stop cycling. The saddle should be level with the floor. A saddle pointed up puts pressure on the groin area and pointed down puts too much pressure on the arms and shoulders. Proper saddle height prevents the hips from rocking back and forth when the user is pedaling. Handlebars should be adjusted to allow for a slightly forward-leaning position. A handlebar that is too high puts pressure on a person's seat and one that is too low can cause lower back soreness and arm and shoulder fatigue.
- Rowing machines provide low-impact exercise that gives a total body workout, focusing on the muscles of the arms, abdomen, back, and legs. A good rowing machine mimics the smooth motion of rowing on water. The seat must slide back and forth smoothly and allow for full extension and flexion of the arms and knees. Users should learn proper rowing techniques to prevent back injury. The combination of stroke rate and resistance determines the workout, which can range from fat-burning, aerobic exercise to high-intensity strength training.

Recommendations for Daily Aerobic Exercise

People should select enjoyable aerobic activities and establish a weekly schedule that accommodates three to five workouts ranging from 20 to 60 minutes each. They should monitor their heart rate and keep the activity within the target heart rate range. To be effective, low-intensity workouts should extend for a long period of time. If time is a limiting factor, people should choose a high-intensity workout. People should establish realistic goals and monitor progress for all fitness programs.

The key to a successful program is to make aerobic exercise a fun habit. Many aerobic activities can be done with family, friends, and even pets. Having an exercise partner can increase a person's commitment to the program and provide a social outlet. Instead of looking at the family dog as a "dog with a leash," look at him or her as an "exercise machine." He or she will not forget when it's time to go for the next walk or run! Identify a variety of enjoyable activities and combine the workout with recreation. Great activity choices include:

- Ice skating
- Rollerblading
- Dancing
- Hiking
- Snowshoeing
- Cross-country skiing

People who work out at home should make the area inviting and conducive to success. It should be well lighted and have good ventilation and cooling. Accessories such as TV, stereo, and reading stands can make the workout seem to go faster.

For improving cardiovascular fitness, the exercise session can last continuously (20–60 minutes) or intermittently in sessions of no less than 10 minutes. Scheduled physical activity can supplement with changes in lifestyle choices; walking can be incorporated into daily fitness activities. Some suggestions include:

- Walking to work
- Finding an errand to do each day on foot
- Going for a 15-minute walk for a break instead of taking a coffee or snack break—a midday walk can be rejuvenating
- Unwinding after work with a walk around the neighborhood
- Wearing a pedometer to track the number of steps and set goals to increase it

The recommendation for scheduling strength training and aerobic activity on the same day is to strength train before doing a cardiorespiratory workout. The strength training uses the anaerobic energy system by using creatine phosphate and glucose as fuel. This readily available energy is for short duration activities that don't depend on oxygen. The strength training session can be used to warm up and move into fat burning sooner in the cardiorespiratory workout.

Warm-up and cool-down phases that consist of stretching and light endurance activity should always be part of workout. They provide a psychological adjustment and a physiological transition that reduce the risk for injury. Stretching and light endurance activities should focus on the core and the muscles involved in the workout. The duration of each should be in proportion to the training period but should last for at least 5–10 minutes. Several benefits of warming up follow:

- Increases flow of blood and nutrients to active structures
- Prepares soft tissue and muscles for the activity
- Allows for a gradual increase in metabolic requirements
- Enhances cardiorespiratory performance
- Reduces risk of injury
- Facilitates neural transmission for motor unit recruitment
- Provides screening instrument for potential musculoskeletal problems that could occur at higher intensity

Some of the benefits of the cool-down period are:

- Prevents venous pooling and rapid drop in blood pressure
- Decreases the risk for fainting and/or lightheadedness
- Reduces muscle spasms and cramping
- Helps to flush the metabolic by-products produced during exercise from the muscles

Clothing should be appropriate for comfort, regulation of body core temperature, and foot support. Loose-fitting clothing allows for better ROM. Moisture-wicking clothing and/or layering properly dissipate heat. Avoid rubberized or plastic clothing because they prevent necessary evaporation of perspiration for cooling. Quality footwear appropriate

for the activity cannot be stressed enough. Bodyworkers should remember that they are on their feet for extended periods, so extra care of the feet is essential.

Both strength training and cardiorespiratory exercise are necessary to obtain optimum performance as a bodyworker. This combination results in muscle balance, corrects postural alignment, and decreases risk of injury.

STRETCHING

The incorporation of stretching in a fitness program increases flexibility and ROM and reduces the risk of injury. Flexibility develops and is maintained as a result of a relationship between the musculoskeletal system and the nervous system. Two separate reflex systems are known to operate; the muscle initiates one and the tendon the other. Muscle spindles activate the **stretch reflex** when a muscle is stretched, to keep the muscle within a preset length, and reduce the danger of muscle strain (torn muscle). A sudden or prolonged stretch causes the muscle spindles to trigger the muscle to contract and its antagonist to relax. This sensitivity of the muscle spindles to the stretching of the muscle sets and maintains muscle tone throughout the body. In chronically tight muscles, this set point is off. The second reflex system is the **Golgi tendon reflex**, which can also be referred to as an **inverse stretch reflex**. Upon contraction, muscle tension is transmitted to the tendon and detected by the Golgi tendon organs. Initialization of a signal causes the muscle to relax, preventing unusually high and potentially damaging muscle tension and torn tendons.

A flexible body is less likely to experience pain, stiffness, and repetitive motion injury than a body that is stiff and tight. Thus, by maintaining flexibility, bodyworkers increase career longevity. Working as a massage therapist requires the constant use of muscles that leads to shortened, tightened muscles. The shortening should be reversed and the implementation of a good stretching program can help.

Types of Stretches

Three different types of stretching techniques can increase flexibility. The oldest form is **ballistic stretching**, which is performed with repetitive bouncing movements that work to extend the muscles. However, there is risk for exceeding the extensibility of the muscle leading to muscle injury, especially in sedentary individuals. Highly trained athletes are unlikely to experience that injury, but the risk has made the technique obsolete.

The second form is known as **static stretch**. Hatha yoga is a good example of it. This stretch takes a muscle to a point of comfortable tension and holds it for a designated period of time, usually 15–30 seconds. Maintaining the stretch is important to reset the stretch reflex pattern of tightened muscles. A fundamental rule of static stretching is to avoid overstretching the muscle because this can cause tearing. This safe mode of stretching can be done on a daily basis. The benefit to bodyworkers is to reduce the tension from their workday and maintain and/or increase flexibility.

The last type of stretching is called **proprioceptive neuromuscular facilitation (PNF)**. It was developed in the 1940s as a treatment protocol for patients who were paralyzed to increase their strength, coordination, and flexibility. Static stretching is a simple technique that focuses on tight muscles and operates through the response of the muscle spindle reflex. On the other hand, PNF is a comprehensive approach to working with movement patterns of multiple muscle groups. It consists of various combinations of alternating muscular contractions and stretches such as hold-relax and contract-relax methods. A fundamental tenet of PNF is that the greater the muscle contraction, the greater the relaxation response. This inverse stretch reflex is believed to facilitate a greater stretch of the muscle(s) by using neuromuscular responses involving the Golgi tendon organs and spindle cells. PNF also incorporates the reciprocal action of pairs of agonist and antagonist muscle groups, as in biceps/triceps, which curb the stretch reflex and thus increase flexibility (Voss, Ionta, & Myers, 1985). The muscles contracting in the direction of their shortened state (concentric contraction) is the agonistic pattern, and the muscles approaching their lengthened state (eccentric contraction) are the antagonistic pattern. PNF is used primarily in a rehabilitation setting to improve strength and range of motion but is experiencing widespread popularity. Many bodyworkers incorporate this type of stretching into practice with their clients. PNF is beneficial to people who have postural distortions. PNF can retrain patterns of movement after development of faulty patterns of movement (weakness, incoordination, joint immobility, and muscle tightness). We recommend that people who have a physical disability consult a professional for PNF treatment.

Recommendations for Stretches

The goal of a stretching program should be to improve the flexibility of the musculotendinous unit surrounding a joint, thereby increasing its ROM. Performing either static or PNF stretches one to three times a day at a minimum of 3 days a week helps to achieve this goal. The number of stretches performed and the number of days of stretching should be directly related to the restrictions surrounding a particular joint. A tight joint requires more attention: more reps more frequently. Stretching is safe to do on a daily basis.

People can have differences in flexibility on each side of the body. Usually, the dominant side is more flexible than the nondominant side. Also, females are generally more flexible than males. Many other factors can affect flexibility, such as environmental temperature, age, injury, and muscle mass.

Watching for hypermobility while performing a stretching routine is important. **Hypermobility** is excessive movement around a joint as a result of overstretching the

musculotendinous unit and from too much stretching and/or a lack of strength around a particular joint. This can lead to joint instability and dislocation. People who have hypermobility should refrain from stretching those areas and modify their movements to prevent extending into the hypermobile position.

USING SUGGESTED STRENGTHENING AND STRETCHING EXERCISES BY BODY AREA

A tailored exercise program must consider the individual's current physical condition and sets reasonable goals for increasing cardiovascular fitness, muscle strength, and flexibility. It will simultaneously help the person to achieve and maintain a healthy weight.

Before designing an exercise program, people should evaluate their posture to identify any of the distortions covered in Chapter 4. The program should include strengthening and stretching exercises to correct any distortions they notice and to prevent developing them. The most common for bodyworkers include hyperextended knees, forward pelvis, kyphosis, lordosis, elevated shoulders, protracted shoulders, hyperextended wrists, flexed wrists, and forward head. Problems with these areas usually result from weak, overstretched, or inflexible muscles around the body area in question. See Table 7.2 ■ for a summary of the PDs common to bodyworkers and specific exercises to stretch and strengthen these areas. A variety of methods can strengthen muscles (i.e., free weights, machines, and exercise bands). A variety of exercises can be beneficial both mentally and physically. Each individual should find a particular combination that works best for her or him and that keeps her or him interested in the activity. See Helpful Hint 7.4 for ways to improve program success. Below we discuss a few exercises that will help the area involved, with some precautions noted. Keep in mind, however, that a large number of exercises can be done to work the same area. It is wise to change the routine often to work the muscle in new ways and also to avoid boredom. Refer to Worksheet 7.1 for a checklist for developing a fitness plan and to Worksheet 7.2, a one-week exercise log that can be photocopied for developing a fitness plan and tracking its activities.

Arms

Bodyworkers subject their arms, wrists, and hands to a variety of physical stresses. Any repetitive or forceful motion is potentially harmful; therefore, stretching and strengthening the arms are important. The following sample exercises are helpful in starting a program.

1. *Hand and wrist flexor stretching:* Stretch the arms by interlacing the fingers while the arms/hands face out at shoulder height. Press the hands forward. Hold for 20–30 seconds and repeat two or three times. This stretches flexors, wrist, and hands. Precaution: People

TABLE 7.2   Exercises for PDs Common to Bodyworkers

Area of Concern	Potential Causes	Muscle Areas for Focus and Action Needed	Stretches/Exercises
Hyperextended knees	Weak or overstretched calf/hamstring muscles; tight quadriceps	Strengthen gastrocnemius, soleus, hamstrings	Toe raise; heel raise; hamstring curl
Anterior tilt	Tight low back or weak abdominals	Maintain neutral spine while working; stretch low back/hamstrings; strengthen abs	Bridges; low back stretches; hamstring stretch; abdominal curls
Posterior tilt	Tight hamstrings or weak low back and abdominals	Stretch hamstrings; strengthen low back and abdominal musculature	Hamstring stretch; bridges; abdominal curls
Lateral tilt (lumbar)	Tight and/or weak quadratus lumborum; tight and/or weak transverse abdominals	Focus on either stretching or strengthening affected muscle group	Lateral flexion stretch; weighted lateral flexion for strength
Kyphosis	Forward head posture; weak rhomboids and trapezius muscles; tight pectoralis muscles	Stretch the posterior neck musculature; strengthen upper back; stretch chest	Chin tucks; seated and upright rows; lateral pull downs; wall stretch
Lordosis	Tight low back extensor and/or hip flexor muscles; tight lumbar fascia; overstretched/weak abdominals	Maintain neutral spine; stretch low back and hip muscles; tighten abdominals	Bridges; hamstring stretch; hip flexor stretch; knees to one side stretch; abdominal curls; reverse curls
Elevated shoulders	Tight trapezius; deltoid; levator scapulae muscles	Stretch and strengthen to keep them flexible and able to handle high demand	Trap; deltoid; levator scapula stretches; shoulder shrugs; upright row; shoulder abduction; shoulder extension
Protracted shoulders	Short chest musculature; lengthened upper back muscles	Stretch pectoralis; strengthen rhomboids and trapezius	Standing wall stretch; seated/upright row
Hyperextended wrist/flexed wrist	Fatigued wrist extensors; shortened/tight extensors; lengthened wrist flexors	Maintain neutral wrist position; strengthen wrist flexors and extensors; stretch wrist extensors/flexors	Wrist extensor/flexor strengthening to prevent fatigue; flexor strengthening to help shortening; forearm stretching
Forward head posture	Shortened muscles on the anterior neck; lengthened posterior neck musculature; possible cervical nerve impingement	Stretch SCM and scalenes; strengthen upper trapezius; scalenes; paraspinals	Chin tuck and isometrics for all head positions
Lateral tilt (cervical)	Tight scalenes or upper trapezius	Stretch affected muscle group	Scalene and/or upper trapezius stretch

SCM = Sternocleidomastoid muscle.

HELPFUL HINT 7.4

Tips for Success in an Exercise Program

People are naturally social and habitual. They seek enjoyment and variety and work well toward realistic goals and rewards. Therefore, to have a successful exercise program:

- Vary the modes of exercise and type of equipment you use.
- Pick activities you enjoy.

- Exercise with a partner or join a class.
- Pick a specific time and day for the activity.
- Set realistic, achievable goals for yourself.
- Reward yourself when you meet a goal.

who are prone to wrist hyperextension shouldn't do this activity. See Figure 7.4 ■.

2. *Forearm, wrist, and hand strengthening:* Grasp a broomstick with a rope and with a 2-pound weight attached to it. With elbows at the sides, flex the forearms to 90 degrees and use the hands to wind the weight up the rope with a flex action of the wrist until it reaches the broomstick. Reversing the action: Repeat this two to three times. Precaution: Keep the arms close to the body to stay within the safe zones. This exercise is good for addressing hyperextension. See Figure 7.5 ■.

Upper Back and Neck

The nature of bodywork puts practitioners at risk for protraction of the head, which stresses the neck and creates upper back tension. Working at a computer or doing desk work of any kind also promotes head protraction. The following activities help with neck and upper back tension.

1. *Neck stretch:* Stand or sit with the head centered and as neutral as possible. Slowly lower the chin *toward* the chest. Hold for 20–30 seconds and return to neutral. Precaution: Don't force the chin *to* the chest. For lateral neck tension, begin with the head centered and slowly lower the ear toward the shoulder. Hold for 20–30 seconds and return to neutral. Repeat on the opposite side. See Figure 7.6 ■.

2. *Contract-relax neck stretch:* Do the exercises in (1), but apply resistance with the hand/arm pressing against the forehead while slowly tucking the chin toward the chest. Repeat two to three times, holding 20–30 seconds, and notice the gradual increase in range of motion by the third stretch. See Figure 7.7 ■.

3. *Diagonal raise:* Work to strengthen the trapezius and latissimus dorsi muscles by lying in the prone position with legs straight and together but not locking the

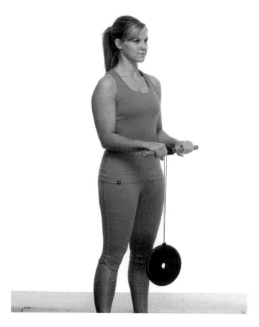

FIGURE 7.5

Secure a weight to the middle of a broomstick or dowel with strong twine or a small rope; make sure the twine or rope is tightly secured. Hold the stick at each end with your elbows at your side and your arms flexed 90°. Rotate the stick to wind the rope and move the weight upward, then rotate the stick to unwind the rope and lower the weight. This works the flexors of the forearms during both concentric and eccentric contraction.

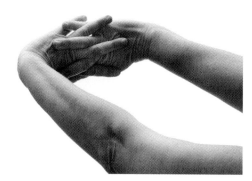

FIGURE 7.4

After interlacing your fingers, rotate your hands so that the palms face outward. Stretch your arms outward to stretch the flexors of the hand and wrist.

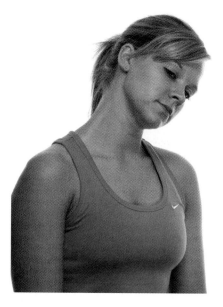

FIGURE 7.6

The photo demonstrates the proper alignment for a lateral stretch. A slow lowering of the head and maintaining the stretch lengthens the muscle on the opposite side and reprograms the stretch reflex of the muscle.

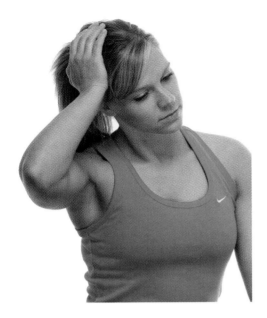

FIGURE 7.7

Stretching the neck against resistance as demonstrated triggers the Golgi tendon receptors of the flexor muscles which in turn causes relaxation of the muscle.

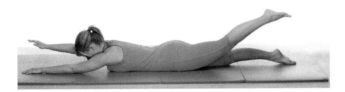

FIGURE 7.8

Lie on your stomach with arms outstretched and legs parallel and not braced. Raise the diagonal arm and leg, starting with the right arm and left leg, slowly to a comfortable position. Lower the limbs slowly, and then repeat with the left arm and right leg.

knees. Slowly lift the right arm and the left leg from the floor. Slowly, lower them to the starting position. Switch limbs and repeat the exercise. Count 2–3 seconds to lift. Do 8 to 15 reps for each pair. Precaution: Lifting too high can cause back strain. See Figure 7.8 ■.

Chest

Bodyworkers' pectoral muscles are often tight as a result of the forward position required of their hands and arms while working. The necessity of this position for many of the stroke applications causes the muscle fibers to shorten. The wall stretch exercises should help. Bodyworkers should stand beside a wall and place their arm/hand behind them on the wall, palm side down. If they feel the stretch in their pectoral muscle and anterior deltoid, they should hold this for

20–30 seconds and repeat two or three times. If they don't feel much of a stretch, they should then slowly turn their torso away from the wall while maintaining their arm/hand and shoulder beside the wall. Precaution: Bodyworkers who have a shoulder injury should not do this exercise. See Figure 7.9 ■.

Shoulders

Shoulder protraction is common among bodyworkers because of the forward motions of their work. This creates shortened chest muscles and lengthens the upper back muscles. They can use the wall stretch exercise for the anterior deltoid. Refer to the exercise for the chest. A good shoulder strengthening exercise includes these steps:

1. *Front barbell raises:* With a barbell in each hand, stand with the feet shoulder wide and the knees slight flexed to protect the low back. Use a weight that can be comfortably raised. Pull in the abdominal muscles to further protect the back. Raise one barbell at a time slowly. Do two to three sets of 8–12 repetitions. If you do not have barbells, make your own weights by using a half gallon milk or juice jug partially filled with sand or water. See Figure 7.10 ■.

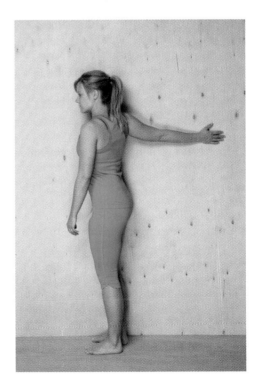

FIGURE 7.9

Stand perpendicular to a wall with your arm at your side and your palm flat on the wall. Slide your arm behind you, keeping the palm flat to produce a stretch of the pectoral muscles. You may increase the stretch if necessary by keeping that position and rotating the torso away from the wall.

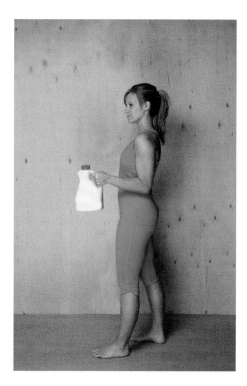

FIGURE 7.10

Adjust the weight of a juice jug with either sand or water with what you can lift for 8–12 reps (8–12 RM load). Hold the jug by the handle with arm down and forearm extended. Flex the forearm, raising the jug with a count of "1, 2," and then lower the jug with a count of "1, 2, 3, 4." Repeat for the recommended number of repetitions.

2. *Plank pose:* To work the shoulders and build core abdominal strength, lie in the prone position, place the arms ulnar surface down, and clasp the hands, forming a triangle. Slowly, raise the body off the floor, keeping it flat to look like a plank or board perched on the toes and forearms. See Figure 7.11 ■. Hold for 15 seconds and repeat three times. Build the time to 1 minute. Precaution: Keep the abdominals contracted to prevent low back sway (lordosis), and keep the elbows under the shoulder joints to avoid strain.

Abdominals

The sedentary lifestyle common in society is a major reason for weak abdominal muscles. Prolonged sitting also contributes to shortened, hypertonic hip flexors, mainly the iliopsoas. Strengthening the abdominals will help correct or prevent abnormal pelvic tilts.

Many aerobic activities, including brisk walking, jogging, and cross-country skiing, are excellent for strengthening the core body muscles including the abdominals. On the other hand, isometric abdominal exercise can be performed intermittently throughout the day in a daily routine. For isometric activity to be effective, it should start with an exhale

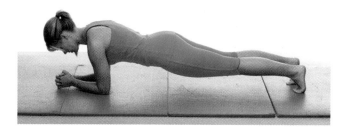

FIGURE 7.11

Begin by lying prone. Raise your head and chest and slide your arms under you so that you are resting on your ulnar surfaces. Clasp your hands to form a triangle. Dorsiflex your feet so that you are resting on your toes. Raise your body upon exhalation so that your body is straight like a plank, resting on your toes and forearms. Hold for a minimum of 15 seconds while breathing. Lower and repeat.

and mentally focus on the lower abdominals to slowly pull them as tight possible. Hold for several seconds and then relax. During this time, breathe to remain relaxed and to be able to hold the contraction longer. Work up to 10 repetitions and/or repeat several times a day.

Abdominal crunches (i.e., sit-ups) are the best known of the abdominal workouts, but they must be done with caution. Straight leg sit-ups should not be done because they develop the hip flexors rather than the intended abdominal muscles. Overdeveloping the hip flexors actually contributes to lordosis and low back problems, which are already common PDs for bodyworkers. Double leg raises are also not a good choice for the same reason. These exercises should be modified in the following ways to be more beneficial.

1. *Abdominal crunch with flexed knees:* Lie on the floor with the knees flexed. One way to do this is to support the lower legs on a low chair seat or footrest while lying on the floor (Figure 7.12 ■). The thighs should be perpendicular to the torso, and hip flexors should be relaxed. Keep the hands beside the head or resting on the shoulders to avoid thrusting them forward. Flex the torso to slowly raise the shoulders off the floor as far as possible without flexing the neck. The amount of movement should be less than 30 degrees with the spine flexing and the pelvis stationary. Avoid flexing

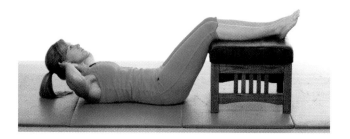

FIGURE 7.12

Lie supine with your lower legs supported by a low bench or stool. With your hands at your shoulders or alongside your head, raise your torso while maintaining neutral alignment.

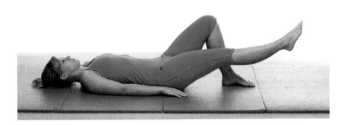

FIGURE 7.13

Lie supine with your legs straight. Bend one knee, keeping the sole flat on the floor, and raise the opposite leg up to 8 inches off the floor. Hold, lower, relax, and repeat at least 5 times. Reverse your position and repeat with the other leg.

the neck in an attempt to pull the shoulders up. The rectus abdomininis is efficiently worked with this activity.

2. *Cross knee crunch:* This exercise works the obliques. Start with the same position as for the abdominal crunch, but do the crunch diagonally as if you were attempting to touch each shoulder to the opposite hip. As you crunch, both the shoulder and the opposite hip will rise off the floor. Avoid pressing the leg against the chair to raise the hip.

3. *Single straight leg raise:* The straight leg raise will strengthen both the abdominals and legs, but do only one leg at a time. Lie on your back with one knee bent with the sole of the foot flat on the floor. Keep the other leg straight and slowly raise it 8 inches off the floor (Figure 7.13 ■). Hold for 5 seconds and slowly lower and relax. Initially start with five reps. Repeat with the other leg.

Lower Back and Hips

Exercise routines developed to prevent or rehabilitate low back pain target the abdominal, back, and hip muscles. When performing back exercises, doing them slowly and stopping any activity that causes pain to the back are important, especially for people who have a history of injury or pain. Also note that swimming, which is an aerobic exercise, is excellent for strengthening the back.

Back-strengthening exercises include the following:

1. *Wall squats:* Stand with the back against a wall and the feet 12–14 inches from the wall. Keeping abdominal muscles tight, slide down into a crouch with the knees bent at 90 degrees while keeping the lower back straight (Figure 7.14 ■). Count to five and slide back up. Keeping the lower back straight and against the wall rather than arched works the erector spinae muscles effectively.

2. *Prone leg raises:* Lying on the stomach, tighten the abdominal muscles, and raise one leg approximately 8 inches off the floor while keeping it straight (Figure 7.15 ■). Hold to a count of 10 and lower the leg (remember eccentric contractions). Do the same routine with the other leg. Repeat 5 to 10 times depending on the level of fitness.

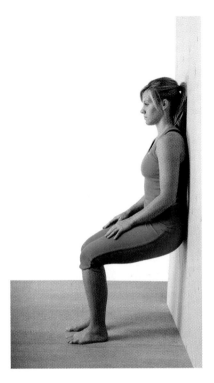

FIGURE 7.14

Stand with your back against a wall. Slide into a crouch with your knees bent 90°. Hold for a count of 5, then slide back up the wall and repeat.

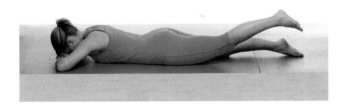

FIGURE 7.15

Lie prone, tighten your abdominal muscles, and raise one leg approximately 8 inches off the floor while keeping it straight. Hold for a count of 10, lower, relax, and repeat with the other leg.

Stretching exercises are best accomplished by stabilizing the body and focusing the mind on stretching the muscle or body area. The stretch should be controlled, so care needs to be taken with exercises in which gravity can have an effect, such as the toe touch from a standing position. Remember that stretching too rapidly actually elicits a reflex contraction in the muscle and that a stretch that is not maintained long enough will not allow the muscle to conform to the new length. Maintaining this for less then 15 seconds is not helpful. About 20–30 seconds is considered the minimal stretch time. Stretching exercises include the following:

1. *Lumbar and gluteal stretch:* Lie on the back on a padded floor or mat. First pull the knees to the chest and flex the upper torso and head to roll up into a ball

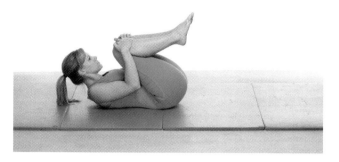

FIGURE 7.16

Lie supine and roll into a ball by pulling your knees to your chest and flexing your upper torso and head until your feel a comfortable stretch in the lumbar area. Hold for 20 seconds and relax.

(Figure 7.16 ■) until you feel a comfortable stretch in the lumbar area. Hold for 20 seconds and then relax. Follow this by lying on the back and flexing one leg. Cross the other leg over the flexed leg with the ankle slightly above the knee (Figure 7.17 ■). Clasp the hands around the flexed leg above the knee. Pull the knee toward the chest to stretch the gluteal muscles on the side of the crossed leg and hold for at least 20 seconds. Relax and then reverse the leg positions and repeat.

2. *Psoas stretch:* Stand facing a wall with the hands against it and the elbows slightly flexed. To stretch the right psoas, place the left leg in front of you and slide the right leg directly behind you to a position that you can comfortably stretch. As you shift your lower body forward, push your upper body backward with your

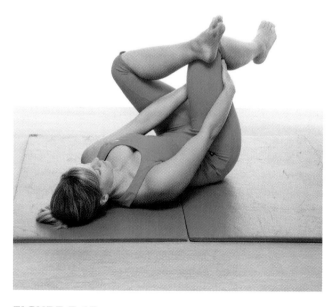

FIGURE 7.17

Lie supine; flex one leg and cross the other leg with the ankle slightly above the knee. Clasp your hands behind the flexed leg and pull the knee toward the chest. Hold for at least 20 seconds, relax, and repeat on the other side.

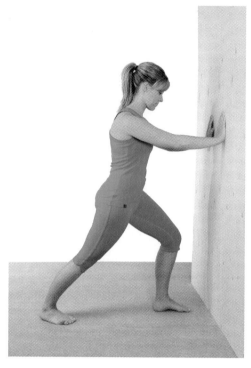

FIGURE 7.18

Stand facing a wall with your palms against the wall. Stretch one leg back and shift your lower body forward while you push your upper body backward to achieve a stretch of the psoas of the outward stretched leg.

arms (Figure 7.18 ■). When you feel a good stretch of the psoas of the outstretched leg, hold for 20–30 seconds. Repeat for the left leg.

Legs

A program of leg exercises should be designed to achieve a balance of strength and flexibility. In regard to PDs, recall that hyperextended knees can result from either weak or overstretched hamstrings or tight quadriceps. The condition of the thigh muscles also affects the back, especially in the case of tight hamstring, which pulls on the pelvis so that stretching the hamstrings not only loosens the leg muscle but also reduces strain on the back. The following are samples of strengthening and stretching exercises for the legs.

1. *Supine hamstring stretch:* This stretch can be worked into the routine described earlier for floor stretches. While lying on the back with both legs bent, grasp one thigh with both hands behind the knee. Straighten the leg slowly until you feel a full stretch to the hamstrings (Figure 7.19 ■). Hold for 20–30 seconds, relax, and repeat with other leg.
2. *Hamstring curl:* This exercise is often done with an exercise machine but can be accomplished using ankle weights. Lie in a prone position. Flex one leg at a time for 10–20 repetitions (Figure 7.20 ■). Repeat with the other leg.

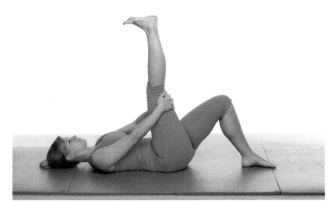

FIGURE 7.19

Lie supine with both knees flexed. Grasp the back of one thigh and extend that leg into a stretch. Hold for up to 30 seconds, relax, and repeat with the other leg.

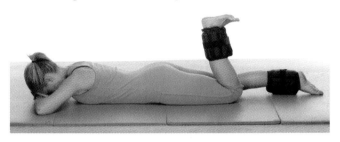

FIGURE 7.20

Attach ankle weights. In a prone position, flex one leg at a time for up to 20 reps. Repeat with the other leg.

3. *Heel and toe raise:* Stand with equal weight distributed between both feet. Slowly rise, transferring the weight to the balls of the feet, elevating the heels. Then lower back down. Repeat 10 times. Follow this by a series of toe rises. As you raise your toes, your weight will be transferred to your heels. To do this slowly and keep your balance at first, you could need support by keeping a hand on a wall or chair.

Tips for Success

Whether individuals work out at home, join a fitness club, hire a personal trainer, or do a combination, they should stay with their program plan to give it time to become a habit. Everyone has had the experience of jumping into a new activity with enthusiasm but finding that after a few days, normal daily demands may call into question whether the time or energy to stay with the activity is available. People should set their goals, give themselves at least 3 weeks to establish a new habit. Those who "drop-out," shouldn't give up but redirect themselves to their goals. They should award themselves as they make progress. In time, as fitness improves, they will feel better, have more energy, and better-fitting clothes, and others will begin to notice the changes and make positive comments. Those are the best awards of all!

CHAPTER SUMMARY

- An exercise program should incorporate elements of strength training, muscle endurance, cardiovascular endurance, and stretching.
- Before starting an exercise program check, people who are over 35 years of age or have underlying health concerns should consult their physician.
- Strength training helps maintain muscle tone and muscle balance to prevent PDs as well as improve the ability to do physical tasks.
- Muscle strengthening can be accomplished through isometric or isotonic contractions, but for increased strength over time, the force generated should continually increase.

- Aerobic exercise improves health of the cardio-respiratory systems and the tone of core muscles. It also assists in weight control. Effective cardiovascular activity requires maintaining a target heart rate for a period of 20–60 minutes three to five times per week.
- Flexibility improves range of motion and reduces injury from repetitive motion. Static stretching and PNF are the recommended stretching techniques.
- When designing an exercise program, people should consider their health history, physical condition, and any identified PDs.

REVIEW QUESTIONS

1. Increased muscle tone and force are achieved through _____ training.
2. Stretching results in increased muscle _____.
3. A muscle contraction during which the length of the muscle stays the same but the force in the muscle increases is known as:
   a. concentric contraction
   b. eccentric contraction
   c. isometric contraction
   d. positive contraction
4. The calculation of an individual's heart rate is based on:
   a. age
   b. physical condition
   c. weight
   d. height
5. The presence of which of the following indicate(s) the need to consult a physician before starting an exercise program?
   a. family history of early stroke or heart attacks
   b. dizziness
   c. joint problems
   d. all the above
6. True or False? One day of rest should be taken after strength training for a given area of the body.
7. True or False? Ballistic stretching is the most recommended form of stretching.
8. Name and compare the three types of stretching techniques.
9. Explain why rapid overstretching of a muscle is detrimental.
10. List three general activities that are important components of a fitness program.

REFERENCES

American College of Sports Medicine. (2010). *ACMS's guidelines for exercise testing and prescription* (6th ed.). Philadelphia: Lippincott Williams & Wilkins.

Voss, E. D., Ionta, K. M., & Myers, J. B. (1985). *Proprioceptive neuromuscular facilitation patterns and techniques* (3rd ed.). Philadelphia: Harper & Row.

SUGGESTED READINGS AND WEBSITES

American College of Sports Medicine. (2010). Retrieved September 10, 2010, from http://www.acsm.org

American Heart Association. (2006). Tips for exercise success. Retrieved January 24, 2006, from http://www.americanheart.org

Arnheim, D. D., & Prentice, W. E. (1993). *Principles of athletic training* (8th ed.). St Louis: Mosby.

Beil, A. (2001). *Trail guide to the body* (2nd ed.). Boulder, CO: Books of Discovery.

Fritz, S., Paholsky Maison, K., & Grosenbach, J. M. (1999). *Mosby's basic science for soft tissue and movement therapies*. St. Louis: Mosby.

Centers for Disease Control and Prevention. (2006). Physical activity for everyone. Retrieved April 1, 2006, from http://www.cdc.gov/nccdphp/dnpa/physical/activity/everyone/guidelines/index.html

Consumer Reports. (2006). Health and fitness. Retrieved February 5, 2006, from http://www.consumerreports.org/health/healthy-living/healthyliving.html

Golding, L. A. (2000). *YMCA fitness testing and assessment manual* (4th ed.). Champaign, IL: Human Kinetics.

Howley, E. T., & Franks, B. D. (2003). *Health and fitness instructor's handbook* (4th ed.). Champaign, IL: Human Kinetics.

Nicholas Institute of Sports Medicine and Athletic Trauma. (2005). Low back exercise program. Retrieved August 14, 2005, from http://www.nismat.org/orthocor/programs/lowback.html

President's Council on Physical Fitness and Sports. (2005). Fitness fundamental—Guidelines to personal exercise programs. Retrieved August 2, 2005, from http://www.fitness.gov/fitness.html

U.S. Department of Health & Human Services. (2006). Small step program. Retrieved April 1, 2006, from http://www.smallstep.gov

Voss, E. D., Ionta, K. M., & Myers, J. B. (1985). *Proprioceptive neuromuscular facilitation patterns and techniques* (3rd ed.). Philadelphia: Harper & Row.

Zatsiorsky, V. M. (1995). *Science and practice of strength training.* Champaign, IL: Human Kinetics.

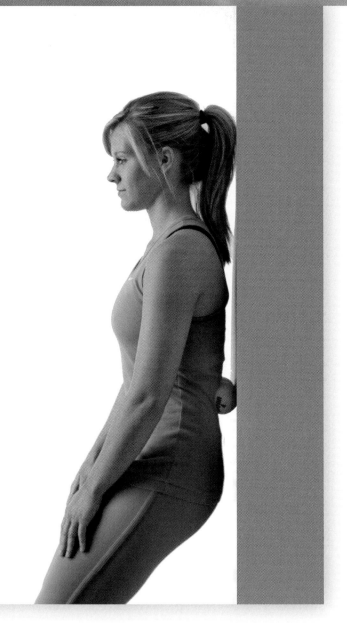

Self-Care: Self-Massage

 CHAPTER OUTLINE

General Benefits of Self-Massage

Overview of Techniques

Self-Massage Techniques for Specific Body Regions

Chapter Summary

Review Questions

LEARNING OBJECTIVES

Upon successful completion of the chapter, you will be able to:

1. Recognize and explain the benefits of self-massage.
2. Identify and select the appropriate technique for the different conditions: ischemia, hypertonicity, tension, pain, adhesion, and inflammation.
3. Identify tools and their uses and limitations.
4. Distinguish the value and use of hot and cold treatments.

5. Discuss the efficacy of topical treatment.
6. Identify useful techniques for body region most applicable for your needs.
7. Apply various treatments on yourself to relieve muscle conditions while maintaining good ergonomic technique.

KEY TERMS

As health care providers, we focus on the relief of discomfort of our clients by applying our specialty, be it massage, energy work, or other modalities. This chapter focuses on how we can perform these modalities on ourselves, with the primary focus being self-massage. It reviews the benefits of various massage techniques and how they can be self-delivered. The challenge of this self-care is applying it ergonomically correctly. The discussion emphasizes how to accomplish this by suggesting tools that many practitioners would not necessarily use in their everyday practice with their clients.

GENERAL BENEFITS FOR SELF-MASSAGE

As professionals in the field of bodywork, you are acutely aware of the overall benefits of body therapies, but many therapists don't take time to take advantages of these therapies for themselves. Self-massage cannot substitute for a professionally delivered massage for thoroughness and relaxation, but it is a practice that can provide immediate care. Whether you are doing reflexology, energy work, the Swedish technique, Yamuna body rolling, or neuromuscular techniques, the benefits of self-massage (see Table 8.1 ■) are many: It eases the aches and pains of everyday life, changes negative patterns by reeducating muscle memory, prevents injuries from overuse, reduces scar tissue, and restores balance. Regular use of massage techniques can help prevent muscles from becoming hypertonic and help maintain good circulation to prevent the development of postural distortions (PDs). On the other hand, if you have an established PD associated with muscle imbalance, such as protracted shoulders, which is common for massage therapists, a combination of professional massage and self-massage can be used to restore and maintain normal muscle balance.

TABLE 8.1	General Benefits of Massage
1.	Massage brings about improved nutrition and increases cellular activity (i.e., metabolism) and blood supply to the organs of locomotion: muscles, ligaments, and bones.
2.	Massage increases circulation; the contractions of the heart become more complete and forceful, developing the heart muscle, and the blood pressure in the veins are reduced which in turn reacts beneficially on the heart and arterial circulation.
3.	Massage develops the respiratory muscles, increasing the mobility of the chest and promoting lung expansion.
4.	Massage stimulates the organs of elimination (i.e., skin, lungs, and kidneys) to increased activity.
5.	As a result of the increased circulation with massage, the brain and nervous system also receive an increased supply of blood, and thus increasing their vital activities.

A significant advantage of self-massage is that we know immediately the efficacy of each stroke or movement and can adjust the location, direction, or pressure to gain the greatest benefit. As a therapist, you are aware of the importance of communication with your client so that you can provide a good massage. When the client is yourself, you are in immediate control.

Self-massage is nothing new. We all have an innate, unconscious response to rub or apply pressure to an area of the body that is sore, tired, or overused. If you watch others, you probably have often observed this behavior, for example rubbing the palm of the hand following prolonged manual activity.

The recommendations and techniques described in this chapter provide a more deliberate and planned approach to self-massage. Short periods of massage inserted throughout the day will be beneficial for excessively tired muscles. Such massage also helps to restore balance between antagonistic pairs of muscles by relaxing the hypertonic muscle. The palpation of muscles makes us more aware of those prone to hypertonicity. This helps us to become aware of our inner awareness of our body and improve our ability to maintain a more neutral balance in our posture and motion.

OVERVIEW OF TECHNIQUES

Techniques we include here are only a few of those that can be applied as self-massage. The two emphasized are Swedish massage and neuromuscular techniques, which are more familiar and are the mainstay of many massage programs throughout the country. In addition, we selected modalities that are easily performed while maintaining good body mechanics and have identified tools to help target specific areas. The chapter provides an overview of the terminology and general descriptions of techniques and modalities in the event that you are not familiar with them.

Swedish Massage

Swedish massage, developed by Per Henrik Ling at the turn of the nineteenth century, is perhaps the most popular form. D. Baloti Lawrence and Lewis Harrison (1983) described the Swedish technique as an exercise regimen that includes bending, stretching, flexing, and rotating the muscles and joints to stimulate circulation. It contains 47 positions and over 800 movements. In Swedish massage, the practitioner imitates these exercise positions by using kneading, stroking, friction, tapping, and sometimes shaking or vibrating parts of the body. These modalities, also known as *medical gymnastics* or strokes, can stimulate or relax the body. The Swedish strokes and their physiological effects are identified below. These strokes can be applied individually; however, they are most effective when administered sequentially.

Effleurage is a long superficial or deep stroke, usually used with the entire palm of the hand but can be done by using the ulnar surface, olecranon, and the fist. It increases circulation and blood flow to the area. It is relaxing and aids sleep.

Petrissage uses small circular movements to stimulate muscle structure in circumscribed areas to bring nutrients (i.e., blood) to the area and can be applied with fingers, thumbs, and elbows.

A *friction stroke* stimulates heavy muscle structure and areas around bony prominences. The hands can go in a clockwise motion, like kneading, or back and forth. Friction brings more nutrients to the muscle and increases cellular and nerve activity. This stroke helps to break down adhesions and relieve **stasis,** which is stagnation of the fluid flow in the tissue.

Tapotement is a percussive stroke applied in rapid succession. It can be administered in many ways such as hacking, tapping, clapping, and cupping. It is beneficial for increasing blood to an area that is **ischemic,** which is a lack of blood supply to the tissues as a result of vasoconstriction or local obstruction to arterial flow. This technique stimulates muscles and soothes or stimulates nerves, depending on how it is used. Moderate percussion (tapotement) increases the excitability of the nerves and is an excellent way to stimulate sluggish sensory or motor nerves. When applied for local purposes, follow with kneading to prevent soreness and inflammation of the superficial tissues. Prolonged use can cause dilation of the blood vessels. This stroke can remove or produce **hyperemia,** an increased amount of blood in any part of the body.

Tapotement is used to drive the blood out of parts that can't be reached by other procedures; it is valuable for flushing a region with blood as a means of enhancing the resorptive effects of kneading and other manipulations promoting circulation. Different surfaces of the hand are useful and recommended for the desired result.

- Use the palms of the hands in a cupped shape (cupping) for cutaneous (surface) vessels.
- Use the ulnar surface for deeper vessels.
- Use a clenched fist for heavy muscles such as quadriceps.

Vibration is a trembling motion applied to the tissues and can be performed using the palm of the hand, fingers, ulna, and fist. This movement stimulates the nervous system via nerve centers. It can be applied to any part of the body (such as over the abdomen to stimulate peristalsis of the colon) to stimulate nerve and muscle activity.

A *nerve stroke* is a light feathery stroke applied away from the heart with the fingertips to both soothe the nerve endings in the skin and relax the nervous system.

Neuromuscular Technique

Neuromuscular technique (NMT) is often synonymous with deep tissue massage. Like most of today's body-centered therapies, NMT has ties to ancient times. It can be traced back to the eighth century A.D. and has ties to India, China, Korea, and Japan in the form of **Shiatsu.** Some of the modern day gurus of NMT are Dr. Janet Travell, Dr. David G. Simons, Dr. Leon Chaitow, Bonnie Prudden, and Paul St. John.

The three primary strokes used in neuromuscular technique are fascia release, cross-fiber, and trigger point. They can be used sequentially or individually but are more effective when used sequentially. Start with a fascia release stroke to help determine where the trigger points are, and then apply a cross-fiber stroke to break down the adhesions and follow-up by isolating the trigger point(s). It is good to end with a light nerve stroke to soothe the nerve endings, which is part of the Swedish protocol and is a nice ending to techniques that are more invasive.

The physiological basis of NMT is that it triggers neurotransmitter release by neurons. Neurotransmitters are the chemical agents released by a neuron upon excitation, which then crosses the synapse or in this case, the motor end plate for the stimulation of muscle fibers.

Fascia release is similar to effleurage in that it is usually a long stroke commonly applied the length and direction of the muscle fibers. It is very effective with ischemic tissue and is the precursor to trigger point work. Ischemia is reduced blood flow to a tissue causing it to be in an oxygen-deprived state (**hypoxia**). It can be pathological as in a narrowing of the arteries, or anatomical, such as the typical lower vascularity of some muscles as in the supraspinatus. It can also result from trigger points, which we will discuss shortly. The fingers, thumbs, and elbow can be used to lengthen restricted fascia, increase blood flow, help restore balance to opposing muscles, and help to determine the location of trigger points.

Cross-fiber is most beneficial if you are trying to break up scar tissue, adhesions, or ease and alleviate muscular tension. This is applied by crossing the direction of the muscle fibers at a right angle as shown in Figure 8.1 ■. Fingers, thumbs, ulnar surface, and tools can be used.

A *trigger point* is a spot that demonstrates any of the following signs: tenderness, change in temperature from

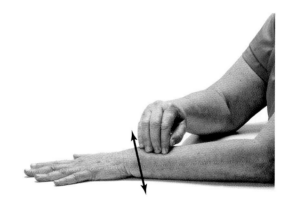

FIGURE 8.1

The cross-fiber stroke is perpendicular to the direction of the muscle fibers as shown by the arrows.

the surrounding area, or adhesion. It develops as a result of injury, disease, repetitive motion, and emotional trauma or can be birth related as with the use of forceps during child delivery. Trigger points can be electrical (amplified input to the spinal cord) or chemical (cellular waste) in nature. Travell and Simons' *Myofascial Pain and Dysfunction: The Trigger Point Manual,* published in 1983 by Williams and Wilkens is one of the most definitive resources on the study of trigger points. Microtrauma and/or muscle overuse leads to a pain-spasm cycle. The excessive amounts of acetycholine (ACh) released by the somatic nervous system leads to hypertonicity and calcium overload within the myofibers. The muscle tension restricts blood flow and results in ischemia. Trigger point therapy is performed by applying pressure to the points with your knuckle, elbow, thumb, or a tool. The theory behind the efficacy of trigger point work is that the isolated point is deprived of oxygen for the duration that the point is held, usually 8–12 seconds. Upon releasing the point, a cascade of impulses occurs, causing vasodilation and restoring blood flow to the area. It also leads to the release of endorphins and enkephalins that reduce or eliminate the pain. Both are endogenous opioid compounds or natural painkillers (analgesics), which give you a sense of well-being.

It is important to follow up NMT with stretching to allow the muscles to maintain the benefits of the work. Refer to Chapter 7 on exercise and stretching to review the stretches most beneficial for your needs.

Energy Work

The field of energy work is vast today and includes Reiki, Shiatsu, Shen, healing touch, Qi Qong, polarity, and therapeutic touch. In reality anytime someone touches someone else, an exchange of energy occurs. All energy work systems begin with the premise that a flow of life-giving energy circulates throughout the body. Some refer to this flow as *Ki, Qi, Prana,* or *Chi.* Energy can be thought of as life force. The flow or current of energy moving through our bodies at any given time can easily become distorted by everything from our thoughts, our body mechanics while we are working, accidents, to disease. Energy work is a great way for practitioners to recharge themselves between clients or at the end of their day.

Energy work can be administered on areas of the body easily reached by laying on of hands to send healing energy to the specific site. Props, such as pillows, towels, and blankets, can support the hands and arms to maintain neutrality while holding the site. An alternative approach that provides an ergonomic benefit is the use of positive thoughts. These thoughts can be projected to deliver healing energy to the area. We can't adequately emphasize the mind/body connection and its value in any type of bodywork.

The section on tools explores some tools and equipment that direct energy to areas such as the Infratonic™ Chi machine. It and other tools can make doing energy work easier, but props could be necessary.

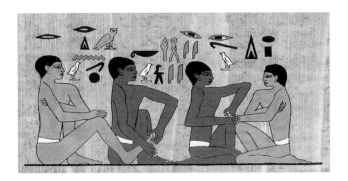

FIGURE 8.2

Pictograph in the tomb of the physician Ankhmahor in Saqqara, Egypt, dating from 2330 BCE.

Reflexology

Reflexology is another ancient healing art with ties to Egypt, India, and China. Inscriptions found on tombs and the translations of hieroglyphics depicting the feet give evidence to what we know as reflexology today (Figure 8.2 ■).

The precursor to reflexology is zone theory therapy that began when Dr. William H. Fitzgerald, supported by his colleague Dr. Edwin Bowers, published papers on zone analgesia in 1917. Dr. Fitzgerald was an ear, nose, and throat specialist; he discovered that pressure applied to an area of the body would result in pain relief, or analgesia. Some of the tools he used were:

- Elastic bands
- Combs
- Clothes pegs
- Surgical clamps

He developed the first chart on longitudinal zones of the body (Figure 8.3 ■). Furthermore, Dr. Fitzgerald found that the application of pressure on the zones not only relieved the pain but also alleviated the underlying cause. The same is said of reflexology today, which is based in part on zone theory.

Dr. Shelby Riley further developed zone therapy by adding horizontal zones. Eunice D. Ingham, a physical therapist working closely with Dr. Riley, began developing her foot reflex theory in the 1930s based on the zone theory premise. Her theory states that the feet and hands serve as blueprints for the internal organs and glands of the body. She wrote her first book *Stories the Feet Can Tell* in 1938.

There is a significant difference between zone therapy and reflexology in that zone therapy uses only the zones to determine the areas for pressure but reflexology uses the zones and anatomical model as the blueprint for where to apply pressure. Today Eunice Ingham's nephew Dwight Byers is responsible for furthering the field of reflexology through the International Institute of Reflexology.

Reflexology is an extensive field of therapy. For a comprehensive treatment, consult a certified practitioner. Nevertheless, we recommend a basic approach for assessing the need for professional help and establishing a day-to-day

FIGURE 8.3

The zone theory chart shows the longitudinal lines on the body that depict the areas to apply pressure for pain relief.

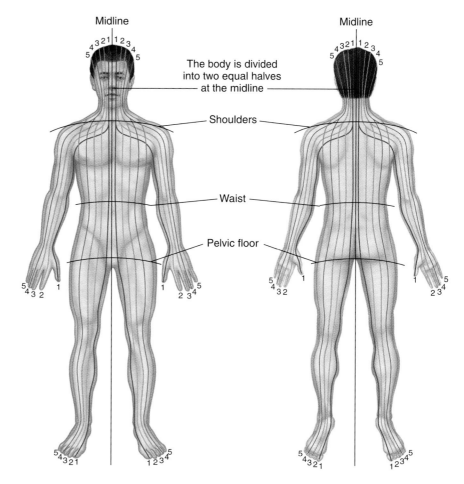

protocol. Although the starting point on the foot is not critical, a sequential approach will ensure that you do not miss any points. When a tender or adhered point is encountered, apply deep, circular pressure in both directions or use a criss-cross motion. Adjust pressure to your comfort level. The use of a pencil eraser can help accurately locate these typically small areas. Several tools that allow for a hands-free treatment, such as the foot roller, are available today.

Ball Techniques

Balls can be used to massage various areas of the body, release tension, and stretch fascia and can be used for toning. See Figure 8.4 ■ for one type of activity using a ball. Medicine balls, miracle balls, and yamuna (ya-men-ah) body rolling are among several popular brands, each of which has its own protocol for use.

Yamuna Zake, a bodyworker, yoga instructor, aromatherapist, and herbalist, created Yamuna body rolling (YBR), a system to take care of her body and remain free of injuries. *Yamuna* means "river," which is appropriate because her work focuses on flow. YBR is a form of deep tissue self-massage that uses dense, plastic balls that range from 6 to 10 inches in diameter and entails progressive routines of rolling on the ball to unwind tension and improve body alignment. YBR reeducates muscles, stimulates bones, and facilitates positive changes in the body. The muscles are worked from origin to insertion, and each ball

has different levels of density, elasticity, and resistance designed to give the best results for the individual. The balls are color coded with each color representing the level of intensity. Going inward to feel, assess, and move through fascia restrictions with the help of gravity is intrinsic to YBR. We recommend looking for a trained practitioner for an assessment and evaluation. For more information about the YBR technique of self-care, visit www.yamunabody rolling.com.

Thermotherapy and Cryotherapy

Heat and cold affect the circulation. Heat dilates blood vessels, which increases blood flow to an area and helps to speed healing. Heat is effective for muscle strain, sprains, soreness, and arthritis and has a relaxation effect. Cold, on the other hand, constricts blood vessels and is effective for reducing inflammation and inhibiting pain stimuli. It is the preferred treatment for acute injury to reduce inflammation. The use of thermotherapy and cryotherapy needs to be selected based on the conditions one is experiencing at the time of treatment to determine the best protocol. The means of delivery can vary from hydrotherapy, compresses, and paraffin baths to stones. Contraindications for the use of thermotherapy or cryotherapy include heart conditions, high or low blood pressure, and neuropathies.

Hydrotherapy has been used for centuries and depicted in most cultures. Hippocrates prescribed it for its curative

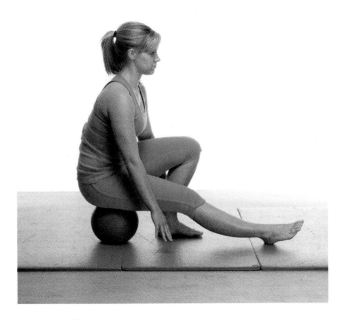

FIGURE 8.4

Balls can be used in a variety of ways for exercise and massage. Here a larger ball is being used to massage the hamstrings.

effect. Romans were known for their communal baths. Today health spas all over the world tout the benefits of hydrotherapy. Among the several types of baths are foot-bath, sitz bath, and full emersion bath; the temperature of the water (hot or cold) depends on your needs.

Many people prefer a hot shower in the morning, which certainly can help ease tight and sore muscles. Even more soothing is a long soak (20–30 minutes) in a hot bath, whether it is in a jacuzzi or tub. Herbs and oils can be added to increase the benefits, but only those safe for water use should be added. Other suggested tools for hot/cold treatment include compresses, which are effective for site-specific treatments. These can be commercial gel packs, heating pads—moist or dry, rice or flax seed bags; if none of these is readily available, a bag of frozen peas work great. Moist heat usually penetrates deeper and so is more efficacious for treatment of tendon or ligament injuries. Cold therapy is effective in reducing inflammation and is used immediately after a trauma for the first 48–72 hours. It can also be used for chronic pain for migraines, tension headaches, and tendon injuries.

Another source of heat is infrared light. Infrared is a form of radiant heat, similar to the energy released by the sun. Its use increases blood flow, brings Qi to the area to promote healing, and can raise the white blood count, thereby increasing immunity. Infrared lamps should be positioned at least 12 inches from the treatment site to avoid burns and should not be used near flammable materials. Therapeutic oils can be applied before, during, or after treatment, but read the product guidelines before using infrared light.

Another thermotherapy approach is the paraffin bath. The paraffin contours the afflicted area to hold in the heat and stimulate circulation. As with other heat methods, it provides relief to pain caused by arthritis, bursitis, and chronic joint pain. By relaxing muscles, paraffin bath relieves stiffness and spasms. An additional benefit is its softening and soothing effect on dry skin. We recommend buying a paraffin wax unit from a reputable source and one with a history of serving the bodywork community, salons, and spas. Continuously check the temperature on the inside surface of the wrist to avoid burns. Contraindications for use include cuts, wounds, warts, inflamed skin, peripheral vascular disease, and any condition that reduces sensation.

Stones can be used for either thermo- or cryotherapy as well as self-massage. The application for each is the same; however, granite stones are used for thermotherapy and marble for cryotherapy. Granite stones can be heated by placing them in hot water, a warm oven, or the sun. Marble stones are refrigerated or frozen. Strategically place the stone(s) on areas of tension or pain for a therapeutic effect. Various sizes and shapes are available, or you can go outside to find your own. If climate allows, simply place the stones in sand warmed by the sun. Complete your kit by purchasing a crock pot or electric roasting pan.

Guidelines for Selecting Techniques

Assessing your condition to determine which technique(s) will be most effective is important. Worksheet 8.1 can be used to document your conditions and chart your progress. Once you have determined the body area that needs work, you can select the technique that would be most efficacious for the specific condition, keeping in mind contraindications.

Earlier chapters discussed many conditions we as bodyworkers address. Most often the wrist, shoulder, cervical area, back, and feet are subjected to tension, pain, and inflammation. These conditions can be either chronic or acute, and each requires its own treatment approach. A common cause of many chronic conditions is reduced circulation. Use of ice on an injury can immediately reduce inflammation. Use of petrissage or cross-fiber stokes can increase lymphatic flow, and friction and petrissage are effective for sprains to prevent joint stiffness. However, these techniques should not be used on the immediate site of acute injuries, especially if the skin is abraded or inflamed.

For people who suffer from sciatica or other nerve impingements, we recommend friction and vibration at the points along the junction of the affected joint and over the nerve. Self-treatment to the sciatic nerve is difficult without being a contortionist, but later sections provide some helpful tips.

Muscle atrophy, regardless of the cause, benefits from improved circulation and neural stimulation from friction, tapotement, petrissage, cross-fiber, trigger point, and nerve strokes.

When the muscles become adhered because of overuse or injury it is necessary to break down the adhesions and restore balance with a combination of techniques. Fascia release, cross-fiber, and trigger point strokes followed by effleurage and nerves strokes and a stretching program are effective.

WORKSHEET 8.1

Documentation of Tools and Techniques for Self-Massage

After you have identified the area with the most tension, choose a tool and technique. Do daily massage to the area for one week and document the results. Note changes using the following chart and key guide. Points of improvement can include:

- Increased ROM
- Less tension

- Softening of fascia
- Reduced pain

If improvement does not occur, try another technique. If the condition worsens, seek professional help.

Body Region	Technique/Tool	ROM	Tension	Fascia	Pain
Feet and ankles					
Lower extremities					
Pelvis					
Back and neck					
Face and head					
Chest and abdomen					
Upper extremities and hands					

+ = improvement; O = no change; − = deterioration

Safe ergonomics are somewhat challenging when doing self-massage. The specific body area and your ability to reach it could limit a technique. Some modalities could also be affected by anthropometrics. For example, if your arms are short and your condition is hypertonicity of the extensors of the forearm, performing fascia release using the olecranon of the opposite arm will be challenging. In this instance, you will have to adapt by using one of the recommended tools. The tools discussed in this chapter can be adapted and applied to other modalities not covered in this book; be sure to practice them in an ergonomically safe way.

As bodyworkers, we have been taught the contraindications to massage, but it is always helpful to review them. The following is a list of common conditions that are contraindicated for massage:

- Inflammation and abrasions
- Fever
- Skin disorders
  - Boils
  - Acne
  - Cellulitis
  - Fungal infections (athlete's foot, ringworm)
  - Bruises (severe)
  - Impetigo
- Recent trauma
- Hypertension (severe)

Always be aware of the importance of consulting a professional health care provider. When in doubt about a condition, especially one that is recurrent or chronic, consult a physician.

Tools and Equipment: Uses and Limitations

Many tools for use in their practice or for self-massage are available to bodyworkers. You could already have some that this textbook discusses. If you have a personal favorite that we have not addressed, please let us know. These tools, such as the Backnobber™ for the back, and those for hands-free operation, such as with the foot roller, are designed to make it easier to reach an area.

A wide variety of equipment and tools that massage various regions of the body is available (Figure 8.5 ■). They range from self-massage tables, such as Migun™, to shiatsu massage pads that attach to a chair. The Homedics® brand of shiatsu pad is reasonably priced under $100. Infratonic™ chi machine and Pointer® Excel II are handheld energy tools. The list of websites in Helpful Hint 8.1 can help you in selecting equipment. The following are additional manual tools that we recommend.

- *Backnobber™:* Excellent tool for working trigger points on the back. Avoid endangerment sites.
- *Bongers™:* Great for heavy muscled areas such as the quadriceps. Don't use on bony surfaces.

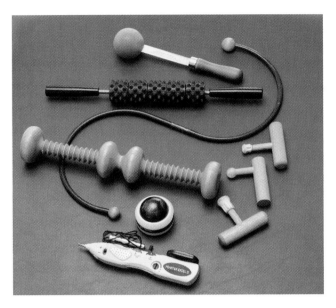

FIGURE 8.5

Tools for self-massage. Beginning with the bottom of the photo and going counterclockwise: Pointer Plus (point finder), Omni Roller (ball), Backnobber, Acu-reflex systems, Bonger, Bodos-3 neuromuscular tools, Ma Roller.

- *Foot roller:* Primarily for the feet, but useful for tight flexor muscles of the arm. Avoid over bony surfaces.
- *Thumper® MiniPro 2 Massager (electric vibrator):* Good for hard-to-reach areas and to give your hands a break.
- *Omni roller:* Great tool for petrissage and applying direct pressure to numerous areas of the body.
- *Compression bars (T-bars):* Primarily used for trigger point technique.

Topicals: Liniments and Analgesics

The topic of self-massage isn't complete without discussing topical ointments. A plethora of ointments and rubefacients is available to reduce swelling, increase circulation, ease painful joints, and soothe muscular aches and pains. They are packaged as gels, crèmes, aerosols, ointments, oils, and liniments and are available over the counter (OTC) or by prescription. The main drugs used in topical analgesics are salicylates (aspirin), nonsteroidal anti-inflammatory drug (NSAIDs), and a variety of herbal-based medications including menthol, camphor, arnica, and capsaicin.

Topical NSAIDs block enzymes that cause inflammatory responses. Some topicals act as counterirritants, which means they counter pain. **Rubefacients** act as counterirritants and cause the skin to turn red by dilating the skin's blood vessels. The underlying muscle and joint are served by the same sensory nerves; therefore, irritation of the skin offsets the deeper pain. Some common OTC topicals analgesics are:

- BenGay™
- Icy Hot™
- Aspercreme™
- Zostrix™, a capsaicin product

SELF-MASSAGE TECHNIQUES FOR SPECIFIC BODY REGIONS

Self-massage techniques have no set protocols. The techniques discussed here are basic for most massage therapists and have been selected to target common problem areas for bodyworkers and are easily adapted to self-massage. In addition, many tools that assist with these techniques are on the market; however, common cost-effective household items can be adapted. We encourage you to use your imagination and skills to develop other approaches for self-massage while applying ergonomic principles.

Feet and Ankles

Standing on our feet for long periods of time makes them and the ankles prone to fatigue. Fortunately, these areas are readily accessible for self-massage. The foot and ankle are easily reached by supporting the ankle on the opposite knee. If physical limitation prevents this, tools for applying the techniques with your feet on the floor are available. The Footsie Roller™ is a well-known tool for foot massage. Its raised ridges and overall shape allows you to easily access any part of the plantar surface. Because it is a hands-free device, your hands can rest, and gravity and the foot's

HELPFUL HINT 8.1
Websites for Suggested Tools and Equipment

- http://www.migunworld.com
- http://www.massage-tools/com/prpo.html
- http://www.shopzilla.com/8B--Massagers
- http://www.massagewarehouse.com

- http://www.reflexology-usa.net/
- http://www.lhasaoms.com/infrared_heat_therapy-43-page.html

pressure of bearing down on the roller gives a good massage. Some household items that can be adapted for self-massage are:

- Rolling pin
- Tennis or racquetball
- Tin can with or without ridges (make sure there are no sharp edges)
- Wood dowel or smooth stick

Search your household! We discovered a rolling pin that can be filled with water and when frozen works great for ice massage.

When selecting a tool, make sure it rolls easily on the floor and will not break, causing injury. You could need to change tools if you are working on a hard floor versus a carpeted surface. Experiment until you find what works best.

Hydrotherapy is another option for the feet. A number of commercial models are available, some of which include massage and/or heat. A common footbath with Epsom salts is a good substitute.

The oldest modality for working the feet and ankles is reflexology. This technique not only targets the foot and ankle but also the organ and gland reference points (map) (see Figure 8.6 ■). In addition, basic massage of the foot/ankle can alleviate tired feet. With either modality, placing the ankle on the opposite knee or thigh with a slight inversion (Figure 8.7 ■) positions the foot for accessibility. The approach is similar for reflexology and basic massage.

Once your foot is in a comfortable position, begin palpating the plantar surface. Work the entire plantar surface and around the ankle using the strokes that are most effective for your condition. Depending on the degree of inversion, you could elect to use your thumbs, fingers, or knuckles. Keep your wrist in neutral alignment. With the foot inverted to the point that the plantar surface points superiorly, the thumbs or knuckles can be used. However, if that degree of inversion is uncomfortable, keep the plantar surface pointed laterally and adjust by using the fingers. To work the lateral dorsal side of the foot, place the plantar surface flat on the floor.

A variety of tools (Figure 8.5) can be used to help reduce the impact on the hands.

- A pencil eraser for compression
- Compression bar (T-bars)
- Omni ball

If you do choose to use the Footsie Roller™ or other tool, you will need to practice to achieve the best angle and degree of pressure.

Lower Extremities

The combination of standing, moving, and sitting while we are massaging can impact our legs in a number of ways. Improper sitting position can impair circulation. Tight hamstrings occur when we hyperextend our knees, and our knees can be affected by twisting motions. Whether it is your calves, quadriceps, or knees, the legs are fairly easy to access to administer self-massage. As with the foot, the lateral aspect of the ankle can be propped on your leg to work on its medial side. Any of the Swedish, neuromuscular, and energy techniques can be applied.

All of the tools used for the foot can be applied to the lower extremities. A great tool for working these muscles is the Bonger™.

All aforementioned strokes can be readily used on the legs. A seated position is best for working on the lower leg and the quadriceps. While seated, you should work with the leg either on the floor or propped on a chair (Figure 8.8 ■). Apply the modality of your choice above the ankle and work toward the knee on the lateral and medial side of the lower leg. Remember to work toward the heart. If blood pressure or other contraindications are a factor, use the propped method.

The quadriceps don't present much of an ergonomic challenge for self-massage; however, be aware to keep your hands and wrists in neutral alignment. While seated, work the quadriceps from the proximal end toward the knee. See Figure 8.9 ■ (page 152) for the hand positions that enable you to keep neutral alignment and exert deep pressure. Repeat with overlapping strokes until you have covered the area of tension. The fists work well on the heavily muscled area. You can also use your ulnar surface or olecranon in this area, but you will have to bend over your quadriceps to do so. Experiment with the other modalities and use what feels ergonomically safe. Rolling on your hip to one side gives access to the lateral aspect of your upper leg.

The hamstrings are the most challenging for self-massage, and you will likely want to use a tool such as a rolling pin, tootsie roller, or tennis ball. Although a single tennis ball can be used, placing two balls in a sock with a knot tied next to them to keep them secure can be a simple tool that can work a larger area. While seated in a chair, place the balls or other tool under your leg just above the knee and rest your leg on the tool with your feet on the floor. By shifting your body, you can glide your leg forward/backward and right/left to work the tight points along the muscle's length. Readjustment of your position in the chair allows you to cover the muscles from above the knee to the gluteal fold. Experiment using different style chairs (with or without arms, cushion or hard seat) to find what works best for you.

Pelvis

The pelvis is a common area for postural distortions (PDs). Whether you have a lateral, anterior, or posterior tilt, all of which impact your body with time, self-massage techniques can alleviate the tension in the muscles that these PDs affected. Remember that when the pelvic muscles are tight and one of these tilts occurs, it will impact the back and lower extremities.

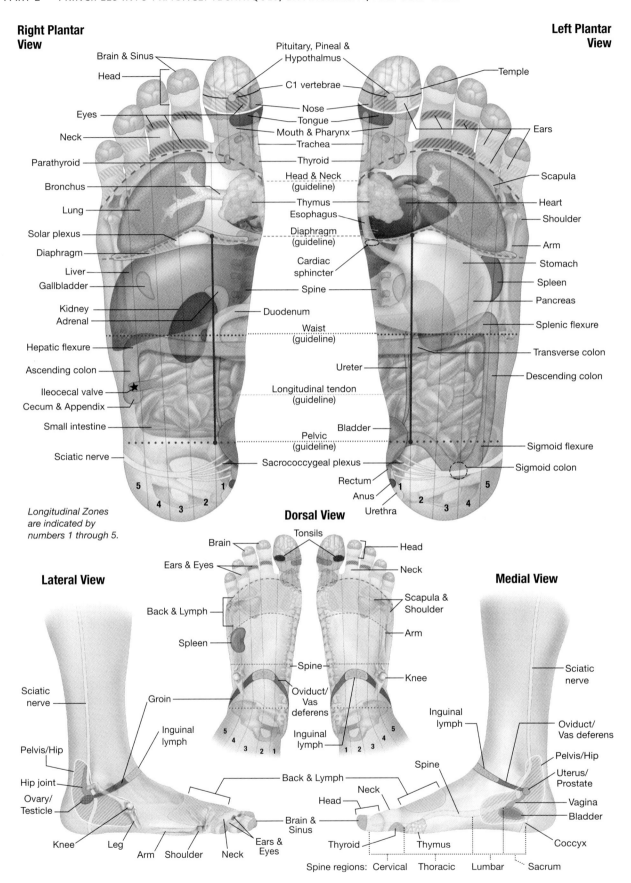

Right Plantar View

Brain & Sinus
Head
Eyes
Neck
Parathyroid
Bronchus
Lung
Solar plexus
Diaphragm
Liver
Gallbladder
Kidney
Adrenal
Hepatic flexure
Ascending colon
Ileocecal valve
Cecum & Appendix
Small intestine
Sciatic nerve

Longitudinal Zones are indicated by numbers 1 through 5.

Pituitary, Pineal & Hypothalmus
C1 vertebrae
Nose
Tongue
Mouth & Pharynx
Trachea
Thyroid
Head & Neck (guideline)
Thymus
Esophagus
Diaphragm (guideline)
Cardiac sphincter
Spine
Duodenum
Waist (guideline)
Ureter
Longitudinal tendon (guideline)
Bladder
Pelvic (guideline)
Sacrococcygeal plexus
Rectum
Anus
Urethra

Left Plantar View

Temple
Ears
Scapula
Heart
Shoulder
Arm
Stomach
Spleen
Pancreas
Splenic flexure
Transverse colon
Descending colon
Sigmoid flexure
Sigmoid colon

Dorsal View

Tonsils
Brain
Ears & Eyes
Back & Lymph
Spleen
Spine
Oviduct/ Vas deferens
Inguinal lymph
Head
Neck
Scapula & Shoulder
Arm
Knee

Lateral View

Sciatic nerve
Pelvis/Hip
Hip joint
Ovary/ Testicle
Knee
Leg
Arm
Shoulder
Neck
Ears & Eyes
Groin
Inguinal lymph
Back & Lymph
Brain & Sinus
Head
Neck

Medial View

Sciatic nerve
Inguinal lymph
Spine
Thyroid
Thymus
Oviduct/ Vas deferens
Pelvis/Hip
Uterus/ Prostate
Vagina
Bladder
Coccyx

Spine regions: Cervical Thoracic Lumbar Sacrum

FIGURE 8.6

Foot reflexes.

FIGURE 8.7

Resting the ankle on the opposite knee or thigh with inversion of the foot makes the plantar surface easily accessible for reflexology or massage.

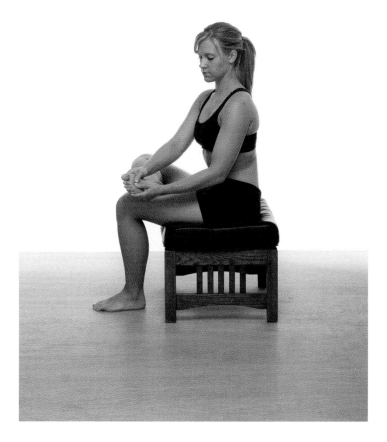

Because of the location of this area, working without the aid of tools is more challenging. Some of our favorite tools and props for working these areas are:

- Bongers
- Tennis balls
- Wall edges or door jam

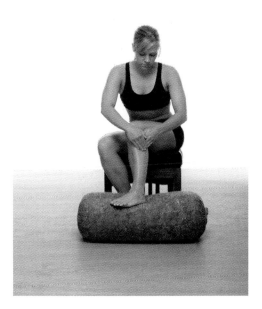

FIGURE 8.8

Propping the leg for working below the knee reduces flexion and maintains a more neutral spine.

- Doorknobs
- BacKnobber®

If you are flexible or have a daily yoga practice, try some of the recommended techniques using only your hands. While seated in a chair, cross your leg and rest on one hip. Use the hand to massage the gluteal area (see Figure 8.10 ■). Make a fist to maintain neutral wrist position. Massage the gluteal muscles using either an effleurage stroke or tapotement. You can also apply a cross-fiber stroke with the fist, but doing so is not recommended if you have shoulder problems as a result of the angle and range of motion required. This is a great place to use the Bonger™ for tapotement.

If you want hands-free technique, several options by which you can apply controlled pressure to this area are available. You can use a stable structure such as a doorknob, stair railing, rounded end of a counter, or a ball against the wall to apply localized pressure while in a standing position. Find one that is at the right level for you to be able to apply pressure without putting your body in an awkward position—out of neutral alignment. If you are too tall, you can squat, but be aware of your body mechanics so you don't hurt your knees. See Figure 8.11 ■ for positioning the gluteal muscle against a ball placed between the wall and the gluteal muscle to allow you to apply pressure that mimics fascia release, effleurage, or cross-fiber or to isolate a trigger point. Keep the torso in neutral alignment and squat with a wide enough stance to prevent the knee from extending beyond the toes. Another option is to apply the pressure while you are lying down with a tennis ball positioned

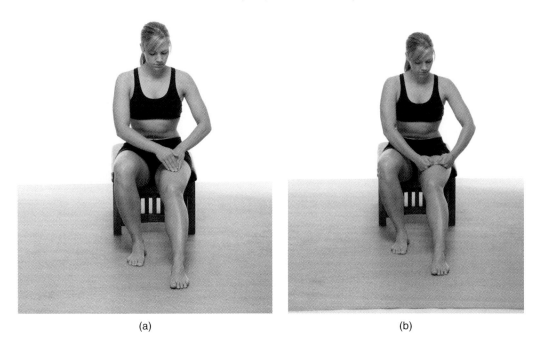

(a)   (b)

FIGURE 8.9

A triangle is created when the hands are overlapped or fists are adjacent to one another. By keeping neutral alignment, maximum force can be generated with minimal ergonomic impact.

under the gluteal area and to work it as described for the hamstrings.

While using these tools, props, and techniques, it is important to remember your body mechanics. If any of the positions take you out of neutral alignment or cause discomfort, stop immediately.

Anyone with an anterior tilt of the pelvis (lordosis) is at risk for a hypertonic psoas muscle. The psoas requires considerable care while treating it because of its location and the presence of vital organs in this region. Therefore,

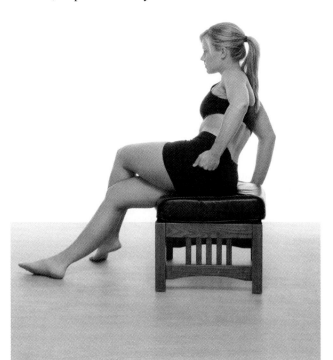

FIGURE 8.10

With legs crossed and weight on one hip, the gluteal region is positioned for massage. The figure shows the use of the fist. Note to keep the wrist in neutral alignment.

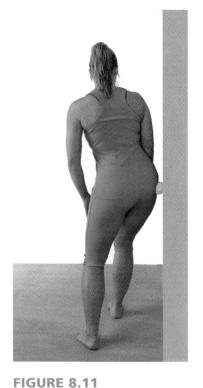

FIGURE 8.11

Align your buttock against the tennis ball. Maintain neutral alignment by keeping the torso straight. A wide enough stance will keep the knees from extending past the toes.

HELPFUL HINT 8.2
Trigger Pointing the Psoas

Before beginning this technique, use the other recommended modalities, such as energy work, that provide a more moderate and less invasive approach. These techniques will warm up and prepare the muscle for deeper work. The next step is to palpate the area and make sure you are on the muscle to avoid injury to the large intestine. You can do this technique lying down. A tool can be used to reach the deep trigger point sites. If you don't have one of the tools specifically marketed for trigger point technique (i.e., compression bar), a rolling pin works well because its length provides good leverage to apply pressure to the trigger point.

While lying down, measure approximately 2–3 finger widths down from your ASIS and then 2–3 finger widths medially. Check the site with your fingers to confirm the trigger point before placing the tool. Position the tip of the tool on the trigger point and apply pressure. Recheck the position of the tool on the muscle by raising the extended leg an inch or two. The flexion of the muscle should be felt through the tool. If you are in position, relax the leg and maintain the appropriate pressure for the recommended time, typically 8–12 seconds.

we limit this area to gentle techniques such as energy work, effleurage, and petrissage. This deep muscle that extends from the lumbar vertebra and ilium to the proximal end of the femurs can be accessed only at its distal end along the inguinal line. Initiate the treatment with energy work by placing both hands over the muscle, directing healing warmth to the area. Follow this by gentle effleurage and/or petrissage. These techniques frequently eliminate the tension in the muscle. However, if the psoas is extremely tight and you are confidant in your skills, apply trigger point technique. Because of the depth of the muscle, a tool is necessary. See Helpful Hint 8.2 for information about this technique.

Back and Neck

As bodyworkers, the neck and back are subjected to significant muscle strain throughout the day. This is compounded by treating too many clients or having a traveling business that requires constantly hauling equipment. PDs of the neck and back cause additional limitations.

The neck is easily accessible for self-massage. Begin while seated by placing both hands on your upper trapezes, palms down and cupped. Compress the muscle and allow your arms to relax against your chest as your fingers/hands glide off the trapezes. Then move to the neck by placing your fingers on either side of cervical vertebra C7 and repeat the gliding motion as you lower your arms to the chest. Repeat this until you cover the entire neck from C7 to C1.

A nice treatment is to gently roll a tennis ball up and down the posterior neck muscles followed by light tapotement using a Bonger.

Various tools are available to work the back. Specific back tools, such as the shiatsu massager by Homedics, come with instructions. Simple, inexpensive tools, such as tennis balls and foam tubing, are personal favorites and are available at local stores. Tennis balls are effective in those tight, hard-to-reach spots. Use a wall free of wall hangings. Stand with your back toward the wall, feet approximately

1 foot away and shoulder width apart. Lean against the wall while slightly squatting and place a ball on either side of the spine on the erector spinae (Figure 8.12 ■). You can choose to do both sides of the spine at once or one at a time. Apply pressure against the balls and slowly roll up and down. When you find a tight spot, shift to rolling side to side or apply straight pressure. Reposition the balls higher up the back, adjust your stance as needed, and repeat the rolling. Repeat this technique until you have covered the erector spinae group from the lumbar region to the top of the thoracic region.

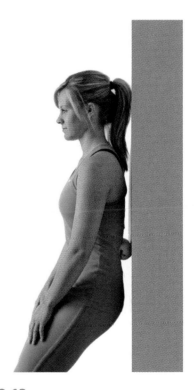

FIGURE 8.12

Rolling tennis balls sandwiched between the back and the wall relieves muscle tension.

To apply self-massage to a broad area of the back, foam tubing is an exceptional tool. Using a length of foam pipe insulation approximately the width of your back, lie supine with your knees flexed. Place the tube horizontally under your back at L5. Relax for a minute or two and then using your feet, lift your buttocks and begin rolling against the tube. Reposition the tube and repeat the rolling. Continue this cycle until you have covered the entire back. If at any point this feels too invasive or causes pain, discontinue it. Rolling on a body ball such as the Yamuna technique uses is excellent for opening up restricted areas and has the added benefit of stretching. Many systems that incorporate the use of balls have balls of varying density to adjust the depth of the massage.

Use of a Backnobber™ facilitates the release of trigger points and can be used for cross-fiber strokes where indicated. The s-shape of the tool (Figure 8.13 ■) reaches to the back and gives leverage for applying pressure.

Try all of these suggested techniques and choose the one that works the best for you.

Face and Head

The face and head can be host to many maladies, such as temporomandibular joint dysfunction (TMJD), migraines, tension headaches, and sinus conditions, that can manifest when we are stressed, rushed, or have poor body mechanics. Several techniques are effective for these conditions.

Cross-fiber and fascia release techniques can alleviate the muscle tension within the masseter and pterygoids associated with TMJD. The masseter can be worked by placing three fingers just below the zygomatic process. With the jaw relaxed, apply pressure and glide across to the ramus of

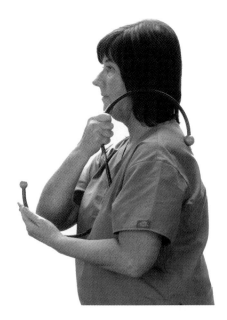

FIGURE 8.13

The Backnobber™ reaches the back for applying a variety of techniques.

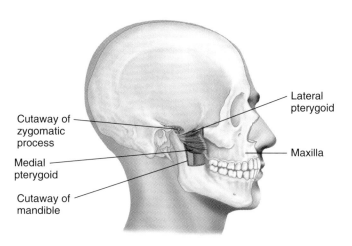

Cutaway of zygomatic process

Medial pterygoid

Cutaway of mandible

Lateral pterygoid

Maxilla

FIGURE 8.14

The pterygoid muscles lie on the medial surface of the mandible and require intraoral technique.

the mandible. For adhered areas, use trigger point or deep petrissage.

The medial and lateral pterygoid attachments to the TMJ capsule and articular discs make hypertonicity of these muscles central to TMJD. These muscles lie medial to the mandible and require intraoral palpation to be thorough (Figure 8.14 ■). To reach the lateral pterygoid, run your index finger along the lingual side of the upper teeth until you reach the back molars. Keeping the jaw relaxed and open, apply pressure posterior and superior. Your finger will be positioned between the mandible and maxilla as you apply pressure. If you are in the correct position, you will feel contraction of the lateral pteryoid upon lateral deviation of the jaw. Palpate the medial pterygoid by placing the finger along the buccal surface of the lower teeth until you reach the back molars. Verify the position of the medial pterygoid by clenching your teeth to feel the muscle contract. Compress posterolaterally against the inside wall of the mouth and apply cross-fiber or trigger points.

Compression of the mid-saggital suture helps relieve tension headaches and sinus pressure. Begin by placing your fingers together on your mid-saggital suture and apply pressure (see Figure 8.15 ■). A useful tool for the head is a neuromuscular T-bar with a flat rubber tip.

Self-massage of the face is easy to do and releases generalized tension. Typical massage tools are not recommended for the face because of its more bony nature and thinner, more sensitive skin. However, tools of the cosmetology industry are suitable. Following are recommended techniques:

- Petrissage and light tapotement of the facial muscles
- Cross-fiber and fascial release of the frontalis
- Cross-fiber of the corrugators
- Isolate and cross-fiber the skin along the supraorbital ridge (eyebrow)
- Compression of the supraorbital foramen
- Compression of the infraorbital foramen

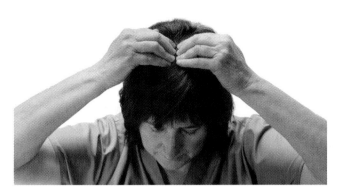

FIGURE 8.15

Fingertip compression of the mid-saggital suture can relieve tension.

Chest and Abdomen

The pectoral muscles in bodyworkers are often hypertonic because of their job demands. Our arms are most often extended, naturally leading to tightened chest muscles. Abdominals weaken unless we are aware of strengthening or holding some tension to maintain a certain degree of core stability. Most of the previously suggested tools work well in the pectoral area; however, you must be careful in the abdominal area because of the vital organs. Whether you are using your hands or a tool, check the ergonomics of your hands and wrist before applying the modality of choice.

Effleurage, cross-fiber, and trigger point can be easily performed on the pectoral muscles. For effleurage, start either seated or lying comfortably and place the right hand on the left pectoral immediately lateral to the sternum just below the clavicle (Figure 8.16 ■). Glide your fingers/hand from this point along the clavicle to the shoulder (humerus). Return to the sternum, lower your hand, and repeat this stroke until you have covered the entire muscle. When treating the right side, use the left hand.

Apply cross-fiber by using both hands with fingers cupped and adducted. Slide the fingers from just below the clavicle along the length of the sternum. Reposition just lateral to the first stroke and repeat, continuing until you cover the whole muscle.

To work the distal end of the pectoralis that forms the anterior portion of the axilla (armpit), abduct and laterally rotate the upper arm (Figure 8.17 ■). Use your other hand to isolate the muscle between your fingers and thumb and compress. Readjust, moving around the muscle to identify trigger points. Opposition of the thumb and fingers provides better compression and at the same time, the thumb and fingers will be able to isolate separate trigger points.

When treating the abdominal area, lie down and begin by focusing on your breathing. Once comfortable and relaxed, place both hands on your abdomen below the sternum and hold this point until you feel an increase in heat. Begin with a gentle stroke—effleurage or petrissage—moving clockwise around the abdomen. With each circle, move your hands closer to your navel and repeat the clockwise motion until you are over the umbilicus. Hold this point for a few minutes and absorb the healing energy and heat from your hands.

FIGURE 8.16

Position for cross-fiber of the pectoral muscle. Note the fingers are cupped and adducted to provide more support.

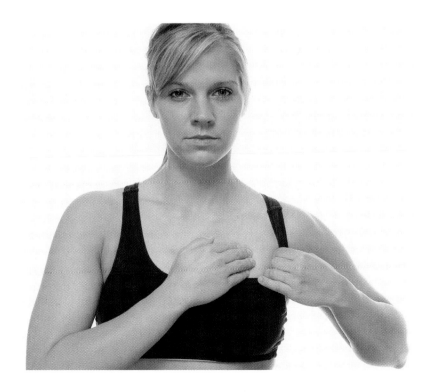

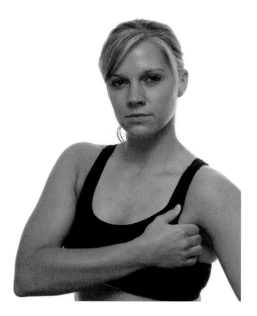

FIGURE 8.17

Opposing thumb and fingers provide compression and isolation of trigger points.

Upper Extremities and Hands

Overuse of the hands, wrists, and arms are common for all people, and practitioners' work compounds it. A good foundation in ergonomics and awareness allows us to participate in our favorite activities that require the use of our arms and hands, be it sports, crafts, or music, and still allow us career longevity. We emphasize the use of tools to relieve the hands. If your fingers need a break after a day of work, use some suggested tools:

- Electric massager (follow product instructions)
- Tennis ball
- Foam tube
- Bongers

The upper and lower arm can easily be worked with the Bonger™ to apply tapotement or friction. Try improvising with a tennis ball by rolling it with the palm of the hand for the extensors or against a table surface for the flexors to simulate effleurage, petrissage, or cross-fiber. It is easy to keep the wrist in neutral position with this technique (Figure 8.18 ■). A small wallpaper roller is another option for effleurage of the larger muscle groups, such as the biceps brachii, triceps brachii, or bra-chial radialis.

One of the best treatments for the hand is a paraffin bath. Dipping the hands in the wax 4–6 times and leaving the wax on until it cools (approximately 20 minutes) can help aching hands. Follow all manufacturers' recommenda-tions. Neuropathy is a contraindication because the loss of sensation makes you less aware of heat. The tennis ball or similar tool is effective for massaging this area relatively hands free.

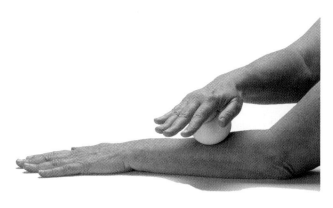
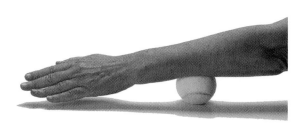

FIGURE 8.18

(a) For treating the extensors, place a tennis ball over the muscle; stabilize it with the palm of the hand. The ball can be moved to simulate effleurage, petrissage, or cross-fiber. (b) For the flexors, stabilize the tennis ball between the wrist and a hard surface.

CHAPTER SUMMARY

- Self-massage provides immediate and daily care for tension, hypertonicity, circulation, and pain.
- The advantage of doing self-massage is the awareness of the efficacy of each stroke and self-awareness.
- Self-massage can incorporate a variety of techniques, including Swedish massage, neuromuscular technique, energy work, reflexology, Yamuna body rolling technique, thermotherapy and cryotherapy, hydrotherapy, and the use of topicals.
- Body area and present condition determine the best approach for self-massage.
- Ergonomics can be more challenging when doing self-massage.
- Tools play an important role in self-massage for hard-to-reach areas and hands-free applications.

REVIEW QUESTIONS

1. Identify three benefits of self-massage.
2. Which Swedish stroke breaks down adhesions and relieves stasis?
3. Identify the Swedish stroke most effective for increasing blood to an ischemic area.
4. True or False? Tapotement can remove or produce hyperemia.
5. True or False? Vibration is best used when you want to increase peristalsis.
6. True or False? Nerve strokes relax the nervous system.
7. The flow of energy can be distorted by thoughts, _____ , and _____.
8. Zone theory consists of horizontal and _____ zones.
9. During trigger point therapy,
   a. compression deprives the points of blood flow and oxygen
   b. release triggers vasodilation
   c. triggers release of endorphins and enkephalins
   d. all the above

10. Each of the following is a contraindication for massage except:
    a. abrasions
    b. recent trauma
    c. hypertonicity
    d. inflammation
11. The benefits of using tools include:
    a. reaching hard-to-access areas
    b. reducing impact on the hands
    c. facilitating and supporting good ergonomics
    d. all the above
12. Match the tool with their special uses:

_____ Tapotement	A. Tennis balls
_____ Compression and trigger point	B. Bonger™
_____ Effleurage, petrissage, cross-fiber	C. Stones
_____ Heat or cold	D. Backnobber™

REFERENCES

Lawrence, D., & Harrison, L. (1983). *Massageworks: A practical encylopedia of massage techniques.* New York: Putnam.

SUGGESTED READINGS

Byers, D. C. (1990). *Better health with foot reflexology: The original Ingham method.* Saint Petersburg, FL: Ingham.

Fowlie, L. (2006). *An introduction to heat and cold as therapy.* Toronto: Curties-Overzet.

Lett, A. (2000). *Reflex zone therapy for health professionals.* New York: Churchill Livingstone.

9 Self-Care: Stress and Stress Busters

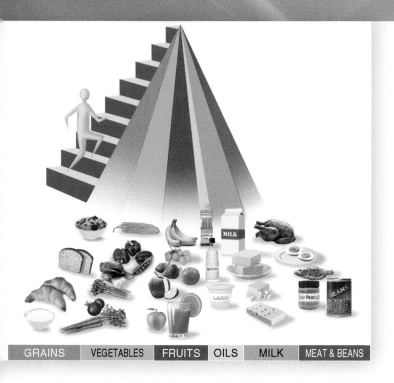

| GRAINS | VEGETABLES | FRUITS | OILS | MILK | MEAT & BEANS |

 CHAPTER OUTLINE

Causes of Stress

Recognition of Stress

Physiology of Stress

Ergonomic Impacts of Stress

Techniques for Managing Stress

Summary

Review Questions

LEARNING OBJECTIVES

Upon successful completion of the chapter, you will be able to:

1. Define stress and differentiate between the different types of stress.
2. Identify the cause/s of stress in general and specific to the field of bodywork.
3. Identify and recognize the signs of stress.
4. Discuss the physiology of stress.
5. Differentiate between emotionally, mentally, physically, and spiritually stress.
6. Identify the regions of the brain tied to the mind-body connection.
7. Compare acute stress to chronic stress.
8. Describe how the hormonal changes associated with chronic stress leads to chronic disease.
9. Identify how stress can affect ergonomics.
10. Select lifestyle and techniques for managing stress.

KEY TERMS

Acute stress 162

Chronic stress 163

Distress 162

Emotional intelligence 160

Episodic acute stress 163

Eustress 162

Fight or flight response 164

General adaptation syndrome 164

Limbic system 163

Reticular activating system (RAS) 164

Stress is a word we hear frequently today. As a part of the equation of health, this concept gained foothold in the 1960s. With the recognition that it contributes to chronic illness, many books and programs have become available that focus on stress management, which clearly recognizes mind-body connection. Stress relates to ergonomics in two ways. *Job stress* is a form that most of us encounter and that influences our personal lives. In addition, *stress from our personal life* affects our work performance and can directly contribute to body tensions, headaches, and fatigue. The purpose of this chapter is to provide an overview of the stress response, explain how it relates to ergonomics for the bodyworker, and offer practical guidelines on how to recognize and reduce stress to improve the quality of our lives.

CAUSES OF STRESS

Stress happens for a variety of reasons, some of them specific to each individual. Self-appraisal allows us to identify stressors in our life and is the first step toward reducing stress and learning to adapt. Some stress factors are common in society, others are distinctive to careers, and others are very individualized.

Most of us attempt to find balance in our lives on a daily basis. The culture of our society doesn't support relaxation; rather it bases success on work and performance. Add events such as marriage, divorce, responsibility for dependants, death of loved ones, moving, loss of job, and so on, and the balancing act becomes more challenging. Some people believe that stress is not an external factor, but rather it is an individual's perception and response to circumstances. Ultimately, each person's perception is the important factor because what stresses one person might not stress another.

Stress results from a web of underlying factors. However, we can learn more about it by separating it into its different types.

Physical Stressors

Stress occurs when our bodies are subjected to conditions that push their physical limits. Not being in the physical shape necessary for required activity is one cause. Other causes of physical stresses include illness, insufficient sleep/rest, malnutrition, obesity, and excessive alcohol use. Maintaining a healthy lifestyle is crucial to reducing these stresses. Some challenges that bodyworkers face are both physical and emotional. Overscheduling, shortage of time between appointments, imbalance between work and downtime, injury, illness, and aging can have both a physical and emotional impact.

Emotional and Mental Stressors

Emotional and mental stressors can be distinguished from one another, but they are both neurological and often go hand in hand. Mental stress directly relates to intense mental activity, such as studying for exam and making complex decisions. Following intense mental activity, we commonly feel exhausted much the way we feel after a physically strenuous day. Emotional stress kicks in when we begin to feel overwhelmed or out of control of situations.

A recent school of thought in the field of psychology is the notion of **emotional intelligence,** introduced by Daniel Goleman in 1995 in his book *Emotional Intelligence.* Today it's referred to as emotional intelligence quotient (EIQ), which differs distinctly from intelligence quotient (IQ). Someone can have a high IQ and not be emotionally intelligent or visa versa. EIQ measures our ability to be self-aware, self-motivated, empathic, and to deal with our moods. Awareness of our emotional maturity is necessary to create a positive emotional environment in our personal and professional lives. Recognizing that an emotional pattern can underlie stress in our life can help us redirect our feelings and energy in a positive direction. The inability to do this sets the stage of chronic stress.

Stressors of Bodywork

People choosing to enter the field of bodywork do so for a variety of reasons but one common theme is the desire to help others. This caretaker theme is part of why the work is rewarding. However, it comes with a price. Bodyworkers need to be aware of the physical and emotional stressors as health care providers. If they are private business owners, maintaining a client base compounds the stress.

Bodyworkers and health care providers have the best of intentions. It is easy to become invested in their client's health, and their concerns for the outcomes can create an emotional investment. This can be devastating for them if the client's health declines and/or she or he dies. Even with healthy boundaries, it is easy to care deeply and therefore be deeply impacted by the loss of a client.

Bodyworkers have the option of self-employment or employment. Each has its own stressors. See Table 9.1 ■ for the pros and cons of each. Most things in life are negotiable, so these pros and cons don't necessarily apply in every given situation. The best work environment is one that gives choices. To achieve well-being, the bodyworker needs to pay attention to the number of clients seen, how closely they are scheduled, the work environment, and the balance between work and relaxation.

Between what happens in our professional life and what occurs in our personal life, we have all experienced feelings of anger, sadness, frustration, and remorse. We need to recognize our feelings and be in tune with those of others to avoid unnecessary conflict and stress. A congruency between our mental and emotional state can occur when we are focused on a goal while keeping our social obligations and perceived expectations in balance. At times we can feel like jugglers, tossing several objects into the air and managing them all but only through concentration and dexterity.

TABLE 9.1	Employment versus Self-Employment: Pros and Cons
Employment	**Self-Employment**
Pros • Paid time off (pto) • Benefits: medical, dental, pension plan • Structured environment	Pros • Be your own boss • Make your own schedule • Create the environment you want • Schedule free time for relaxation, exercise, etc. • Work within your physical capacity (i.e., number of clients treated)
Cons • Has too much structure • Is a subordinate position • Has no control of your schedule • May not be able to dictate the environment	Cons • No paid time off (vacation and sick leave) • No employee benefits (401k, pension plans) • No medical, dental plans

RECOGNITION OF STRESS

Knowing the signs of stress is the first step in creating a plan to alleviate and/or manage stress. The road to stress is paved with events that, depending on our perception, determine mental, emotional, behavioral, and physiological outcomes for us. The signs of stress can manifest physically, emotionally, cognitively, and behaviorally, or in all of these. See Table 9.2 ■ for the more common signs of stress.

PHYSIOLOGY OF STRESS

Stress is a complex physiological process that depends as much on the individual as the situation triggering the response does. The stress response is a natural mechanism of survival that involves many elements of the body. A certain amount of stress is normal and necessary for us to stay in tune with our surroundings; however, when stress becomes chronic, it impacts our health and quality of life.

Definitions of Stress and Health

Our understanding of stress has evolved over the last several decades, resulting in the emergence of a number of related definitions. The word *stress* was first used in the field of physic to refer to a force or tension placed on an object. The psychologist Richard Lazarus used the word in reference to anxiety produced when events and responsibilities go beyond a person's coping ability. Hans Selye expanded the definition: a nonspecific response of the body to any demand placed on it. The demand could be physical or psychological and can occur regardless of whether the demand/stressor was negative (pain) or positive (pleasure) and whether the person recognized the stressor. Now research has shown that

TABLE 9.2	Signs of Stress		
Physical Symptoms	Emotional Symptoms	Behavioral Symptoms	Cognitive Symptoms
Weight gain or loss	Irritability, quick temper	Bruxism (teeth grinding)	Anxious thoughts
Backaches	Restlessness	Changes in food and alcohol consumption	Loss of creativity
Sleep problems	Crying	Procrastination	Fearful anticipation
Stomachache	Overwhelming sense of pressure	Overly critical attitude	Constant worry
Lack of libido	Difficulty relaxing	Fist clenching	Poor concentration
Tense muscles	Lack of meaning to life and pursuits	Ruminating over the situation	Difficulty thinking
Shakiness or tremors	Sense of loneliness	Taking up smoking or excessive smoking	Difficulty remembering things
Frequent urination	Unhappy with no clear cause	Difficulty completing assignments	Indecisiveness
Dizziness or fainting	Depression	Withdrawing from others	Loss of sense of humor

although the body responds to both positive and negative stressors, the type of response seen differs and can include the types of neurotransmitters released. A positive change is called **eustress,** whereas a negative change is called **distress.** We are referring to distress when we talk about stress and its impact on our health.

The most current definition of stress upheld by the holistic medical community is that it is the inability to cope with a perceived threat to one's physical, mental, emotional or spiritual well-being, resulting in a series of physiological responses and adaptations. Each component of well-being is distinct.

- *Physical well-being* refers to the body's physiological processes that provide optimal body performance and the ability to adjust to a variety of environmental factors. It includes adjusting blood flow, respiratory rate, nutrient storage or mobilization, body temperature, and all of the many other physiological processes that keep our body functioning.
- *Mental (intellectual) well-being* refers to the cognitive function and includes the ability to process information, communicate, recall memory, and make decisions. These processes take place in the higher cerebral cortex regions of the frontal, parietal, and temporal lobes. Stress can overload the cognitive process, impairing our thoughts and ability to communicate, as when we are upset and lose focus.
- *Emotional well-being* (or *emotional intelligence*) comes from the ability to successfully manage emotions. It includes the state of mind and expressions of emotions without being controlled by them. The most basic emotions, including anger, fear, and pleasure, are processed by the limbic system of the brain, an area considered the primitive, mammalian brain. However, other regions of the cortex involved with personality and behavior influence the limbic system. Processing within these higher regions produces more complex emotional patterns or overtones and provides individuals the ability to learn to keep their emotions in balance. Stress can impair the processing between the higher regions of the cortex and the limbic system with the result being expressions of anger and fear.
- *Spiritual well-being* is the higher consciousness including personal value systems, a sense of a purpose of life, and the relationships individuals have with themselves and others. Embedded in spiritual well-being is social well-being (i.e., the relationship within the social structure). Woolfolk and Lehrer (1993) state that Western society has become less communal and spiritual compared to the past and has become more centered on the individual and materialism. The result is the stress of the lack of social support.

Although each of these contributors is a separate element of well-being, the four are connected, interwoven, and synergistic. This is reflected in psychosomatic illness in which emotional imbalance can cause or aggravate a physical disorder.

The perspective of health care changes when one considers the definition of stress just provided and recognizes that stress directly or indirectly affects many disorders. For years, health care has followed a mechanistic model with physicians playing the central role in treatment of the physical body, sometimes treating the direct cause of disease, other times treating only symptoms. Before 1950, the leading cause of illness and death in America was infectious based; influenza, pneumonia, tuberculosis, and gastroenteritis were the most prevalent causes. The advent of antibiotics has helped to better manage these conditions, and the average life span has increased.

Today, chronic illnesses, often with insidious onset, are more common than ever. The Centers for Disease Control (CDC) (2007) reports that cardiovascular disease and cancer have become the leading causes of morbidity and mortality. Research has begun to establish a correlation between stress and cardiovascular disease, and some link between stress and cancer has been suggested. With these insights, a wellness model for health and health care is emerging; it specifies that health is the balance, integration, and harmony of the physical, intellectual, emotional, and spiritual aspects of the human condition (see Figure 9.1 ■). Note the parallel between the wellness model and the earlier definition of stress. This paradigm shift places each person at the center of their own health care, which has been expanded to include preventative as well as prescriptive measures. Allopathic medicine has joined complementary medicine, and everyone needs to become more self-reliant in achieving health.

The American Psychological Association (APA, 2008) has identified three forms of stress based on their patterns of development: acute, episodic acute, and chronic. **Acute stress,**

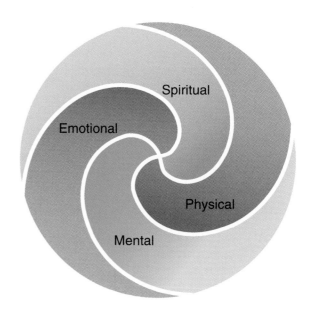

FIGURE 9.1

Wellness is an integration of the physical, emotional, mental, and spiritual body, with each component superimposed on the others.

the most common, is a sudden, often unexpected, emergency that occurs (for example, getting into a fender bender accident, realizing two clients are scheduled at the same time, having to cancel a day of appointments because of a sick child, and making a presentation to a group with butterflies in the stomach). These acute stressors trigger an arousal response but are relatively quick to resolve, and the person goes on with their life.

Some individuals, however, tend always to have a life of turmoil and to daily face a series of minor emergencies, whether real or perceived; this is considered to be **episodic acute stress.** This condition is typically self-induced because of overcommitment, poor organization and time management, and/or the tendency to perpetually worry and have a pessimistic attitude about the future (i.e., people with this stress have a low emotional IQ). The extended overarousal results in long-term effects on the body. These individuals can have severe difficulty in realizing what they are doing to themselves because of their ingrained lifestyle and personality. Instead of taking responsibility for how their life is unfolding, they often blame others and external factors for their lives of upheaval.

Chronic stress is insidious and occurs as a result of being caught in a long-term situation that a person cannot resolve or doesn't see a way to do so. It is a form in which a person has unrelenting demands and experiences pressure from which they can't escape, such as major debt, poverty, a dysfunctional family, or being caught in an unhappy relationship or work environment. It can also result from chronic illness or disabilities that impact our expectations of life, such as someone previously physically active becoming disabled and unwilling to accept his or her new limitations.

Episodic acute stress and chronic stress are most instrumental in leading to chronic disease patterns and decreased quality of life. Learning to recognize the patterns

of stress will help us learn how to handle them and prevent overreacting to the point that stress dominates our lives.

The Body's Response to Stressors: Neural and Hormonal

The stress reaction is a complex process based on (1) a neurophysiologic response, (2) the qualities of the stressor, and (3) differences between individuals. Early research by Selye examined the uniform pattern of physiological changes that occurred in animals and in humans during illness or physical stress; his observations identified a clear connection between the nervous system, endocrine system, and immune response. The emotional circuit carrying the stress input is routed through the brain's limbic system. It and associated structures serve as the headquarters for regulating the response to stress. The first reaction is a flight or fight response that prepares us for an emergency. When stress is chronic, additional physical adaptations occur mediated by hormones that virtually affect all areas of the body. The correlation between stress and its many effects on the body can be understood by examining the functions of the areas responsible for the mind-body connection: the limbic system, the cerebrum, and the midbrain regions.

LIMBIC SYSTEM

Although Brocca first described the **limbic system** and by the late 1880s had associated it with olfactory integration, it began to be linked to emotional experience and expression in the 1930s by researchers such as James Papez and Paul MacLean. Stress triggers strong emotional responses, so the area of emotions is central in the stress response.

The hypothalamus sits anatomically and physiologically in the center of the limbic system. The hypothalamus is surrounded by the amygdale, hippocampus, fornix, and limbic cortex (Figure 9.2 ■). Each has a role in emotional

FIGURE 9.2

The limbic system includes the thalamus, hypothalamus, hippocampus, amygdala, and the limbic cortex, with the hypothalamus at the center of the system. The RAS, indicated by the arrows, is a network of nerve fibers that regulates the rate of incoming information. It both influences and is influenced by the limbic system.

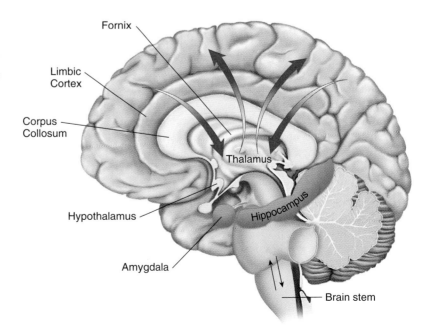

response and stress. Also associated with the limbic system is the **reticular activating system (RAS),** which extends through the brain stem and is the neural connection between the spinal cord and upper regions of the brain.

The hypothalamus is the key integration point from the limbic system. It links the conscious and involuntary nervous systems as well as the neural and endocrine responses. In this capacity, it both receives signals associated with stress and sends other signals that influence broad areas of the body. Some of the functions of the hypothalamus include being the:

- Relay point between within the cerebrum, the area of consciousness and autonomic nervous system, which controls the body's involuntary responses
- Site of the feeding and satiety centers that regulate appetite, digestive secretions, and motility
- Site of the thermoregulatory center that adjusts blood flow to the periphery, sweat gland activity, and shivering
- Regulator of the pituitary gland and thus an integration point between the nervous and endocrine systems
- Contributor with other regions of the limbic system in wake and sleep cycles

Neural output from the hypothalamus includes an extensive dispersal to the visceral organs, which control basic bodily functions, and it influences somatic motor output to the skeletal muscles. Neural output from the hypothalamus also regulates the pituitary gland, which releases a variety of hormones that influence many bodily functions. As a result, stress response mediated through the hypothalamus affects many areas of the body.

The amygdale controls a person's overall pattern of behavior and is strongly affected during stress and anxiety because it is involved in the perception and response to fear-based stimuli and aggressive responses. The amygdale processes potential threatening conditions from input received from the high-level processing areas of the cortex. These signals can be from something seen or from abstract thought.

Output from the amygdale reaches many brain regions. Signals to the frontal cortex help to make judgments about incoming stimuli and initiate behavior. Signals to the sensory cortex regions enhance the sensory sensations. Signals sent to the hypothalamus, midbrain, and brain stem regions influence the output of the autonomic nervous system and trigger the physiological changes that occur during fear and anxiety.

The hippocampus receives most sensory stimuli and in turn transmits signals to the hypothalamus and other portions of the limbic system. The area that receives the signal determines the response to it. When the information is channeled to the reward centers, we feel gratification, but when it is channeled to the punishment centers, we feel anxiety or disappointment. The hippocampus determines our ability to maintain our attention and can influence what we learn or remember. Memory is enhanced when the stimulus is sent to either the reward or punishment centers. We

often remember strong emotional experiences including those that occurred during acute stress. However, long-term stress impairs memory. The elevation of the stress hormone cortisone causes atrophy of the hippocampus and results in impairment of memory production (Sapolskyl, 2003).

The limbic cortex is the junction between the areas that provide emotional experience, memory, and ability to think and reason and the lower centers that control behavioral patterns. This crossroad links conscious thought processes to behavioral patterns through a two-way path. At times, the body can trigger a stress response merely because of our thoughts and feelings stemming from chronic emotional stresses without being confronted with immediate threats. The limbic cortex can trigger a broad spectrum of physical responses via the hypothalamus (i.e., gastric, respiratory and cardiovascular activity) and affective reactions (i.e., rage, docility, excitement, and alertness).

An enormous amount of sensory input comes to the brain at any one time. These signals must reach the cerebrum to provide conscious awareness. The input signals travel through the RAS, which works as a filter for incoming sensory stimuli. During sleep, RAS activity is very low, and we are unaware of our surroundings. The level of activity increases when we awaken and fluctuates during the day according to changing levels of alertness. When awake, nonessential information, such as the pressure of clothes on the body, is filtered out and does not reach the cerebrum. However, when something new occurs, such as a watch falling from the wrist, the information does pass through, and the individual becomes conscious of the event. This allows one to be attentive to the most important information within their surroundings.

Several factors determine the level of RAS activity: the daily rhythms established by the limbic system, the amount of stimuli being received, and feedback from the cerebral cortex back to the RAS. With emotional arousal, the amygdale triggers an increase in RAS activity, causing sensations to become more vivid. A feedback loop from the cerebrum to the RAS also increases activity. Inability to fall asleep at night when someone has something on his or her mind can be a result of an overactive cerebrum stimulating the RAS, thereby keeping him or her awake. Learning relaxation techniques helps a person to learn to control this to improve their quality of sleep.

GENERAL ADAPTATION SYNDROME

The **general adaptation syndrome** proposed by Hans Seyle considers the body's response to stress in stages: acute, resistance, and exhaustion.

The acute stage of stress is the **fight or flight response,** which refers to the physiologic changes that occur during an emergency. The response is from the sympathetic nervous system (SNS), which is one side of the autonomic nervous system. Its counterpart is the parasympathetic nervous system (PSNS). These two systems operate to keep the body in correct balance to deal with stress (triggering the fight or flight response) and to promote rest and restoration

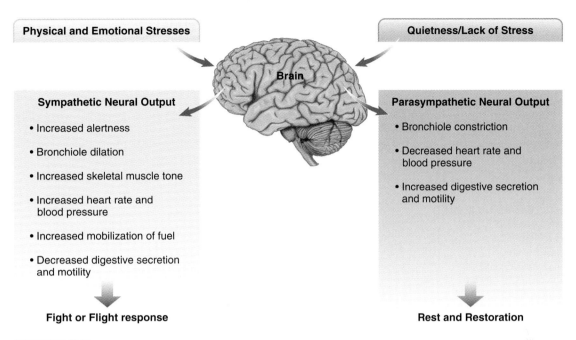

Physical and Emotional Stresses

Quietness/Lack of Stress

Brain

Sympathetic Neural Output

- Increased alertness
- Bronchiole dilation
- Increased skeletal muscle tone
- Increased heart rate and blood pressure
- Increased mobilization of fuel
- Decreased digestive secretion and motility

Fight or Flight response

Parasympathetic Neural Output

- Bronchiole constriction
- Decreased heart rate and blood pressure
- Increased digestive secretion and motility

Rest and Restoration

FIGURE 9.3

The sympathetic and parasympathetic neural controls operate to keep our body responses in balance based on the situation at hand.

of the body. See Figure 9.3 ■ for a comparison of the functions of the sympathetic and parasympathetic systems.

When someone perceives a threatening condition, a network of neurons scattered throughout the body releases norepinephrine. The resulting fight or flight response prepares him or her to physically handle a threatening situation. The heart rate quickens and additional blood flow is sent to the skeletal muscles, heart muscle, and brain. He or she breathes more deeply and quickly, and the bronchioles dilate to increase respiratory volumes. The eyes dilate, and we become more alert because of the RAS's increased neural activity. At this point, neural excitability increases, and the muscles tense. These changes allow a person to think and run more quickly and to fight more fiercely. Metabolic changes occur: fat is released back into the circulation to provide tissues with fuel, and glucose/carbohydrate levels increase for use by the nervous system. At the same time, activities promoted by the PSNS system, such as digestive secretions and motility, are blocked. This is why the mouth feels dry or indigestion is experienced during stress.

The release of epinephrine into the blood from the adrenal medulla backs the neural stimulation of target organs with norepinephrine. The circulating levels of epinephrine prolong the effect of the response, which does not subside until well after one is out of harm's way. As the SNS response declines, the PSNS activity increases to bring on rest and restoration of the body (i.e., digestion, tissue repair, and fuel storage).

If the stressor continues and/or the individual is unable to adapt to it, output from the amygdale establishes a more

prolonged effect known as the *resistance stage,* which is endocrine based. The hypothalamus mediates this response (see Figure 9.4 ■). The pituitary gland boosts its output of hormones, which work collectively to increase the physical ability to meet the stressor's demands. The changes include increased blood pressure, blood coagulation in the event of injury, and mobilization of more fuel for metabolism to meet the body's energy needs.

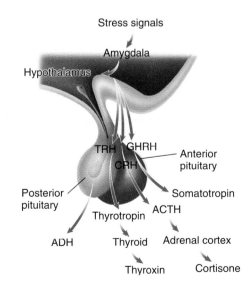

Stress signals

Amygdala

Hypothalamus

TRH   GHRH

CRH

Anterior pituitary

Posterior pituitary

Somatotropin

Thyrotropin

ACTH

ADH

Thyroid

Adrenal cortex

Thyroxin

Cortisone

FIGURE 9.4

The body's response to a longer, sustained stress involves hypothalamic control of several hormones.

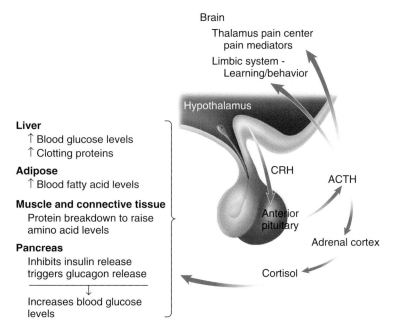

Brain
Thalamus pain center
pain mediators
Limbic system -
Learning/behavior

Hypothalamus

Liver
↑ Blood glucose levels
↑ Clotting proteins

Adipose
↑ Blood fatty acid levels

Muscle and connective tissue
Protein breakdown to raise
amino acid levels

Pancreas
Inhibits insulin release
triggers glucagon release
—————————————
↓
Increases blood glucose
levels

CRH

ACTH

Anterior
pituitary

Adrenal cortex

Cortisol

FIGURE 9.5

The principle function attributed to ACTH is its action to stimulate cortisone release. However, both hormones affect other target areas in the stress response.

Of the hormones involved, cortisol is commonly known as the *stress hormone*. Although a baseline level of cortisol is always present, when the amygdale perceives stress, the hypothalamus responds by increasing output of corticotrophin releasing hormone (CRH), which triggers the pituitary axis. Both adrenocorticotropic hormone (ACTH) and cortisol have their specific effects (see Figure 9.5 ■). In addition to ACTH's direct stimulation of the adrenal cortex for the release of cortisol, it also affects learning and behavior and, in conjunction with beta-endorphins, pain. However, the most recognized hormone response to stress is cortisol, which mobilizes energy stores and raises blood glucose, fatty acid, and amino acid levels. This shift in fuel availability provides the body the energy to meet the stress condition.

In addition to the pituitary stimulus, an immune response triggers cortisol release. During an infection, certain white blood cells release a chemical messenger known as *interleukin-1;* it triggers the secretion of cortisol. It is thought that the purpose of cortisol during infection is to mobilize fuel within the body to help meet its need during a stressful time when the person isn't eating enough. These same white blood cells also have receptors for cortisol. Cortisol inhibits the actions of the lymphocytes and macrophages and blocks further release of cytokines. This completes a negative feedback control over the release of cortisol (see Figure 9.6 ■). The result is cortisol has an immunosuppressive effect over the long term with increased risk for infections (discussed later).

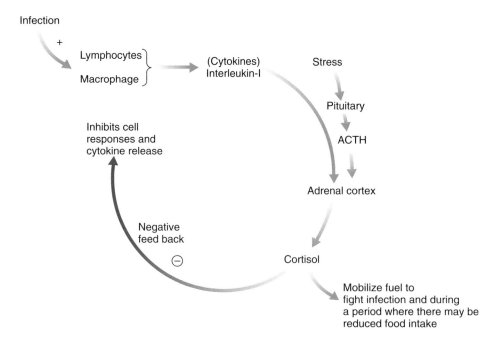

Infection

+

Lymphocytes
Macrophage

(Cytokines)
Interleukin-I

Stress

Pituitary

ACTH

Inhibits cell
responses and
cytokine release

Adrenal cortex

Negative
feed back

⊖

Cortisol

Mobilize fuel to
fight infection and during
a period where there may be
reduced food intake

FIGURE 9.6

During inflammation, the immune system triggers cortisol through chemical messengers released by white blood cells. The elevated cortisol in turn inhibits the immune cell response. The pituitary response during stress elevates cortisol and leads to inhibition of immune cells and an immunosuppressive effect, which can have an undesirable effect in the body.

Cortisone does not work by itself during stress. Other hormones of the hypothalamic-pituitary axis also become elevated (refer to Figure 9.4). Each hormone in the following list contributes to the resistance stage by mobilizing fuel and boosting circulation.

- *Thyroxin* increases metabolic rate throughout the body and increased neural excitability. A part of this broad effect is an increased heart rate, which in turn increases blood pressure and circulation.
- *Growth hormone (GH)* increases fat mobilization and conserves glucose, which is complementary to the effects of cortisol as discussed.
- *Antidiuretic hormone (ADH)* acts on the kidneys to conserve water and maintain blood volume to keep proper blood pressure for good circulation. At high levels, ADH is often referred to as *vasopressin* because of its effect to cause vasoconstriction of arteries and veins. It also increases blood pressure and circulation. The higher levels of ADH released during stress contributes to increased blood pressure.

Although the response during the resistance stage keeps the body prepared to fend off the stressor, at some point physiologically (the *exhaustion stage*), the system begins to shut down. Recent research has found that it is due to a process known as *down regulation response to cortisol* (Hayes, 2003). When cortisol is chronically elevated, the number of receptors on target cells for it declines. The result is that circulating fuel levels, especially glucose and fatty acids, drop. Electrolyte imbalance occurs, and blood pressure cannot be maintained. The result is severe illness or death.

The Point at Which Stress Becomes Detrimental

Dr. Paul Rosch of the American Institute of Stress points out on the home page of the organization's website (2008) that

> stress is not always necessarily harmful. Winning a race or election can be just as stressful as losing, but it is good stress. Increased stress results in increased productivity—up to a point after which things rapidly deteriorate, and that level differs for each of us. It's very much like the stress on a violin string. Not enough produces a dull, raspy sound and too much an irritating screech or or snaps the string, but just the correct degree of stress creates a beautiful tone. Similarly, we need to find the right amount of stress that allows us to make pleasant music in our daily lives.

Research on physical activity has identified that peak performance lies at a midpoint at which eustress has increased our abilities but before distress begins to impair our abilities. The Yerkes-Dodson principle (Figure 9.7 ■) correlates the level of performance to the level of stress during physical training. Studies have shown that peak physical performance occurs when stress hormones are at their optimal levels. At these levels, muscle strength and endurance are heightened, and we are mentally alert and

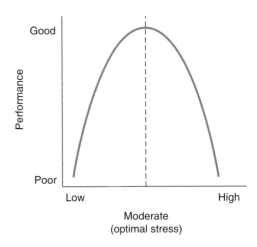

FIGURE 9.7

The Yerkes-Dodson curve correlates that an increase in stress (eustress) can improve performance to a point. After the optimal midpoint, further stress (distress) reduces performance.

focused. Research has also shown that moderate exercise enhances the body's defense system as the result of an increase in antibody levels and natural killer activity. However, training that is too rigorous pushes the body into distress and has detrimental effects. A study of marathon runners comparing those who trained more than 60 miles per week to runners who trained less than 20 miles per week showed that those with the more intense workout had twice as many respiratory infections. Other studies have shown that salivary antibodies, which reduce our susceptibility to respiratory infections, decrease following prolonged exhaustive exercise. As a result, researchers recommend that athletes avoid contact with others who have colds or flu for 6 hours following strenuous activity.

Although measuring psychological stress and its consequences is much more difficult than physical stress, current theory suggests that it follows a similar pattern. Eustress is needed for emotional, mental, and spiritual development. New situations when first experienced can seem very stressful, but after working through the situation, it no longer seems stressful or is at least less stressful if it occurs again. Without eustress, boredom occurs and individuals function below optimum level and do not attempt to "push the envelope." Nevertheless, when a chronic distress situation occurs, the elevated stress hormones have the same effect as when under physical stress. This lays the foundation for chronic illness.

Research has identified a number of chronic diseases and conditions that have stress, whether physical or psychological, as a risk factor. The hormonal changes that occur during the resistance stage of stress can underlie many of the connections. Consequently, debilitating effects of stress are set into place without advancing to the exhaustion stage. Each of the following areas discussed has research that supports correlations between stress and the pathology although it is also recognized that most of these conditions are multifactorial.

CARDIOVASCULAR DISEASES

Atherosclerosis and hypertension are the two principal cardiovascular diseases of concern regarding stress. The combination of hormones, including norepinephrine/epinephrine, ADH, thyroxin, aldosterone, and cortisone that rise during stress increases the risk for hypertension (see Figure 9.8 ■).

Hypertension, in turn, is a risk factor for atherosclerosis, potentially contributing to injury of the vessel wall that initiates the disease. Atherosclerosis is a buildup of a fibro-fatty plaque in arterial walls, which impairs the arteries' normal elasticity and can lead to blockage and ischemia. It is the most common cause of coronary heart disease and is associated with the carotid artery and cerebral vessels that lead to strokes, the aorta that causes aortic aneurysms, and renal arteries that lead to kidney disease. Elevated levels of fat within the circulation increase the fatty accumulation. The fat mobilization effect of cortisone and growth hormone that rises during stress can contribute to the process.

HYPERGLYCEMIA AND DIABETES

Cortisone and growth hormone act to mobilize fat and conserve glucose, and cortisone indirectly inhibits insulin production. As a result, glucose levels become elevated.

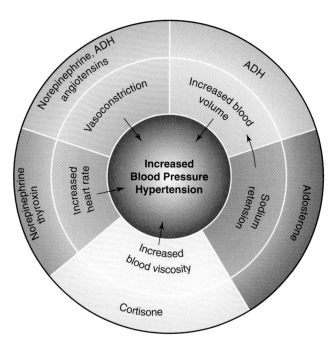

FIGURE 9.8

Essential hypertension is considered to be idiopathic; however, stress is considered to be a risk factor for its development. Correlation can be drawn between the hormonal elevations associated with chronic stress and their influence on blood pressure.

Chronically elevated blood glucose can have a variety of effects in the body:

- Increases risk for glycation of protein, which can contribute to peripheral vascular disease and aging processes
- Can reduce insulin sensitivity and set the stage for noninsulin-dependent diabetes mellitus.
- Aggravates existing diabetes by making managing the disease effectively more difficult.

IMMUNE DYSFUNCTION

As stated earlier, cortisone is noted for its immunosuppressive effects that can contribute to:

- Increased risk for infections and exacerbated symptoms when they occur
- Reduced response to immunizations
- Activation of latent viruses, such as herpes

Chronic stress can have mixed effects, ranging from remission to relapse, on a number of autoimmune disorders, including eczema, lupus, and rheumatoid arthritis. However, it is a major risk factor for flare-up of multiple sclerosis.

Although no evidence currently indicates that chronic stress causes cancer, there is increased evidence to indicate the effect of stress on the immune system can reduce anti-tumor activity and contribute to faster tumor growth and latent cancer growth. Researchers in Sweden and Australia independently correlated increases in colon cancer with serious work-related problems and major illness or death of a close family member. British studies have found a correlation between severe life events and the risk for breast cancer, and it has been hypothesized that long-term, intense grief, despair, and hopelessness can contribute to activation of latent breast neoplasia in some women (Biondi, 2001).

GASTROINTESTINAL CONDITIONS

The parasympathetic nervous system output from the hypothalamus promotes secretion from and motility of the gastrointestinal system. During acute and chronic stress, this output diminishes; hence, blood flow to the gastrointestinal (GI) tract, secretion, and motility decreases. Irritable bowel syndrome, also known as *spastic colon,* is strongly correlated to stress and is thought to be directly related to autonomic imbalance. Symptoms include spastic contractions and irritation of the large intestine with resulting diarrhea, constipation, cramping, and bloating. At one time, stress was thought to be a major factor in peptic ulcer disease; however, it has been shown that either the bacteria *H. pylori* or the use of nonsteroidal anti-inflammatory medications causes this disease. Nevertheless, studies still support stress as a risk factor for ulcers or sustaining existing ulcers. Chronic stress can also cause flare-up of the symptoms of inflammatory bowel diseases (Crohn's disease and ulcerative colitis.)

NEURAL CONDITIONS

Stress-induced tension headaches are perhaps the most well-noted neural response to stress. They occur as a result of strong stimulation of the muscles of the neck, jaw, forehead, and eyes. A similar pain pattern can occur in the lower back. Stress can also generate migraine headaches, which are thought to be triggered by a sympathetic stimulation of the cerebral vasculature causing strong vasoconstriction followed by a rapid vasodilation. The changes in pressure along with other chemical signals released cause the intense pain.

Chronic elevated levels of cortisone have been tied to atrophy of neurons within the brain. Chronic stress can speed the aging of brain. Atrophy of neurons of the hippocampus impairs memory and learning.

Stress affects mood by changes in neurotransmitters in the brain. Early on, anxiety occurs as the result of elevated norepinephrine and cortisone. Over time, however, anxiety typically leads to depression and altered mood and sleep cycles. At that stage, a drop in dopamine causes a decline in the feelings of pleasure.

ERGONOMIC IMPACTS OF STRESS

How stress manifests and its physiological responses will ultimately determine what kind of ergonomic impact it has. Emotional stress commonly leads to increased muscle tension, which can affect breathing, posture, and efficiency of movement. Physical stress can compound other stress factors stemming from the work place and personal life. If left unattended, individuals experience a vicious cycle that impacts them not only physically but also mentally, emotionally, and spiritually. Not only can stress from work affect their personal lives, but stress from their personal lives can affect their work. A holistic approach of evaluating stressors and learning to control/manage stress is necessary to reduce its impact on work performance and reduce the risk for chronic disease discussed earlier. As this overview indicates, the effects of stress on the body are diverse, and many are insidious. Therefore, to effectively manage stress, one must be attuned to its potential causes. Although stress can be only one of several causes of a disease process, the course of the condition can be influenced by managing stress.

TECHNIQUES FOR MANAGING STRESS

Different perspectives can vary the definitions of stress. Eastern philosophies consider stress as an absence of "inner peace" whereas Western culture generally describes it as "wear and tear" or "loss of control." A balanced approach to understanding and managing stress recognizes both. Not all techniques will work for everyone. Each of us needs to try different techniques to find the combination that works for us. An overview of stress management techniques will start you on the path of finding the best techniques for yourself.

Whether you embrace an Eastern or Western approach to life, recognizing that "loss of control" and/or "wear and tear" will disrupt our equilibrium until we make an adjustment is important. This adjustment can occur through an attitude shift or a change in the pattern that creates the dysfunction.

Healthy Lifestyle

We live in a culture that endorses hard work, long hours, and a fast pace. It is no wonder that stress and its effects are rampant. Finding the time to balance work with a lifestyle that promotes well-being is a bit tricky but very possible with good planning and commitment.

DIET

When considering stress, we must recognize three dietary factors: (1) poor diet strips our bodies of necessary nutrients and thus is a physical stress on the body; it can occur alone or with other stress factors, compounding its effect; (2) while under stress, we can stray from healthy to unhealthy eating habits; and (3) nutrient demands can change while we are under stress. Managing stress with proper diet includes considering what and when we eat.

The first guideline in reducing stress is to maintain a balanced diet that is high in vegetables, fruit, and whole grain products as recommended in the FDA food pyramid (Figure 9.9 ■). Changes in nutrient demands during stress triggers an increased demand for protein and carbohydrates, but it is important to stay with complex carbohydrates to avoid the "highs and lows" that refined sugars can cause. Maintaining a good supply of Vitamin B and C, which can become depleted with stress, is important. While under stress, we are drawn to "comfort foods" that contain caffeine and sugars, which can actually make the stress cycle more pronounced. Caffeine increases the feelings of anxiety by raising adrenaline release, mimicking the stress response, and therefore should be avoided or used minimally. Overuse of alcohol as a stress escape is an empty calorie intake that depletes the body of vitamins. Adrenaline release also affects our moods by increasing tension, irritability, and insomnia followed by depression. Remember that stress affects moods; moods affect food choices, which in turn can affect our moods. If you find yourself tempted by comfort foods, begin to make a mental note of why and when you eat. Be aware of emotional states and have healthy snacks on hand when you feel the need to eat.

Foods also affect our moods by altering the production of neurotransmitters in the brain, which can influence how we handle stress. Carbohydrates increase serotonin levels, which has a calming effect. On the other hand, consumption of protein-rich foods causes dopamine and norepinephrine levels to increase, in turn heightening alertness, focus, and reaction time. The optimum is to have a balance of carbohydrate and protein that keeps us focused without becoming anxious, which makes stress worse.

Our daily biological rhythm also affects these neurotransmitters and determines when we are active and when

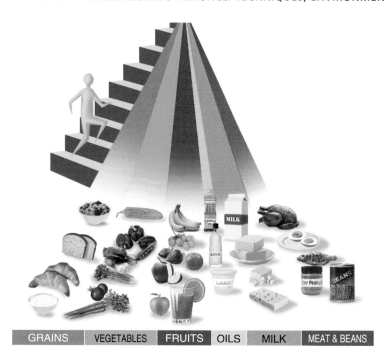

GRAINS   VEGETABLES   FRUITS   OILS   MILK   MEAT & BEANS

FIGURE 9.9

FDA recommendations for a balanced diet are to increase the intake of complex carbohydrates, such as grains, fruits, and vegetables. Refined sugars and fat intake need to be limited. Staying away from processed foods helps in staying within the FDA recommendations.

we are sleepy (Christie, 2004). Some of us are "morning people" and others are "night owls." Morning people naturally wake up early and are more energetic in the morning because they produce a higher level of dopamine and norepinephrine early in the day. By afternoon those levels taper off, and serotonin begins to rise, so morning people begin to slow down and are ready for bed by 9 or 10 PM. The reverse is true for night owls. Getting up early is difficult because of their higher levels of serotonin. The night owls don't become fully engaged until the afternoon but continue to be active well into the evening, sometimes not going to bed until after midnight because of their elevated levels of dopamine and norepinephrine.

Work schedules don't necessarily match our natural rhythms. Selecting the best food to adjust your biological rhythm to your work demands can help. By eating cereals and fruits (carbohydrates) for breakfast, morning people can remain calm as they head to work, and a protein-rich lunch will keep them alert through the afternoon. The night owls, on the other hand, need their protein-rich meal first thing in the morning and as a morning snack to stay alert for the day. The lunch and evening meal should include more carbohydrates to increase serotonin production so they can curb their late-night tendencies.

Proper diet requires regular meals; avoid skipping them. Not eating until the end of a stressful period can cause us to eat the wrong things and too much of them. Eat small meals or healthy snacks every 2–3 hours during the day. Enjoy your meals by eating slowly and being aware of the food. This reduces overeating and can be a relaxing time. Small meals prevent a large shift of blood flow to the digestive system, allowing you to remain more alert to deal with the tasks at hand.

EXERCISE

Chapter 7 discussed the benefits of exercise and offered suggestions for developing and staying on task with an exercise program. Exercise reduces stress and increases the sense of well-being.

Tai chi and yoga have increased in popularity in recent years because of their overall benefits. Both take a mind, body, and spirit approach. Tai chi originated in China as a martial art for self-defense more than 2,000 years ago. It is especially beneficial for older adults because of the ease with which one can perform the movements. Tai chi is often considered a moving meditation, is touted as a stress reducer, and is known to improve balance and agility.

Yoga originated in India thousands of years ago. It is so popular in the United States that almost every club and fitness center offers yoga classes. Of the several styles of yoga, the most popular form, according to the Mayo Clinic website http://www.mayoclinic.org is Hatha yoga. It focuses on poses (asanas) and the breath. There are also different expressions of Hatha yoga (Yoga, 2006). Some focus more on the breathing exercises, otherwise known as *pranayama,* than others. The benefits of yoga are increased flexibility, strength, balance, reduced stress, and overall health. Before enrolling in a yoga class, always check the instructor's qualifications.

Walking is one of the easiest forms of exercise and an excellent stress reducer. It doesn't cost anything and it's easy to incorporate into a workday. Look for ways to increase your walking such as parking farther from your office, the grocery store, and places you visit. A pedometer is a great way to track your steps, distance, and even the calories burned. Refer to Chapter 7 for exercise for specifics for building a program incorporating strength, cardiorespiratory

HELPFUL HINT 9.1
Recommended Web Sites on Stress Management

http://www.acsm.org/
http://www.nsca-lift.org/

http://www.yogaalliance.org/
http://www.mayoclinic.com/health/stress/SR00026

activity, and stretching. See Helpful Hint 9.1 for a list websites for further information about exercise, yoga, tai chi, and other behavioral activities.

Sleep

As with diet, inadequate or poor sleep can cause physical stress or be a consequence of it. Sleep or lack thereof also affects physical and mental performance. Studies indicate a link between lack of sleep and increased appetite because of a decrease in body temperature. The body overcompensates for the loss of heat by refueling with food, resulting in weight gain. According to Dr. Van Cauter (2004), research professor at the University of Chicago, sleep deprivation causes metabolic and endrocrine changes that can cause early aging and age-related diseases, such as diabetes, hypertension, obesity, and memory loss. Lighting, television, and computers have dramatically changed sleep patterns in the last 50–75 years. With modern conveniences available and busy schedules, many working adults try to get by on less sleep. Others find that even when they go to bed at a reasonable time, they have difficulty falling asleep or wake in the middle of the night and are unable to go back to sleep because of worries that plague them. If you find yourself in either situation, you can take a number of steps to ensure that you get sufficient, quality sleep.

You need to be aware of the amount of sleep you need, which varies among individuals but typically is between 6 and 9 hours a night. If you become exhausted toward the end of the day or have difficulty getting up when the alarm rings, you should consider changing your sleeping pattern. The first step is to establish a routine that (1) allows you to wind down several hours prior to bed and (2) maintains a consistent time for going to bed and getting up. Winding down includes forgoing strenuous physical activities during the evening hours as well as avoiding arousing or anxiety-causing activities before bedtime such as talking about family problem, paying bills, working late, or watching disturbing news. Instead, select activities that relax you, perhaps soaking in a hot tub, listening to soothing music, working on a craft, or doing simple chores to prepare for the next day.

Designate the bedroom for comfort and rest. Exclude televisions and do not work in the bedroom. The room should be quiet and dark. If needed, you can wear earplugs or if you need a background sound, pick one that works for you such as a favorite ticking clock or a fountain. The temperature needs to not be too cool or too hot. Although there is not a single optimum temperature for everyone, typically the bedroom temperature should be lower than the general room temperature.

Pamper yourself with a comfortable mattress, bedding, and a good pillow. If you have an old mattress and find that you wake with a sore back or neck, consider purchasing a new one. Take time when buying a mattress to try various types to find one with the correct firmness for your preference. Select a mattress size that gives you plenty of room to stretch and move. Feeling restricted during sleep can cause you to wake up and will reduce the quality of your sleep. Sleeping with a partner demands that you find a bed size to fit both of your space needs. Pets sleeping with you can restrict your movement. If so, train them to sleep in their own bed.

Additional factors identified by the National Sleep Foundation to consider for quality of rest are:

- Avoid eating large meals 2–3 hours before bed; lying down with a full stomach can cause gastric reflux, and the "heartburn" disrupts your rest.
- Avoid caffeine in the evening hours and limit your daily consumption of it.
- Limit alcohol use; the practice of drinking a "night cap" before bed is contradictory.
- Avoid alcohol, which can make you drowsy initially but often causes you to wake up later. Instead, chose a noncaffeinated herbal tea or a glass of milk if you want a beverage before going to bed.
- Avoid overconsumption of liquids including water in the evening; needing to get up in the middle of night interrupts your night's rest.
- Avoid turning on too much light if you do need to get up during the night.
- Get sufficient exercise during the day but avoid strenuous exercise in the hours before bed; cardiovascular exercise 3–5 times per week has been found to improve the quality of sleep.

When waking in the morning, you should typically feel rested and ready for the day. Certainly, each of us has his or her own daily rhythm that accounts for how quickly we wake up, but if we consistently feel tired and unprepared for the day, we need to investigate our sleep patterns and make adjustments to improve our quality of rest.

Behavioral Techniques

Life brings us many challenges. We view some as gifts and others as a curse. We experience joy, sorrow, pain, good health, and many more unusual conditions and emotions. Many techniques are available to help us by influencing our behavior and attitude and empowering us as we navigate the trials and tribulations of life. Many of us are so busy juggling so many tasks and wearing so many hats that we have no idea how to nurture ourselves. Begin by making a list of likes: I like nature, I like baths, I like quiet time, and so on. Commit to doing at least one thing you like per day and build from that point.

SOCIAL INTERACTION

We can't say enough about the importance of social interaction as a means of support and pleasure and what it adds to overall well-being. Daniel Goleman's latest book, *Social Intelligence: The New Science of Human Relationships,* takes a broad look at this subject. "Neuroscience shows our brain's very design makes it sociable; we are wired to connect" (Goleman, p. 4). Studies have shown that a social support system can protect our health and longevity. "Interactions with others create an emotional tango in the brain; it acts like a thermostat as it orchestrates our emotions" (Goleman, p. 5). Goleman says that relationships mold our experience and our biology. Our connection to one another, whether as friend, lover, or acquaintance, can impact our immune system positively or negatively. It is well known that nurturing, positive relationships have a beneficial impact on our health and negative, stressful relationships don't. The relatively new field of social neuroscience is making advances toward increased understanding of how the "social brain" is attuned and responds to what we feel and think about our interactions with others. The word *neuroplasticity* is used to demonstrate that social interactions can reshape our brain through repetitious experiences. Social intelligence is about behavior and "acting wisely in human relationships" (Goleman, 2006, p. 12).

A study in Sweden tracked 17,000 men and women over a 6-year period. The group that felt isolated and lonely and without a social support system had four times the risk of an early demise than those with good social support (Benson, 2006). It is beneficial to think of our confidants, friends, co-workers, peers, family, companions, and pets as life enhancing, immune boosting, and life extending. Sometimes these relationships are negative and can cause stress, but positive ones are quite the opposite. If you think you need to increase you social bonds, try volunteering, taking a class, or visiting a neighbor. Consider fostering or adopting a pet. Many animal shelters need dog and cat foster "parents" until they find a permanent home for the animals. Some hospitals have programs for people to hold premature babies. Dr. Tiffany Field, a massage therapist and founder of the Touch Research Institute, conducted a study several years ago that demonstrated that the weight of premature babies who were massaged increased significantly more than those who were not (2000). Many rewarding and life-enriching experiences await us if we take the time for them.

SPIRITUALITY

As social beings, we depend on our higher consciousness and connection to our surroundings. The field of spiritual psychology utilizes the art and science of human evolution in consciousness. The word *psyche* means "soul." The field of transpersonal psychology embraces the integration of psyche, or soul, and mind. It studies and develops spiritual experiences in a psychological context. The field believes that at the core of every issue—whether it is sorrow, disease, or discontent—is a corresponding root cause. Imbalance in an area of our life can create stress. To achieve balance, we need to assess the root cause of the imbalance.

Self-realization is an expansion of consciousness that leads to self-mastery. Lack of self-esteem is an obstruction on the road of life and can hinder us from growing beyond the limitations set by not valuing ourselves.

Some evidence supports the theory that the more neurotransmitter serotonin we have, the greater is the capacity for spiritual states of experience (Of Serotonin and Spirituality, 2003).

Many people express a spiritual state of being and/or feeling of transcendence by being in nature or spending quality time with their families and loved ones. It is not uncommon for people to leave successful and demanding careers because of stress or a feeling a loss of self or connection to a bigger purpose in life.

JOURNALING AND MINDFULNESS

Of the many tools and techniques available to help us cope with the stressors in life, perhaps one of the most insightful is *journaling.* Keeping a daily journal is a great way to document our conscious and subconscious thoughts. Journaling is a form of mindfulness and attention to the details of our thoughts, feelings, and emotions. Perhaps you can recall keeping a diary when you were an adolescent and your diary was your best friend. It held all of your wishes, dreams, and secrets.

Journaling is a stress management tool and a form of self-exploration. Looking into our inner selves can be an awe-inspiring, enriching experience and a way to grow and expand our consciousness. Journaling provides a way to clarify and define situations in life or conditions such as health concerns that you want to monitor. We can determine after reading a journal entry whether is has clues to a problem we are attempting to resolve. Journaling uses both hemispheres of the brain, allowing the experience to be fully integrated. Writing in our journals can alleviate stress, enhance self-awareness, and aid emotional healing.

Mindfulness can be applied to all situations. We can be mindful through meditation, thoughts, words, and deeds. It is considered a contemplative study of staying in the present. Mindfulness while eating will not only aid digestion but will most likely cause us to eat less. An issue of *Harvard Women's Health Watch* (April 2009, Vol. 16, issue 8) considered how learning to focus the mind can help manage the stressors of everyday living. Mindfulness can increase enjoyment, improve physical and emotional health, and enhance our ability to cope with illness. Some tips for practicing mindfulness include:

- Focus on your breathing, observing each inhalation and exhalation for 10 breaths.
- Chew each bite slowly before swallowing (this aids digestion).
- Practice maintaining your full attention on a daily act such as brushing your teeth.
- Be mindful of what you are saying.

AFFIRMATIONS AND VISUALIZATION

We have approximately 60,000 thoughts per day (Pokea, 2008). That is a lot of thoughts! The popular book *The Secret* written by Rhonda Byrne is about the law of attraction and how thoughts create our reality. Monitoring our thoughts through observation or mindfulness will identify the quality of our thoughts. With awareness and practice, we can replace negative thoughts with an affirmation (positive thought) and visualize a desired outcome. Louise L. Hay states in her book *Heal Your Body* that mental thought patterns form our experience. She uses affirmations as tools for change and healing. Affirmations are statements of acceptance that need to be stated positively and in present time as though what we are affirming that it has already occurred. Negative thoughts such as "I don't like my body" and "I am too fat" would be countered with "I am beautiful and weigh my perfect weight" or "I love and accept myself." Visualizing the outcome that we want adds support and empowers us to make the change we want to see in our lives by picturing it. If you are trying affirmations for the first time, following these guidelines is helpful:

- Use present tense.
- State them positively and maintain a positive attitude.
- Be specific.
- Keep them short and write them down; this adds to empowerment.
- Believe in what you are saying.
- Repeat them (practice your affirmations daily).

Visualization is the formation of mental images or pictures. Countless images occur to us throughout the day, so it is worthwhile to monitor them to affirm that we are creating pictures that we want to come to fruition in our lives. The old adage "seeing is believing" is true: We can visualize our way to the life we want to have because we believe what our eyes see whether mentally or visually.

Our subconscious remembers things such as a lover's glance, a baby's smile, a beautiful sunset that we can play over and over again in our minds, thereby creating the memory and the emotions of these powerful images.

Combining affirmations and visualizations is a powerful tool for creating the life we want. If the affirmation is related to the body, we should see ourselves with the body we want and practice the art of visualizing our way to our heart's desire.

HUMOR

François Voltaire (1694–1778) said, "The art of medicine consists of keeping the patient amused while nature heals the disease." The more current version is that humor is the best medicine. Did you ever notice how good you feel after belly laughing? Bringing a sense of humor to work can ease job stress and make those around you feel better. A sense of humor is a must in intimate relationships. Without one, we are doomed to suffer.

Laughter can boost our immune system and improve our quality of life. Studies in the field of psychoneuroimmunology state that the body responds well to positive thoughts, feelings, emotions, and attitudes. Candace Pert states in her book *Molecules of Emotion* that emotions are stored in the body in a form of chemical messages. These messages can impact our health through neurochemical changes, which determine whether we can get sick or stay well. The key is in complex molecules (neuropeptides) that form a network by which all cells communicate with one another. These messages can be brain-to-brain, brain-to-body, body-to-body, and body-to-brain. The neuropeptides are constantly changing, reflecting variations in emotional states. Pert says, "I believe that happiness is what we feel when our biochemicals of emotion, the neuropeptides and their receptors, are open and flowing freely throughout the psychosomatic network, integrating and coordinating our systems, organs, and cells in a smooth and rhythmic movement" (1997, p. 265).

PROFESSIONAL BOUNDARIES

Most of us have experienced the consequences of having poor boundaries at some point in our lives. Boundary issues come in a variety of shapes and sizes. Whether it is the inability to say no when we already have too much on our plate and we end up feeling used and/or exhausted or an issue such as dating a client. It can be enticing when someone asks for help or advice for us to step outside our scope of practice. A lack of boundaries can create undo stress and lead to potential litigation not to mention emotional suffering. Sometimes we are inclined to become involved with our clients' problems, compounding our stress. The best practice is to know and follow the profession's ethical guidelines. We should post them where they are visible to our clients. People feel safer when boundaries are established, and a safe environment is beneficial to the client and us. The following list will assist you in determining whether you boundaries are slipping.

- Your client feels more like a friend to you than a client.
- You want to be friends with your client.

- You feel sexually aroused when you are with your client.
- Your session with the client is frequently longer than it is for others.
- You want to share your personal problems with a client.
- You borrow money from the client.
- You accept valuable gifts from a client.

Relaxation

Many tools are available to assist us in learning how to relax. We should consider our personality and likes/dislikes before setting course on a particular path to achieving relaxation. Some people find meditation and prayer relaxing; others enjoy reading a book or soaking in a hot tub. Regardless of our chosen path, it is essential that we dedicate ourselves to taking the time on a daily basis to do something that relaxes us. Investigate the following practices to determine whether any or all are helpful in relaxing.

DEEP BREATHING

Breath is integral to life! It is a physiological process that is autonomous (involuntary) and voluntary, so we often forget how important it is to breathe correctly. When we inhale, we are oxygenating tissue and releasing by products from the cell where respiration actually occurs. Upon exhalation, we release carbon dioxide. This important exchange of gases helps to regulate our pH or acid/alkaline balance.

The most efficient way to breathe is diaphragmatic. The diaphragm separates our chest from the abdominal cavity and is a dome-shaped muscle that acts as a bellows; when we inhale, the abdomen should expand and subsequently collapse on exhalation (see Figure 9.10 ■). Other less efficient and potentially harmful breathing patterns occur when we are not conscientious. As bodyworkers, we need to be aware of our breathing while we work on a client because it is easy to hold our breath while focusing on working the muscles. Reversed breathing occurs when the abdomen collapses on the inhalation and expands on the exhalation and when we use chest rather than diaphragmatic breathing. Reversed breathing is shallower and does not inflate the lungs as efficiently.

Inhaling through the nose and exhaling from the nose without external sound is most efficient; however, sometimes exhaling through the mouth seems to more thoroughly empty the lungs. The inside of the nose is lined with mucous membrane and covered with hair that helps to filter dust and debris, direct the flow of air, warm the air we breathe, register our sense of smell, and affect the nervous system (Ballentine, Hymes, & Rama, 1981).

Breathing incorrectly for 3 minutes is enough to decrease the amount of oxygen to the brain and heart by 30%, according to Dr. Courtney Rosalba, an expert in the Buteyko method of "eucapnic" breathing (*eu* means "good,"

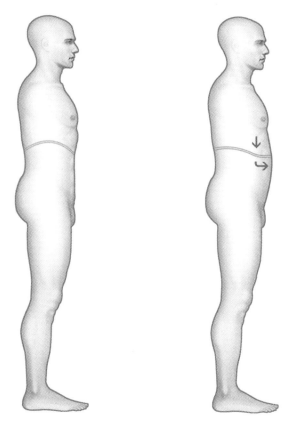

FIGURE 9.10

The dome-shaped diaphragm lies inferior to the base of the lungs. As the diaphragm contracts during inspiration, the lungs expand and the abdomen pushes outward.

and *capnic* refers to carbon dioxide). The Buteyko method is the work of Dr. Konstantin Buteyko, a Russian scientist. In the 1950s in Russia, he conducted many tests before determining that low levels of carbon dioxide is implicated in several diseases, asthma being the most noted. Inefficient breathing can be implicated in 50–70% of all diseases. His method of breathing is used to treat immune dysfunction, circulatory, hormonal, and metabolic diseases with success (Rosalba, 2000).

When we are not conscious of our breathing, our thoughts, feelings, and emotions wreak havoc with it. At any given time we could be holding our breath, breathing shallow, and so on. Refer to Worksheet 9.1 for information on identifying your breathing pattern.

MUSCLE RELAXATION

Most of us feel the effects of stress somewhere on our body in the form of muscular tension. Progressive muscle relaxation teaches us to be aware of the location of the tension and how to release it. We can isolate each muscle individually or sets of them, such as the upper back. As we focus on

WORKSHEET 9.1
Breathing Exercise

Lie comfortably with a pillow under your knees for lumbar support. Close your eyes and place your hands on your lower abdomen. Observe your breath as you inhale through your nose and exhale from you mouth. The mouth should be relaxed with the lips slightly open. Do you feel the rise and fall of your lower abdomen beneath your hands? The rise of your abdomen should occur on the inhalation and the fall on the exhalation. Make a mental note of where you feel the breath in your body. The following breathing patterns are less efficient. Identify any of these patterns that you experienced.

- *Reversed:* The abdomen contracts upon inhalation and expands on exhalation.
- *Chest:* The diaphragm is not used.

Repeat the exercise, only this time focus on the expansion of your abdomen upon inhalation if you are a reversed or chest breather. Feel the rise of your hands with the inhalation. Continue breathing in this manner until you are comfortable. Notice that with each breath, your breathing is deeper, smoother, and more relaxed.

---

the muscle, contract it for a few seconds and then relax. It is best to perform it methodically from head to toe. Progressive muscle relaxation quiets the mind and increases our ability to focus and concentrate. The exercise also includes diaphragmatic breathing and visualization. Try the following exercise in Worksheet 9.2.

MEDITATION

Meditation has been around for centuries and is practiced around the globe by most religions in some shape or form. *Webster's New World Dictionary* defines *meditation* as thinking deeply. Some say it is to empty the mind chatter referred to as "monkey mind" and not think at all. Almost

WORKSHEET 9.2
Progressive Relaxation

Begin by lying or sitting comfortably and breathing diaphragmatically. Inhale through the nose and exhale from the mouth. Continue breathing this way for a few minutes or count 10 breaths. Focus on each breath becoming slower, deeper, and more rhythmic.

Visualize each muscle or muscle set, tighten for a few seconds, and then relax followed by several deep breaths. Move to the next area and repeat until you have progressively covered the body. Follow the steps provided. We suggest making an audiotape of these instructions to guide you on the journey to deeper relaxation and dissolving tension.

- Begin by focusing on the muscles of the forehead, tense them, and then relax.
- Tense and then relax the muscles around your eyes.
- Tense and then relax the muscles of around your mouth.
- Tense and then relax the jaw muscles.
- Tense and then relax the neck muscles.
- Tense and then relax the chest muscles.
- Tense and then relax the abdominal muscles.
- Focus on your left shoulders, then arm, then wrist and hand, tense, and then relax.

- Next focus on your right shoulder, then arm, then wrist and hand, tense, and then then relax.
- Pause and breathe between each area comparing right and left sides. Repeat if there is still tension and you note any differences between the right and left sides.
- Repeat sequence with the muscles of the back and spine from the back of the neck to the tailbone.
- Tense and then relax your buttocks.
- Tense and then relax upper left leg, lower left leg, and left foot.
- Tense and then relax upper right leg, lower right leg, and right foot.

Observe any differences between your right and left sides. Continue deep relaxed diaphragmatic breathing while doing a mental scan of your entire body searching for any remaining tension. If you discover any areas of tension, contract the muscle/s for several seconds and relax. Repeat until the tension is gone or diminished.

every website, book, or article that addresses stress suggests meditation as a form of relaxation or stress reduction. It is up to each reader to discern what meditation means to you.

Meditation can be described as state of concentration, attention, thought, focus, or awareness. It can also be described as letting go, quiescence, and emptying the mind as stated earlier. *Meditation* comes from the Latin *meditatio*, which means "contemplation." Eastern spiritual practices have gained in popularity in the Western culture. Maharishi Mahesh Yogi, a scientist in the field of consciousness, introduced transcendental meditation (TM), one of the more popular forms of meditation. This method is practiced daily for 20 minutes while the person is seated with eyes closed.

Mindfulness is another form of meditation in which the person meditating sits and focuses his or her awareness on an object or process such as breath, sound (mantra), or visualization for a period of time on a daily basis.

Depending on the practitioner's goal and the consistency and duration of practice, meditation can bring about an altered state of consciousness, lower blood pressure, improve cardiovascular health, and bring enlightenment; it can be practiced standing, supine, or seated. Most meditative traditions endorse keeping the spine straight, which means maintaining a neutral spine with the natural spinal curves but no slouching. The straight spine allows the energy to circulate unimpeded. This circulation of energy is referred to as *life force, qi (chi), vital breath,* and *kundalini.*

An article by Albeniz and Holmes (2008) identified the following behavioral components of meditation:

- Relaxation
- Concentration
- Altered state of awareness
- Suspension of logical thought processes
- Maintenance of self-observing attitude

The research and studies discussing its benefits are as vast as the field of meditation itself. Some additional areas of research show that meditation can benefit the following:

- Cardiovascular and respiratory system
- Somatic motor function
- Stress and pain
- Metabolism
- Brain waves
- Immune system

Dr. Herbert Benson, a Harvard Medical School professor and pioneer in the study of physiological changes due to meditation coauthored, "A wakeful hypometabolic physiologic state," in the *American Journal of Physiology* in 1971; he believes that meditation helps us to relax, which in turn produces physiological changes in the body. See Helpful Hint 9.2 for references to meditation that can guide you in investigating some of the many resources for and types of meditation available.

HELPFUL HINT 9.2
Meditation References

http://www.mro.org/zmm/teachings/meditation.php
http://www.t-m.org.uk/differs.shtml
http://healing.about.com/od/meditationtypes/
What_Type_of_Meditation_is_Right_For_You.htm
http://www.shambhalasun.com/index.php?option=content
&task=view&id=2125

Austin, H. James. (1999). *Zen and the brain: Toward a total understanding of meditation and consciousness.* Boston, MA: MIT.
Kabat-Zinn, Jon. (1994). *Wherever you go there you are: Mindfulness meditation in everyday life.* New York, NY: Library of Congress.

CHAPTER SUMMARY

- Causes of stress can be categorized into physical, emotional, and mental. Because perception plays an important role in stress, its causes vary with each individual.
- Bodyworkers face the stresses of being a health care provider and potentially the stress of a business owner.
- Signs of stress can include physical, emotional, behavioral, and cognitive symptoms.
- Stress is the inability to cope with a perceived threat to a person's physical, mental, emotional, or spiritual well-being that results in a physiological response.
- Patterns of stress development include acute, episodic acute, and chronic stress. Of the three, episodic acute and chronic have the most negative impact on health and well-being.
- The limbic system and surrounding area are responsible for the mind-body connection, which explains how mental or emotional stresses can affect the functioning of the body.

- The body's response to stress occurs in stages. Emergencies trigger the SNS (fight-or-flight) response. If the stress does not go away or an individual does not learn to cope, the body goes into a resistance phase with cortisone being the principle hormone maintaining the body. This can lead to the exhaustion phase and death.
- Many chronic disease conditions are thought to be linked to the elevated hormone level during stress: cardiovascular disease, diabetes, high blood pressure, immune dysfunction, and gastrointestinal conditions.
- Eustress improves performance with peak performance reached just before distress reduces performance. This applies to both physical and emotional stress.
- Effective stress management includes maintaining a healthy life style and selecting behavioral and relaxation techniques that match your preferences.

REVIEW QUESTIONS

1. What are the four components of well-being?
2. How is the bodyworker at risk for stress?
3. Identify the disadvantages of self-employment for bodyworkers.
4. True/False? There are physiological signs of stress.
5. True/False? Stress can be good for us.
6. True/False? Stress patterns include acute, episodic acute, and chronic.
7. True/False? Acute stress is short term and does not impact health to the degree that chronic stress does.
8. The following are functions of the hypothalamus.
   a. regulation of hormone release
   b. regulation of body temperature
   c. regulation of apetite
   d. all of the above
9. Fight or flight response occurs in the following:
   a. sympathetic nervous system
   b. parasympathetic nervous system
   c. autonomic nervous system
   d. all of the above
10. Hormones involved with stress are:
    a. cortisol
    b. ACTH
    c. Dopamine
    d. Cortisol and ACTH
11. Important in the management of stress are:
    a. diet
    b. exercise
    c. sleep
    d. all of the above

SUGGESTED READINGS

Romas, J., & Sharma, M. (2004). *Practical stress management: A comprehensive workbook for managing change and promoting health* (3rd ed.). New York: Pearson.
http://www.health.harvard.edu
http://www.mayoclinic.com/health/stress/SR00026

http://www.queendom.com/tests/access_page/index.htm
http://www.usuhs.mil/psy/stressmanagement-health careproviders.pdf

REFERENCES

Albeniz, A., and Holmes, J. (2008). Healthy application and clinical studies of meditation. Retrieved January 9, 2008, from http://peaceandhappy.blogspot.com/2008/01/health-applications-and-clinical.html

American Psychology Association. (2008). Stress: The different kinds of stress. Retrieved January 5, 2008, from http://www.apa.org/helpcenter/stress-kinds.aspx

Ballentine, R., Hymes, A., & Rama, S. (1981). *Science of breath: A practical guide.* Honesdale, PA: Himalayan Publishers.

Benson, H. (2000). Relaxation response. Retrieved January 9, 2008, from http://relaxationresponse.org/

Benson, H. (2006). Stress management: Social support. Retrieved January 9, 2008, from http://www.healthharvard.edu

Biondi, M. (2001). Effects on stress on immune functions: An overview. In R. Ader, D. L. Felten, & N. Cohen (Eds.), *Psychoneuroimmunology* (3rd ed., Vol. 2, pp. 189–226). San Diego: Academic Press.

Centers for Disease Control. (2007, November, 20). Deaths: Leading causes for 2004. *National Vital Statistics Report* [serial online], 916–920. Retrieved September 12, 2010, from http://www.cdc.gov/nchs/data/nvsr/nvsr56/nvsr56_05.pdf.

Christie, C. (2004). Mood and relationships. In: *Nutrition and well-being A to Z.* Detroit, MI: Gale Publishing,

Field, T. (2000). Touch therapy. New York: Churchill Livingstone.

Goleman, D. (2006). *Social intelligence: The new science of human relationships.* New York: Bantam Books.

Hayes, P. (2003, January). Facts about stress. Retrieved September 27, 2010, from http://www.isma.org.uk/about-stress/facts-about-stress.html

Of serotonin and spirituality. (2003). *Psychology Today.* Retrieved December 29, 2006, from http://www.psychologytoday.com/articles/index.php?term=pto-20040206-000004&print=1

Pokea, D. (2008) Whose thought is it anyway? Retrieved January 9, 2008, from http://www.drpokea.com/thought.html

Rosalba, C. (2000, August/September). Breathe easy. *Massage & Bodywork.* Retrieved January 9, 2008, from http://www.massagetherapy.com/articles/index.php/article_id/307

Rosch, P. (2008). The role of stress in health and illness. Retrieved January 6, 2008, from http://www.stress.org

Sapolskyl, R. (2003, September). Taming stress. *Scientific American*: 87–95.

Van Cauter, E. (2004). Effects of sleep deprivation. Retrieved January 9, 2008, from http://www.fi.edu/learn/brain/sleep.html

Woolfolk, R. L., & Lehrer, P. M. (1993). *Principles and practice of stress management* (2nd ed.). New York: Guilford Press.

Yoga: Minimize stress and maximize flexibility. (2006, February). Retrieved January 9, 2008, from http://www.mayoclinic.com/health/yoga/CM00004

Glossary of Terms

Chapter 1   Introduction to Ergonomics

Anthropometry: the study of human body measurement

Ball and socket joint: multiaxial joint in which the spherical end of one bone fits into the cuplike depression of the other; has the greatest range of motion of any joint type

Biaxial: movement along two axes

Biomechanics: study of the action of physical forces on the body, specifically including the actions of muscles and gravity on bones and joints during body movement

Bursa: fibrous, synovial-lined sac that provides a fluid-filled cushion to protect tendons where they pass along bone, ligaments, or other tendons, usually in the area around a joint

Bursitis: inflammation of a bursa, usually due to excessive pressure or repetitive motion

Carpal tunnel syndrome: group of characteristic signs and symptoms including pain, numbness, reduced strength, and motion of the hand; often explained as a result of repetitive motion causing inflammation of the common flexor sheath as it passes under the flexor retinaculum and the median nerve, thereby putting pressure on the median nerve

Cartilaginous joint: joint held together either by hyaline cartilage or by a plate of fibrocartilage; some movement is possible

Chi: concept of life force or vitality driven by the breath in *tai chi*

Ellipsoid joint: biaxial joint in which the oblong, ellipsoid end of one bone fits into the cuplike depression of the other

Ergonomics: science that studies two aspects of how we manage our work, biomechanics, and design of workplace equipment

Ergonomist: scientist in the field of ergonomics

Fibrositis: inflammation of fibrous connective tissue usually caused by muscle fatigue from chronically working muscles beyond their capacity, thereby prompting inflammation and a reflex reaction that creates a hypertonic condition in the muscle; in severe form, a muscle cramp or "charley horse"

Fibrous joint: joint held together by collagen fibers with very little possible movement

Hinge joint: monoaxial joint with one cylindrical, convex articulating surface fitted into a corresponding concave articulating surface

Inflammation: necessary part of the body's healing response to injury in which the injured area experiences vasodilation and an increase in capillary permeability that together bring more nutrients and white blood cells to the area and dilute the toxins; marked by redness, warmth, pain, edema (swelling), and loss of function

Kinesiology: science that studies body movement

Monoaxial: movement along one axis

Multiaxial: movement along more than two axes

Musculoskeletal disorder (MSD):   any injury or disorder of the muscles, nerves, tendons, joints, cartilage, and/or spinal discs not caused by slips, trips, falls, motor vehicle or similar accidents

Neutral: description of a joint that is in proper alignment, thus minimizing joint trauma

Osteoarthritis: inflammation of one or more joints caused by the breakdown of cartilage, which increases friction at the joint and results in pain and limited movement

Pivot joint: a monoaxial joint allowing for rotation along the long axes of the bones involved

Plane joint: a monoaxial "gliding joint" with two opposing, flat surfaces of equal size restricted in motion by ligaments and adjacent bones

Postural distortion: chronic deviations from neutral alignment that are caused by congenital conditions, injury/

disease, or the body's attempt to adapt to ergonomically unsound repetitive motion

Pressure atrophy: degeneration of tissue from the pressure of excess interstitial fluid or other external pressure

Repetitive motion syndrome: (cumulative trauma disorders, repetitive stress injuries, or overuse syndromes): a group of characteristic symptoms including (1) tingling, cold, or numbness due to reduced blood flow or nerve impingement, (2) tightness, stiffness, soreness, burning, or discomfort due to hypertonic muscles, inflammation or nerve impingement, (3) loss of strength or coordination due to muscle weakness or nerve impingement, and (4) pain at night resulting from inflammation, hypertonicity, or nerve impingement; includes osteoarthritis, bursitis, tendonitis, carpal tunnel syndrome, back injury, headaches, sprains, strains, tears, and chronic pain.

Saddle joint: a biaxial joint with two concave, saddle-shaped bone surfaces that fit together at right angles.

Sprain: an injury to a ligament caused by stretching it beyond its capacity

Strain: a tear in the muscle fibers

Subluxation: a misalignment of a joint

Synovial joint: a joint with a complex structure including a joint capsule lined with a synovial membrane that secrets a viscous synovial fluid for lubrication; these joints have a wide range of movement and therefore are of significant ergonomic interest in terms of potential injury

Tendon sheath: a tubular-shaped bursa surrounding a tendon to create a friction-free tunnel for the tendon through which it passes under ligaments or retinacula or through osseofibrous tunnels

Tendonitis: inflammation of the tendon sheath, usually in proximity to a joint, due to persistent friction

Chapter 2   Postural Assessment

Adaptation: the process of developing less than optimal habitual patterns of posture and movement

Anatomical position: the position of the body standing upright with feet parallel, arms at the side with palms forward, fingers pointed straight down, and head facing forward; the traditional position for considering at posture

Balanced approach to neutral alignment: an integration of external and internal approaches; a view that requires the knowledge of anatomically correct neutral positions and a keen awareness of your own body's sensations and energy flow

Base of support: the portions of the body transferring weight and other applied forces down into the earth through contact with the ground, chair, or other support

Carrying angle: the antebrachial deviation from a line running straight with the axis of the humerus

Compensation: the process of developing postural distortions as muscles and ligaments undergo adaptation

External approach to neutral alignment: an objective view of the body's posture and balance

Flow: constant internal awareness even during movement

Internal approach to neutral alignment: a subjective view of the body by tuning into it through sensory awareness

Muscle memory: tensions stored within the neuromuscular system; a body's memory of habitual motor skills

Scoliosis: an abnormal lateral curve anywhere along the spine

Chapter 3   Assessment in Motion

Antagonist: a muscle that opposes an action

Body scanning: monitoring internal sensations of energy: tracking one's state of balance and the flow or stoppage of the person's internal energy in a sequential manner

Contract/relax technique: a tool to achieve neutral alignment by scanning the body to identify tension, contracting the muscle, and then releasing the muscle; a simplified version of positional release and/or proprioceptor neuromuscular facilitation

First-class lever: lever whose fulcrum is located between the force and resistance; for example, a seesaw

Fixator: a muscle that contracts isometrically to stabilize the origin of the prime mover during an action

Focused breathing: increased awareness of the quality of breath; useful in ergonomics to evaluate and adapt to tension during movement

Force system: the sum of all forces involved in any particular movement

Fulcrum: the pivot point of a lever

Isometric contraction: contraction in which a muscle generates tension but the muscle length does not change

Isotonic contraction: a muscular contraction in which muscle tension does not change but muscle length changes

Kinesthetic awareness: sensory awareness of your body while it is in motion

Prime mover: the principal muscle, or one of a group of principal muscles, responsible for an action

Second-class lever: lever in which the resistance is placed between the force and the fulcrum; for example, a wheelbarrow

Synergist: a muscle that prevents unwanted movement at the joint lying between the prime mover muscle and the insertion point where an action occurs

Third-class lever: the most common lever in the body in which force is applied to the middle of the lever, with the fulcrum and resistance at either end; for example, a broom

Vector: a variable having both magnitude and direction

Visualization: creation of a mental image of a physically invisible phenomenon or a desirable future situation

Chapter 4 Common Postural Distortions

Calcaneovalgus: eversion of the hindfoot, associated with pronation

Calcaneovarus: when the distal portion of the calcaneous lies medial to the tibial line; also known as *hindfoot varus*

Forefoot valgus: eversion of the forefoot when the calcaneous is in neutral alignment

Forefoot varus: inversion of the forefoot when the calcaneous is in neutral alignment

Genu recurvatum: hyperextension of the knees

Genu valgus: lateral angulation of the knees in which the distal portion of the leg deviates outward; also known as *knock-knees*

Genu varus: lateral angulation of the knees in which the distal portion of the leg deviates inward; also known as *bowlegs*

Lumbosacral angle: the angle between the long axis of the lumbar part of the vertebral column and the long axis of the sacrum

Pes cavus: exaggeration of both longitudinal arches; also known as *high arches*

Pes planus: a depressed or collapsed medial longitudinal arch; also known as *flatfoot*

Q angle: the angle between a line drawn from the anterior iliac spine through the center of the patella and a line drawn from the tibial tuberosity through the center of the patella; also known as *quadriceps* or *patellofemoral angle*

Screw-home mechanism: the mechanism in which the knee locks in the last 15 degrees of extension

Sesamoiditis: a condition in which pain under the large toe is experienced due to inflammation of the joint and its sesamoid bones

Swing phase: that part of walking in which one foot leaves the ground, lowering the pelvis on that side

Valgus: an indication that the distal component is angled outward from the vertical axis (to the side or "laterally")

Varus: an indication that the distal component of a joint is angled inward to the vertical axis toward the midline

Chapter 5 Ergonomic Techniques for the Bodyworker

Diagonal stance: a stance in which the therapist's feet are parallel, approximately shoulderwide, and staggered; the therapist is at an angle to the body area being worked on

Direct stance: a stance in which the therapist's feet are parallel; the therapist faces the body area being worked on

Martial stance: the standing base of support formed by position of the feet that is ready, poised, and centered; a stance adapted from the practice of *tai chi* in which the therapist is stable, balanced, and able to utilize a shift in weight to administer strokes

Negative space: the empty space between a part of your body and a potential base of support

Triangle of power: an ergonomic concept in which a therapist arranges working parts of his or her body to form a triangle to improve stability and support when applying a bodywork technique

Chapter 6 The Workplace Environment

Building-related illnesses (BRI): diagnosable illnesses in people caused by the individual's place of employment; symptoms can include chest tightness, cough, fever, chills, muscle aches; typically attributed to a specific indoor contaminant

Computer vision syndrome (CVS): the set of eye and vision problems that occur with prolonged computer monitor usage

National Institute for Occupational Safety and Health (NIOSH): A part of the Centers for Disease Control (CDC) responsible for conducting research and making recommendations for the prevention of work-related illnesses and injuries

Sick building syndrome (SDS): a situation in which 25–30% of workers experience poor comfort or health symptoms during working hours that diminish over the weekend or during holidays; symptoms include eye irritation, skin irritation, headache, throat irritation, recurrent fatigue, chest burning, cough, wheezing, nasal congestion, problems with concentration or short-term memory; generally attributed to nonspecific causes but sometimes to tobacco smoke, microbes, volatile organic compounds, particulates, and psychosocial factors; can be associated with a single room, a region of a building, or an entire building

Video display terminal (VDT): an electronic hardware device that displays images, most typically a computer screen/monitor

Volatile organic compounds (VOCs): organic chemical compounds that vaporize relatively easily and can have chronic effects on the environment and human health; workplace sources can include tobacco smoke, upholstery, manufactured wood products, carpets and carpet adhesives, copy machines, pesticides, and cleaning agents

Chapter 7 Self-Care: Exercise

Aerobic exercise: physical exercise that increases the body's need for oxygenated blood and therefore triggers increased circulation (heartbeat) and respiration (breathing); also known as *endurance training*

Ballistic stretch: a method of extending the muscles through repetitive, bouncing movements; is virtually obsolete

Cardiorespiratory endurance: the body's ability to maintain sufficient blood flow to the muscles to provide them necessary nutrients and oxygen and to remove waste products; often described as the body's ability to perform dynamic exercises of moderate-to-high intensity for prolonged periods

Concentric contraction: process in which a muscle shortens while contracting against resistance through the joint's range of motion, typically at the start of a motion; also known as *positive contraction*

Eccentric contraction: process in which the muscle lengthens while contracting against resistance through the joint's range of motion; also known as *negative contraction*

Golgi tendon reflex: process in which a stretch's tension is transmitted to the tendon and detected by the Golgi tendon organs, thereby causing the muscles to relax, thus preventing potentially high muscle tension and damaged muscles or tendons

Hypermobility: excessive movement around a joint resulting from overstretching the musculotendinous unit

Inverse stretch reflex: see *Golgi tendon reflex*

Proprioceptor neuromuscular facilitation (PNF): a comprehensive approach to working with movement patterns of multiple muscle groups, including various combinations of alternating muscular contractions and stretches

Repetition maximum (RM): the maximum amount of weight an individual can lift with proper technique in one and only one repetition of a given exercise

Static stretch: extension in which a muscle is taken to a point of comfortable tension and held for a designated period of time, usually 15–30 seconds

Strength training: the use of resistance to muscular contraction to build the strength, endurance, and size of muscles

Stretch reflex: response in which a sudden or prolonged stretch causes the muscle spindles to trigger the muscle to contract and its antagonist to relax to keep the muscle within a preset length and reduce the risk of muscle strain

Target heart rate (THR): the ideal number of heart beats per minute achieved during a workout, typically between 55–90% of a person's maximum heart rate (MHR = 220 − your age) with the lower part of the range more appropriate for beginning exercisers and the upper range more appropriate for people who have been exercising for a long period of time

Chapter 8   Self-Care: Self-Massage

Hyperemia: increase of blood in a body part

Hypoxia: oxygen deficiency

Ischemic: a body part that experiences a lack of blood

Rubefacients: agents that redden skin, dilate vessels, and increase blood supply locally

Shiatsu: a form of massage that originated in Japan

Stasis: slowing or stopping blood flow

Chapter 9   Self-Care: Stress and Stress Busters

Acute stress: a result of sudden, often unexpected, emergencies that occur during the day

Chronic stress: a result of being caught in a long-term situation that cannot be resolved or for which a way to resolve it doesn't seem to exist

Distress: a painful situation or negative change

Emotional intelligence: the measure of the ability to be self-aware, self-motivated, empathic, and able to cope with varying moods

Episodic acute stress: result of a series of minor emergencies over a period of time, often self-induced

Eustress: positive stress

Fight or flight response: physiologic changes that occur during an emergency, specifically a response from the sympathetic nervous system

General adaptation syndrome: sequence of reactions to prolonged and intense stress consisting of an acute stage, a resistance stage, and an exhaustion stage

Limbic system: area of the human brain that is involved in emotion, motivation, and emotional association with memory

Reticular activating system (RAS): system that extends through the brain stem and is the neural connection between the spinal cord and upper regions of the brain

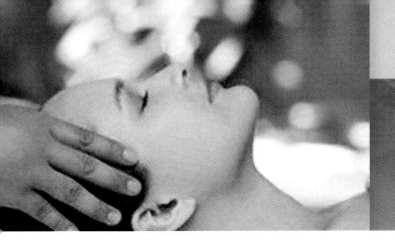

Answer Key

CHAPTER 1
INTRODUCTION TO ERGONOMICS

1. b
2. a
3. a
4. True
5. True
6. True
7. 1. Shape, size, and arrangement of the articular surfaces, 2. Ligaments, 3. Muscle tone around the joint
8. Plane (monoaxial), saddle (biaxial), hinge (monoaxial), pivot (monoaxial), ball-and-socket (greatest ROM, and ellipsoid (biaxial)
9. Redness, heat, pain, edema, and loss of function
10. Neutrality refers to the angles of the body during movement and rest that are most favorable to joint function and health.

CHAPTER 2
POSTURAL ASSESSMENT

1. Posture and balance
2. d
3. d
4. a
5. Helps keep us in balance
6. Endomorph, ectomorph, mesomorph
7. Internal approach
8. True
9. True
10. True
11. False

CHAPTER 3
ASSESSMENT IN MOTION

1. b
2. a
3. a
4. c
5. False
6. True
7. True
8. When a client changes to the side-lying position, he or she presents a higher surface to the therapist, which causes elevation of the shoulders and hyperextension of the wrists unless the therapist modifies posture and attentively maintains neutral alignment.
9. To remain stable during movement, the center of gravity must stay with the base of support (which is those parts of the body in contact with the surface that supports the body).

CHAPTER 4
COMMON POSTURAL DISTORTIONS

1. Scoliosis, exaggerated curves, and reduced curves
2. Genetic, congenital, and acquired
3. Acquired
4. Disease, injury, and chronic misuse
5. Protracted (rounded) shoulders and elevated shoulders
6. e
7. e
8. e
9. Knees should be level, within zero to 5 degrees of flexion, and with no visible rotation.

10. Quadriceps angle
11. Genu recurvatum
12. From an anterior viewpoint, the anterior superior iliac spine (ASIS) should be level. From a lateral viewpoint, the ASIS and the pubic symphysis should each line up on a vertical plane.
13. True
14. False
15. True
16. False

CHAPTER 5
ERGONOMIC TECHNIQUES FOR THE BODYWORKER

1. Evaluating your ergonomics via video can help you identify poor ergonomic habits before you compromise your body's health and well-being.
2. Neutral checkpoints help us work more efficiently by allowing us to recognize when we move out of "neutral," thereby preventing and alleviating repetitive motion injuries and reducing the risk of joint injuries.
3. True
4. True
5. True
6. Joints
7. Tuck
8. Brachium
9. b
10. d
11. d

CHAPTER 6
THE WORKPLACE ENVIRONMENT

1. d
2. False
3. Inadequate ventilation, chemical contaminants from indoor sources, chemical contaminants from outdoor sources, biological contaminants, and particulates
4. True
5. Rest eyes for at least 20 seconds every 20 minutes, blink often, focus on the breath, clean the screen and filter, eliminate or reduce overhead lighting to reduce glare, use low glare lenses and louvers on overhead lighting, eliminate or cover reflective surfaces such as windows, use high-quality monitor with at least 70 Hz and a resolution of between 800 x 600, increase font size, position work within easy viewing distance, position screen perpendicular to the line of sight, wear glasses if necessary, and/or choose slightly tinted glasses to reduce glare
6. c
7. d
8. b
9. True
10. Physical workplace and techniques

CHAPTER 7
SELF-CARE: EXERCISE

1. Strength
2. Lengthening
3. c
4. a
5. d
6. True
7. False
8. Ballistic (repetitive bouncing movements that extend muscles) has become obsolete because of risk of injury, static (holding the muscle at point of comfortable tension for 15–30 seconds), and PNF (proprioceptive neuromuscular facilitation, consisting of various combinations of alternating muscular contractions and stretches).
9. Rapid stretching elicits a reflex contraction in the muscles. Brief stretching does not allow the muscle to conform to the new length. Overstretching can cause hypermobility (which can lead to joint instability and dislocation) and/or muscle injury (when the stretch exceeds the extensibility of the muscle).
10. Strength training, cardiovascular/endurance training, and stretching.

CHAPTER 8
SELF-CARE: SELF-MASSAGE

1. Ease aches and pains of everyday life, change negative patterns by re-educating muscle memory, prevent overuse injuries (including hypertonic muscles and poor circulation that may cause PD's), reduce scar tissue, restore balance between antagonistic pairs of muscles, and/or ward off excessively tired muscles.
2. Friction
3. Tapotement
4. True
5. True
6. True
7. Unhealthy body mechanics and accident/disease
8. Longitudinal

9. d
10. c
11. d
12. b, d, a, c

CHAPTER 9
SELF-CARE: STRESS
AND STRESS BUSTERS

1. The four components of well-being are physical, mental, emotional and spiritual.
2. Bodyworkers experience high physical demands (as therapists), mental demands (as business owners and/or employees), emotional/spiritual demands (as caregivers).
3. The pressure of responsibility for every aspect of the business and no paid time off, no retirement benefits or health benefits.
4. True
5. True
6. True
7. True
8. a
9. d
10. d
11. d

Index

Ligaments
  anterior cruciate, 60
  body mechanics and, 23
  calcaneofibular, 23
  instability of, 59
  joints and, 6, 8
  lateral collateral, 23
  posture and, 23
  pubofemoral, 8
  stabilization by, 8
  talofibular, 23
  tendons under, 10
Lighting, in indoor environment, 103–104
  eye and, 103
  eye strain and, 103
Limbic cortex, 163, 164
Limbic system, 163–64
  amygdala, 163, 164
  hippocampus, 163, 164
  hypothalamus, 163, 164
  limbic cortex, 163, 164
  reticular activating system, 164
  thalamus, 163
Ling, Per Henrik, 142
Liniments, 148
Log, exercise, 125–26
Lower limbs
  checkpoints for, 89
  internal approach, to neutral alignment and, 45
  self-massage techniques for, 149
  working on, 89
Low-intensity workout, 127
Lumbar lordosis, 61, 66
Lumbosacral angle (LS), 60, 61, 66
Lymphatic vessels, 6

M

MacLean, Paul, 163
Magnitude, 37
Martial stance, 84
Massage
  ball techniques, 145
  benefits of, 142
  energy work, 144
  liniments and analgesics, 148
  neuromuscular technique, 143–44
  reflexology, 144–45
  selecting techniques, 146–47
  Swedish, 142–43
  thermotherapy and cryotherapy, 145–46
  tools and equipment for, 147–48
Massage chair, repetitive motion disorders and, 14–15
Mats, in treatment room, 109
Medial epicondylitis, 69
Medicair$_x$ Back Pillo, 106
Medicine balls, 145
Meditation, 175–76
  behavioral components of, 176
  mindfulness, 176
  references, 176
  transcendental, 176
Memory, muscle, 31
Mental (intellectual) well-being, 162
Mental stressors, 160
Metacarpalphalangeal joints, 7, 69
Metatarsal head, 57
Midcarpal joint, 68
Midtarsal joint, 57
Mindfulness, for stress management, 172–73, 176

Miracle balls, 145
Misalignment
  of legs, 24
  shoulder, 67
  skeletal, 52
  of spinal curves, 66
  of vertebral column, 40
Molecules of Emotion (Pert), 173
Monoaxial movement, 6
Morton's neuroma, 58
Motion
  assessment in, 34–49
  balanced approach, to neutral alignment, 45–47
  external activities for maintaining neutral alignment in, 42
  external approach, to neutral alignment, 36–42
  internal approach, to neutral alignment, 43–45
  neutral alignment maintenance in, 46
  of scapula, 68
  sensory awareness tools in, 43–44
Motion ranges, degree of, 6
Motor skills, reflex patterns in, 41–42
Mouse, computer, 107
Movement
  biaxial, 6
  injuries related to, 10–11
  monoaxial, 6
  multiaxial, 6
  muscles involved in, 37–41
  respiratory, 7
MSD. *See* Musculoskeletal disorders (MSD)
Multiaxial movement, 6
Muscle fatigue, 9
  inflammation and, 11
Muscle fibers, 10
Muscle memory, 31
Muscle relaxation, 174–75
Muscles
  abdominal, 119
  as antagonist, 39
  articulation, 9
  atrophy, 146
  contraction, 9
  cramps, 11
  deltoid, 133
  on dominant side, 27
  extensor, 41
  extrinsic, 11
  fast twitch fibers, 118
  fixator, 40
  flexor, 41
  imbalance, 52
  intrinsic, 58, 69
  joint stability and, 9
  limitation of force, 42
  involved in movement, 37–41
  neutral alignment maintenance and, 83
  origination of, 9
  pectoral, 155
  physical conditioning of, 10
  as prime mover, 39
  pterygoid, 154
  resistance and, 38
  skeletal, 9
  slow twitch fibers, 118
  soreness, 120
  spasm, 40
  synergist, 40

  tone, 9, 25, 58
  in vertebral column, 67
Muscle tissue, movement and, 9–10
Muscular endurance, 118
Muscular strength, 118
Musculoskeletal alignment, 6
Musculoskeletal disorders (MSD), 11, 12, 100, 119
Myofascial Pain and Dysfunction: The Trigger Point Manual (Williams and Wilkens), 144

N

National Council on Strength and Fitness (NCSF), 118
National Institute for Occupational Safety and Health (NIOSH), 107
National Sleep Foundation, 171
NCSF. *See* National Council on Strength and Fitness (NCSF)
Neck
  flexion, 14
  self-massage techniques for, 153–54
  stretches for, 132–33
  working on, 82–84
Negative space, 83
Nerve compression, 12, 68
Nerve impingements, 146
Nerve stroke, 143
Nervous system, development of, 41
Neural conditions, stress and, 169
Neuromuscular technique (massage) (NMT), 142, 143–44
Neuromuscular work, 14
Neuroplasticity, 172
Neutral alignment, 13, 95
  assessment for, 30–31, 77
  balanced approach to, 29–31
  complementary modalities for, 46
  ergonomic techniques for, 76, 78–80
  external activities for maintaining, 42
  external approach to, 22–26, 36–42
  feet and, 55
  finding, 14
  head and trunk, 63, 65
  internal approach to, 26–28
  knees, 59
  maintaining, 16, 22
  muscles for maintenance of, 83
  pelvis, 61, 62
  shoulders, 67
  tai chi and, 29
  wringing stroke and, 90
  wrist and hand, 69
Neutral stance, 85
NIOSH. *See* National Institute for Occupational Safety and Health (NIOSH)
NMT. *See* Neuromuscular technique (massage) (NMT)
Nonsteroidal anti-inflammatory drug (NSAIDs), 148
Norepinephrine, 168
Normal posture, 22

O

Obesity
  anterior tilt of pelvis and, 61
  prevalence of, 124
Occupational injuries, basis for, 11–15
  bodyworkers and, 13–15
  improper body mechanics and injury, 13